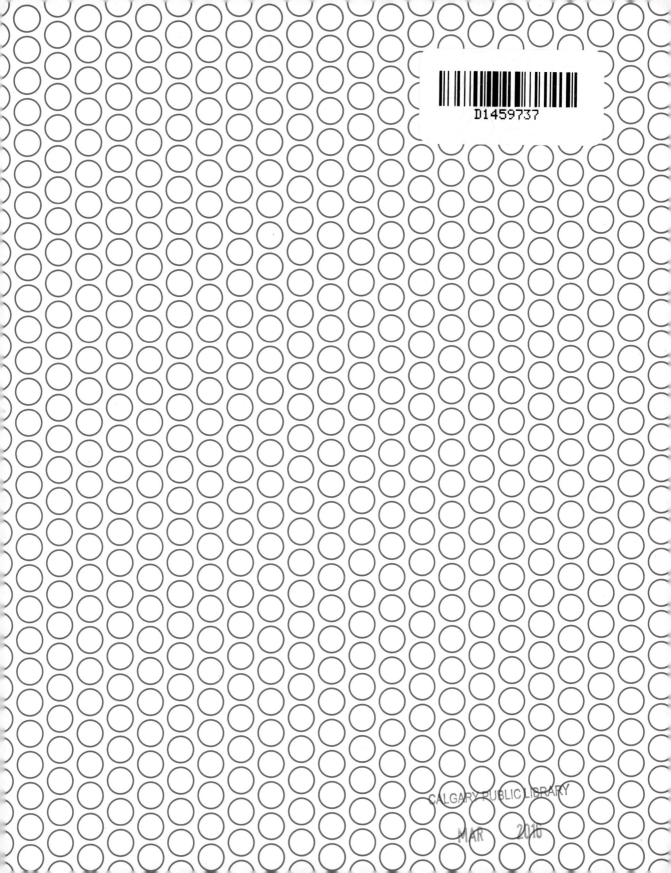

SKINNYSUPPERS

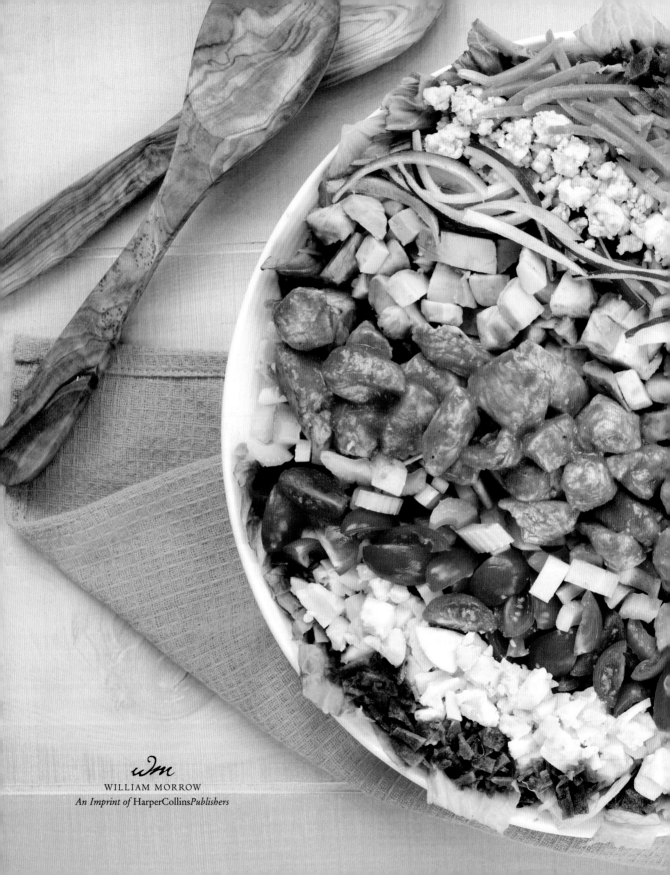

WILLIAM MORROW

An Imprint of HarperCollinsPublishers

SKINNY SUPPERS

125 LIGHTENED-UP, HEALTHIER MEALS FOR YOUR FAMILY

BROOKE GRIFFIN
CREATOR OF SKINNYMOM.COM

HarperCollins books may be purchased for educational, business,
or sales promotional use. For information please e-mail the Special
Markets Department at SPsales@harpercollins.com.

FIRST EDITION

Designed by Ashley Tucker
Photography by Sarah Hone
Food styling by Jen Casperson

Library of Congress Cataloging-in-Publication Data
has been applied for.

ISBN 978-0-06-241915-6

16 17 18 19 20 INDD/QGT 10 9 8 7 6 5 4 3 2 1

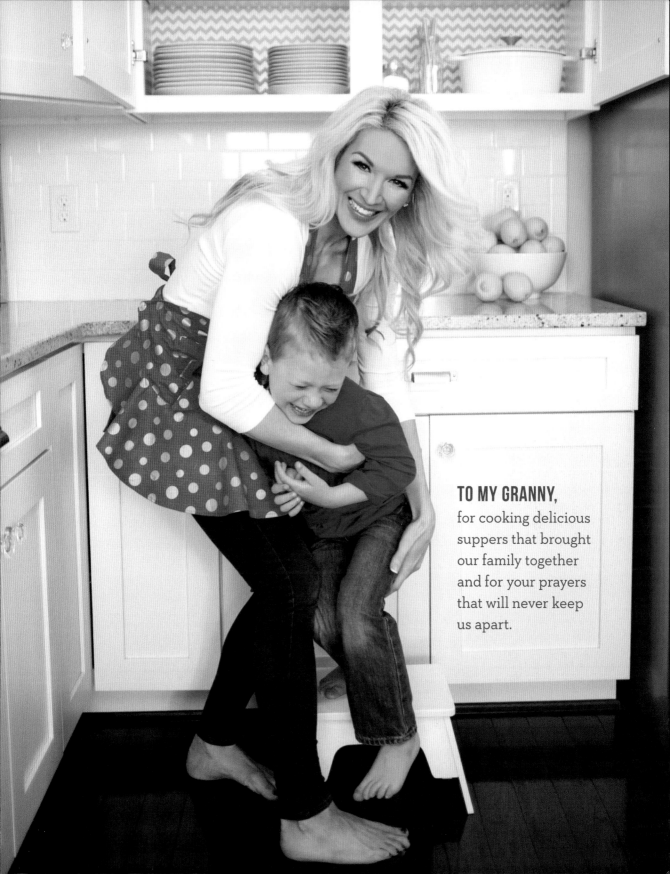

TO MY GRANNY,
for cooking delicious suppers that brought our family together and for your prayers that will never keep us apart.

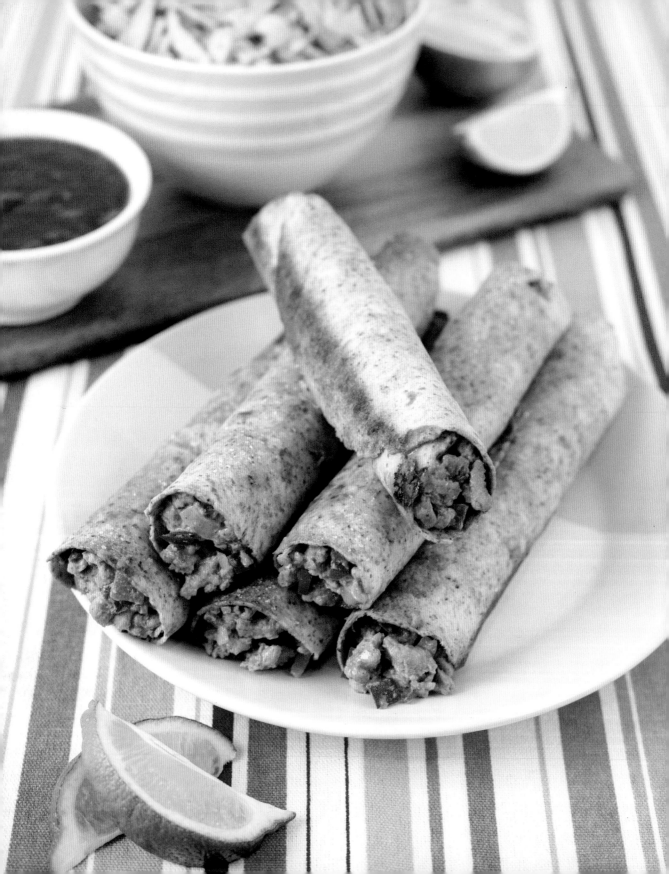

CONTENTS

INTRODUCTION

So you've decided to embark on a new journey. But wait, you've done this before. You've purchased the cookbooks, made the grocery lists, rallied the family, prayed for the wisdom, and then, somehow, less than one week after standing on the kitchen counter pronouncing with fervor your game plan to change the world (or at least your kitchen), you find your supper table is covered in take-out pizza boxes and empty bags of potato chips. Again. What happened? It was supposed to work *this time*. Why does this have to be so hard? When the inspiration hits, you're sure you can make it happen, but somewhere between the purchase of the cookbook and the first trip to the grocery store, there is a disconnect.

Skinny Suppers was created with you in mind—the busy person who juggles so much. This book will guide you through meal planning and prep, grocery shopping, time-management and money-saving methods, and, of course, easy-to-follow recipes. The goal is for you to learn how to pull your family back to the supper table for healthy, balanced meals and more quality time. You can do this! How do I know? Because just a few years ago, I was in the same situation.

In 2011, I found myself going through an unexpected divorce with a newborn and carrying nearly seventy extra pounds! Overwhelmed and quite honestly terrified, I tapped into the two most important characteristics I possess: my faith and my competitive spirit. I leaned on a scripture that has been my favorite for years: "Trust in the Lord with all your heart, lean not unto thine own understanding. In all your ways acknowledge Him and He will make your paths straight." Proverbs 3:5–6. Truly trusting in that verse and all that it said, I did what I do best—took a big leap of faith! I moved back into my parents' home with my little guy, Easton Jack, and began blogging from their basement.

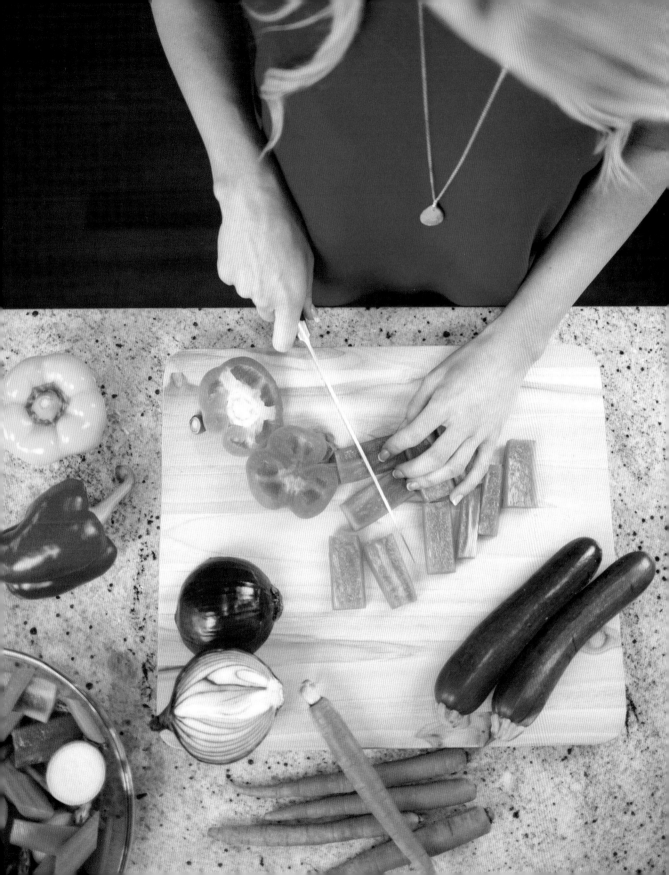

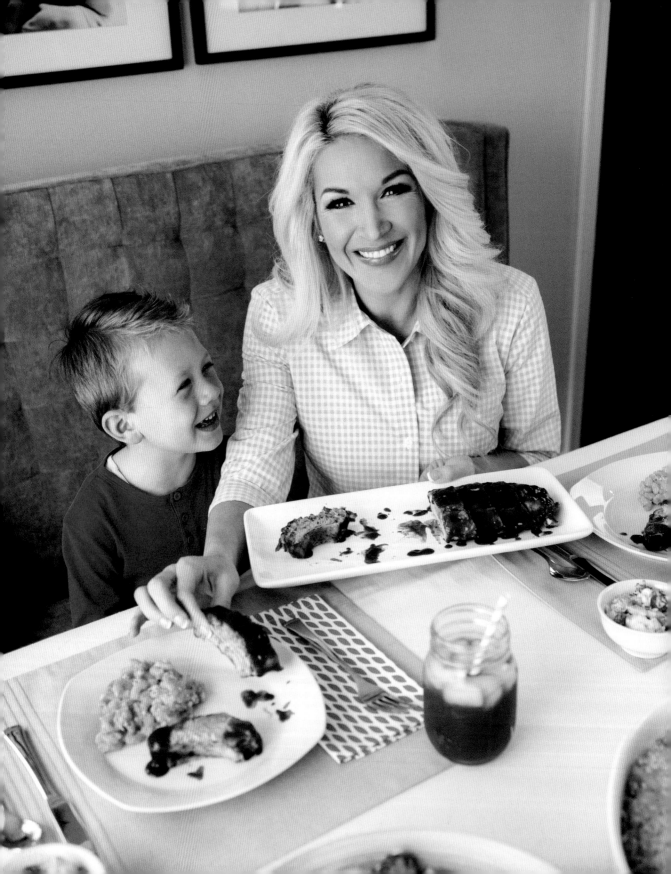

Reaching out to other women in similar circumstances, I set out on a mission to lose the baby weight and inspire others along the way. In 2011, I took the biggest chance of my life: I cashed out my 401K (totaling $20,000), hired my first employee, and built my first website. Skinny Mom was born! An all-out effort to redefine "skinny" and offer an online destination where moms get the "skinny" on healthy living. I was committed to empowering other mothers by helping them realize they can lose weight and lead healthy lives regardless of their circumstances!

I sent my first weekly newsletter to twenty-five people (well, about a hundred if you count the friends and family I took the liberty of including—thanks, guys!) and less than four years later the Skinny Mom weekly newsletter reaches over half a million people. And more than six million people visit our website each month. What's the number one reason this many readers head to Skinnymom.com? Skinny recipes.

In 2013, in response to e-mails and questions, Skinny Mom introduced "The Supper Club," a free monthly meal-planning newsletter to help busy moms prepare a tasty and waist-friendly meal for their families every night of the week. Its overwhelming success has proved that moms want to cook for their families, but convenience and organization are key.

So, if life has sidetracked (or even derailed) your health and wellness goals, you've come to the right cookbook. This book is filled with recipes for suppers you can make in a pinch, using mostly items you have on hand, and you can feel confident that they're all light and balanced. I've searched out my favorite recipes and tweaked, cut, studied, cooked, and tasted them for you. These recipes are simple, satiating, lighter, and lower in fat and calories, and most important, delicious! And guess what? It's going to work this time!

> So, if life has sidetracked (or even derailed) your health and wellness goals, you've come to the right cookbook.

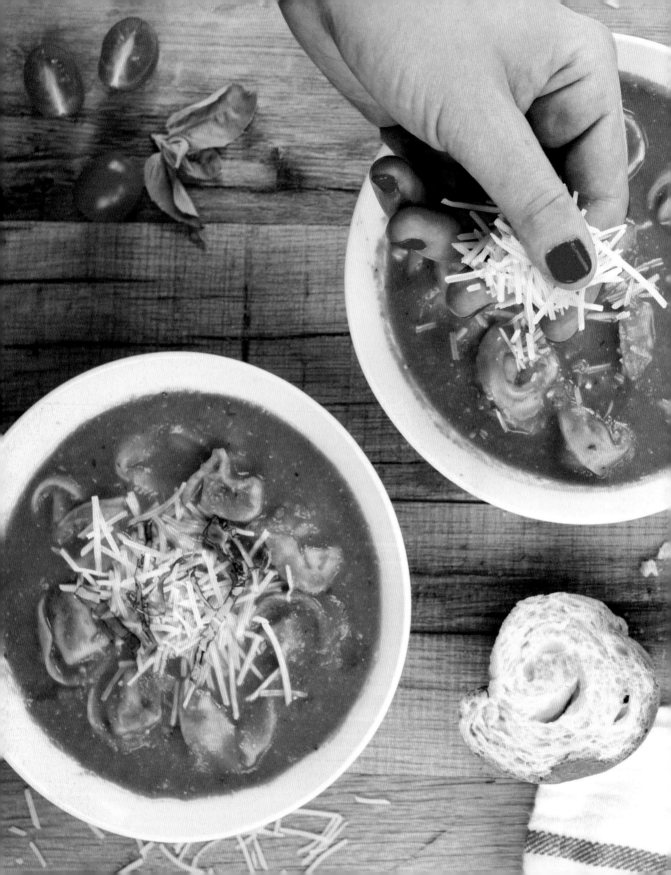

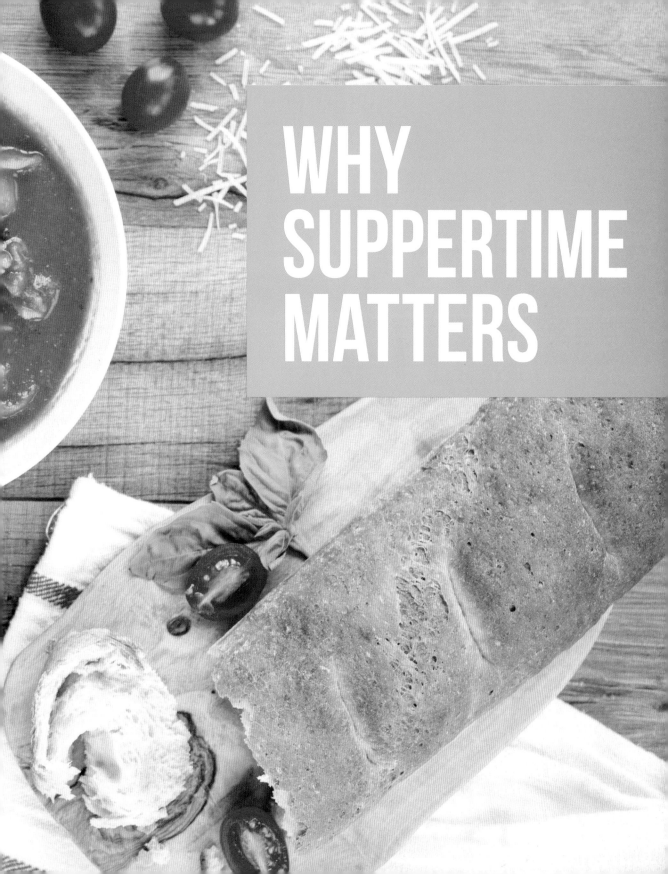

WHY SUPPERTIME MATTERS

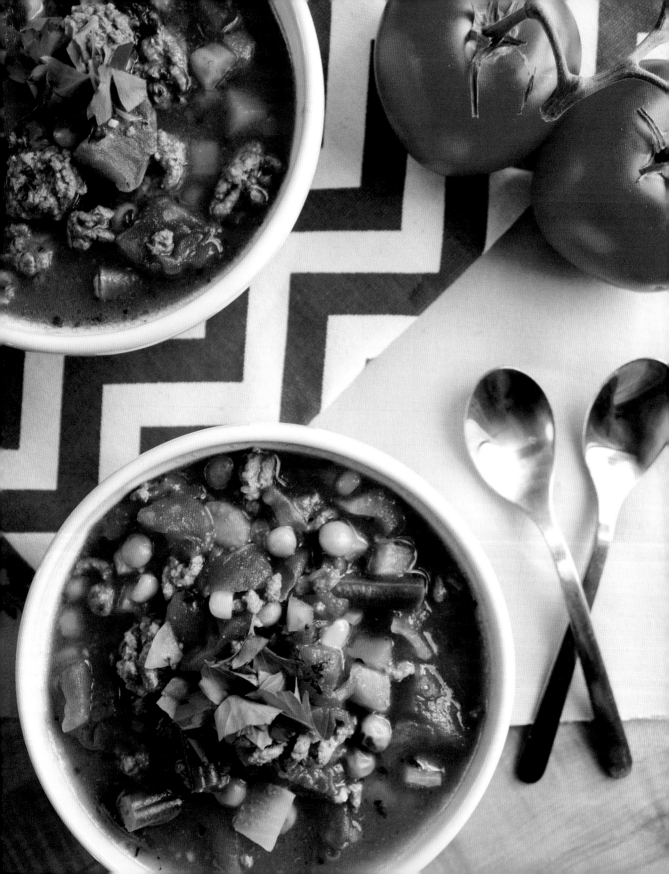

❶ *make time for* SUPPERTIME

I have a burning desire in my heart to teach you how to prepare light, healthy, and tasty suppers that are quick and easy to make. I love to cook—I always have. But I'm also extremely busy and relish simplicity. Even though I love to try new recipes, I'm not a fan of expensive ingredients that I can't pronounce or can't afford. As my son continues to grow, the importance of quality time together has become very real to me. *Skinny Suppers* was inspired by my desire to help families find the time to prepare lighter and healthier meals that they can sit down and enjoy together several nights a week.

Let's face it: everyone is busy. Mom is busy, Dad is busy, and the kids have some crazy schedules to keep, too. Yet we still have to eat. This book is a practical tool that will empower you and help you realize that family mealtime is a wonderful way to reconnect and share stories, all while loving your family and improving their overall health and wellness through nourishing dishes. And yes, prepping, cooking, and enjoying these meals can all fit into your hectic schedule.

FOR THE HOME COOK WITH NO TIME TO SPARE

You might be thinking, *So when in the world do you think I have time to plan meals, much less sit down for them?* I'm glad you asked. If you purchased this cookbook, I'm confident we share the same goals: to eat healthier, lose a little (or a lot) of weight, have the energy we need to successfully navigate through a busy life, and simply feel good (no, make that great) in our skin! The good news is that enjoying suppertime with your family is part of what will help you reach those goals.

I want to ensure that the meals you serve are easy to make, light, and balanced. I want to guide you and empower you in the kitchen in a way that will enhance your family's life, not drain your energy or your time. You, the busy home cook with no time to spare, will find refreshing recipes and tips, inspiration and ideas, encouragement and excitement throughout this book. This is the first step to getting your family back around the table for supper!

WHY SUPPERTIME IS SO IMPORTANT FOR FAMILIES

If you could do one thing that would improve the well-being of your family, would you do it? Of course!

Research shows that families who eat together benefit in more ways than one. Sitting down to share meals boosts communication and strengthens relationships, while the kids statistically perform better in school and tend to make better choices, even under pressure, about alcohol, drugs, sex, etc. This kind of tradition flows into their teen years and adulthood with an emphasis on good nutrition.

Now many of us are already sitting down for supper together. One study found that more than 78 percent of us claim that we eat together as a family on most nights. It's what we do *while* we're eating that has changed drastically in the last twenty years. When I was younger and it was time for supper, you better believe I was sitting at my place at the kitchen table. Coming home for supper was just like coming home when the streetlights came on. There were no TV and no phones at the table. People actually respected suppertime so much they wouldn't call around 6 p.m.—not even a salesperson.

Now we watch the news, talk on the phone, read, text—it's almost like we're doing everything we can to avoid communicating with one another. The influence of technology is overwhelming. Suppertime may very well be our only opportunity to pour into our family the morals, values, and beliefs that we cherish. That's powerful! Our children and teens are desperate for a safe space to discuss ideas within the understanding and nonjudgmental boundaries of family. Having supper together as a family provides the stability and communication that is vital for children and teens.

Health is a major concern, too. In the last decade, there has been a sharp increase in the number of obese parents and children in the United States.

Unfortunately, the numbers continue to increase at a staggering rate. As a result, there has been an increased focus on educating families, especially moms, about how they can help their families eat more balanced diets and live more active lifestyles. This is your "lightbulb moment." Numerous studies are pointing to the fact that regular family meals around the supper table are having positive effects on lowering obesity rates and improving positive eating habits, as well as lessening the risk of food-related disorders.

Suppertime is thirty minutes to one hour without TV, phones, or other electronics. Even if you can have it only a few nights a week, that's better than none. The research is clear. Over the last twenty years, families have become busier, fast food has become more accessible (and more processed), and we have traded the kitchen table for the couch.

We want to get back to the kitchen table, but we don't know where to begin. *Skinny Suppers* has been designed to be your guide. It is my goal to help you get your family back to the kitchen table with light, balanced, and delicious suppers you can prep and cook in about thirty minutes.

TO FIND OUR WAY BACK, WE MUST START AT THE BEGINNING

I love to see the reaction on people's faces when I tell them where I'm from. Of course the accent denotes Southern roots, but few expect to hear that anyone can come from "humble beginnings" these days.

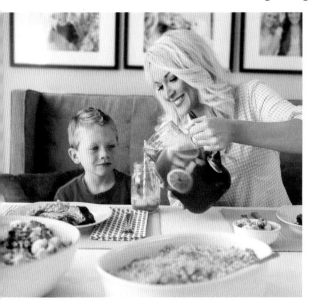

But it's true; I grew up in a small town in eastern Kentucky. It really was a town with just a couple of stoplights where everybody knew everybody else's business.

I was living the simple life most people only read about—school, Friday night football, and big suppers after church on Sunday. And it was the nineties! (Believe it or not, my entire family still gets together as often as they can. More than sixty people gather at my aunt's house now to laugh, chat, catch up, and, of course, eat!) I have since moved, but I haven't missed a holiday or family reunion.

I am the oldest of three girls, the first to go to college, and I am blessed to say that my parents have been happily married for more than thirty years. My life growing up was truly humble. Both my parents worked, and if it weren't for my granny, my sisters and I would have come home to an empty house most days after school. Had it not been for the suppers at Granny's, I would not be the woman I am today. I thank God for grannies like mine, who lived right next door and cooked supper for us almost every day and for our entire extended family on most Sundays and every holiday. And she cooked from scratch. Thinking about her homemade biscuits and gravy still makes my mouth water. I think she spent most of her life cooking.

Even though my granny was the primary cook every day, and my parents both worked, they valued time with their family and made sure they were home every evening to sit down for supper. That's where I want to encourage you. The true value is in the time spent together. So don't get wrapped up in making the perfect meal—get wrapped up in making the memory!

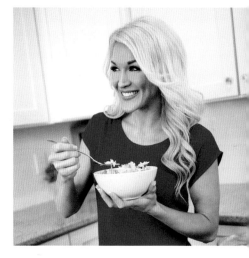

By the time I was a teen, I often had the role of preparing meals for my sisters, and that's where my love of cooking began. Yet more than the food I prepared, I relish the memories. And even though I moved away and my lifestyle shifted incredibly from those humble beginnings, I have never forgotten how the countless hours spent at my granny's house molded and shaped me. Now as my life has come full circle and I am raising a child of my own, I realize the importance of the time spent together and am invested in helping you realize it, too.

However, I am not a chef! I am just a mom who tries to cook the best meals for my family within the craziness of this twenty-first century. This book wasn't designed to make a chef out of you, just to make you a more confident cook in the kitchen, one who can inspire all those around you to be more confident, too!

GET BACK TO BASICS

Have you ever stopped to think about how much "family time" you get on a weekly basis? This does not include watching baseball practice or hosting a sleepover for your daughter for the tenth time this month. I mean hanging out with *just* the family—no friends tagging along and exclusive of extracurricular sports. For many of us, the time together is minimal, and for good reason. We're busy. Although many of us regret not having set aside time to spend with our kids and loved ones, a world of convenience and instant everything pushes us along at such a fast pace. As a result, we become sleep-deprived overachievers and overeaters.

It's time to get back to the basics of what makes a family grow together, and that's spending time together. My prayer for you as you journey through this book is that you will find the determination and motivation to get back to experiencing suppertime most days of the week, reconnecting with the most important people in your life—your family!

But there's one problem. After months (maybe even years) of eating on the go or on the couch, how will we ever get the rest of the gang on board? Here are five ways to get the whole family involved in suppertime:

1 **Let family members take turns choosing what's for supper.** Allowing them to feel some control and responsibility adds to their enthusiasm and desire to take part.

2 **Create theme days.** Believe it or not, kids really do love structure, and knowing that it's "Taco Tuesday" provides them with security and excitement.

3 **Everyone has a place in the kitchen.** Whether it's setting the table or loading the dishwasher, everyone—from toddler to teen—can do something. Turn setup and cleanup into time spent together.

4 **Plan ahead.** You can't get away from supper. Grumbling tummies must be fed. Knowing that the recipes in this book will take around thirty minutes to prepare relieves stress for you and them. (Keep in mind, slow-cooker recipes will take longer to cook but they can be prepped in around thirty minutes and will be hot and ready the second you walk in the door after a long day.)

5 **Keep the atmosphere upbeat!** Background music, fun conversation, and verbal games (like "I spy") all add to the ambiance and mood of family suppertime. This is not the time for scolding about bad grades or messy rooms. Designate a separate time to address those issues.

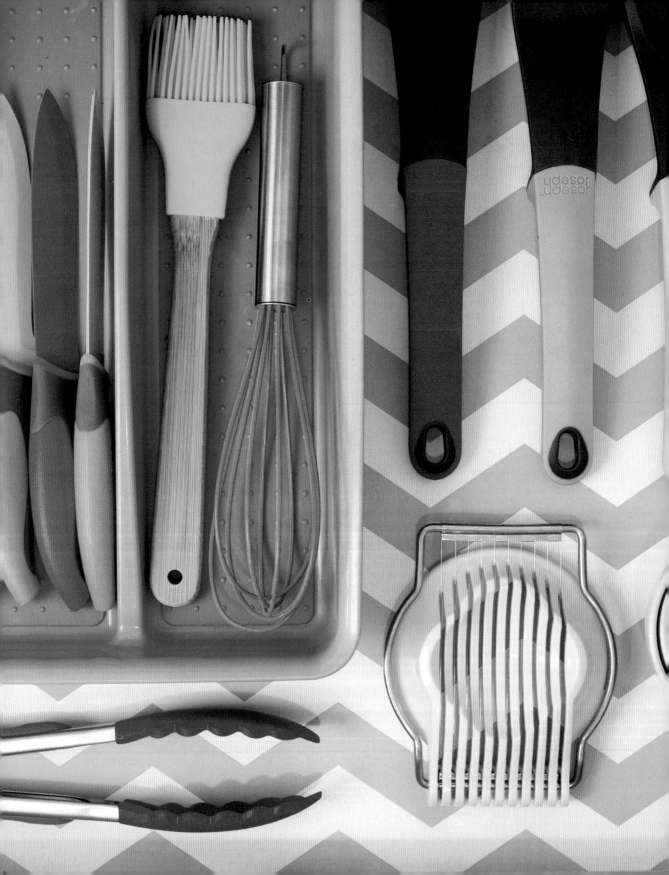

② *prepare for* SUPPERTIME SUCCESS

Nearly everything we do in life requires planning (if we want it to be successful, that is). Weddings take six to twelve months to plan; babies, well, you typically have about nine months to plan for the little bundles of joy. Vacations? The vast majority of us take a year or more to plan our most special getaways. So why is it that we're not taking a few hours out of the week to plan and prep how we will feed the minds and bodies of the most special people in our lives? Prioritize. Eating light and balanced must be a top priority if it is to get our time and attention. *Skinny Suppers* was developed to help you ensure that your waistline gets a little smaller while the bonds in your family grow substantially stronger.

In order to really embrace suppers and time with those you love, you'll probably have to change the way you look at supper just a bit. For many of us, we see making supper and going to the grocery store as chores we can't wait to get finished with. It doesn't have to be that way. View suppertime for what it really is: a way to strengthen the relationships in your family. You'll appreciate the love and work that goes into it. It all starts at the dinner table. And it's my mission to get you back there!

APPROACH GROCERY SHOPPING AND SUPPERTIME WITH A NEW OUTLOOK

Grocery shopping can be a wonderfully relaxing time to recharge, knowing the choices you make will positively impact your family. To help you along, I've compiled a few tips, in the hopes that when you are finished reading you'll be able to approach grocery shopping and suppertime with a new attitude! There are three keys to preparing for suppertime success. Read ahead and commit these to memory.

THREE KEYS TO PREPARING FOR SUPPERTIME SUCCESS

1 **The grocery store is a playground.** It's all about perception. Grocery shopping doesn't have to be brutal. Once we digest why we're there—to purchase foods that will truly "fuel" our minds and bodies, and possibly aid or boost our weight-loss journey—our trips down each aisle can actually be fun. Spend some time in the produce department searching for undiscovered fruits and vegetables, try the whole wheat version of your favorite bread in the bakery aisle, try fresh salmon for the first time—it likely won't be the last.

2 **Good cooking isn't just for chefs.** If you have chosen to purchase this book, you realize that cooking is something you must do. My purpose is to prove to you that you are capable of preparing light and balanced meals while saving time and money in the process. Culinary degree not required!

3 **Prepackaged and frozen foods can be part of light and balanced lifestyles.** Let me be very clear—fresh is always best! I'll never argue with that. However, it's not always economical or efficient. Through the pages of this cookbook I'm giving you permission to purchase frozen, canned, and prepackaged (yes, prepackaged) ingredients, trusting that they are lighter and lower in fat and calories than their traditional counterparts. (I've done the homework for you!) For all intents and purposes, these also make excellent additions to our freezer and pantry.

BUILD YOUR PANTRY, AISLE BY AISLE

Now that you're motivated and pumped up about suppertime again, what pantry staples should you have on hand to prepare these fabulously fun and delicious suppers? I'm a creature of habit, so as you begin to prepare the recipes in the following chapters, you'll see that I like to use some of the same ingredients. In doing so, pulling together lightened-up meals quickly becomes much easier. And it's cost efficient, too. To simplify preparation even more, I've pulled together a little list of pantry staples for you. These are my go-to items. You can use this as a working list at the grocery store. The best thing about it is that once you get used to having your pantry stocked in this way, you will find that cooking lighter becomes easier, less of a burden, and quite possibly even fun!

Note: You may notice that some items have brand names associated with them (for example, Uncle Ben's Ready Rice). I have called out these specific brands for a variety of reasons: because they are lower in fat and sodium than other comparable brands; because I like the variety and flavors offered by the brand; or because I have found them to be easier to cook with. Most are widely available in supermarkets across the country and readily available at your local grocer, too! At any rate, feel free to modify the product according to your needs and availability.

Now, let me take you aisle by aisle to assist you in stocking your pantry with the staples that are the foundation for many of my recipes.

The lists below include almost every single ingredient you will need to make all the recipes in this book.

PRODUCE DEPARTMENT

Spend a little more time in the produce section of your local supermarket every week. Get to know where everything is and play a little game. Choose a new piece of produce to try at home every week. It's a great way to get the kids involved. Allow them to pick a new fruit or vegetable when they come along. Go home, Google how to prepare it, and enjoy! You're likely to be surprised at how many fruits and veggies there are at your local grocery store that you've never tried! Never pass the produce department without buying something.

Vegetables

- Arugula
- Asparagus
- Baby spinach
- Baking potatoes
- Bell peppers: red, yellow, orange, and green
- Broccoli
- Brussels sprouts
- Butternut squash
- Carrots: crinkle cut, shredded, and whole
- Cauliflower
- Celery
- Coleslaw mix
- Corn
- Cucumber
- Eggplant
- Garlic
- Green onions
- Iceberg lettuce
- Jalapeños
- Kale

- Mushrooms: baby bellas (cremini) and portobellos
- Onions: red and yellow
- Parsnips
- Red potatoes
- Romaine lettuce
- Shredded cabbage: red and green
- Spaghetti squash
- Sweet potatoes
- Yellow squash
- Zucchini

Fruit

- Apples: Golden Delicious and Fuji
- Anjou pears
- Avocados
- Blueberries
- Golden raisins
- Lemons
- Limes
- Mangoes
- Oranges
- Pineapples
- Pomegranates
- Raspberries
- ReaLime juice
- ReaLemon juice
- Reduced Sugar Craisins Dried Cranberries
- Strawberries
- Tomatoes: Roma (plum) and grape
- Watermelon

TIP: When purchasing fruits and vegetables, aim for fresh (in season), frozen, and then canned, in that order.

BREADS, BAKED GOODS, AND PASTA

The bakery and bread aisles are wonderful places to glean knowledge about whole grains. Serving size is key in every area but especially in breads and pastas. Just keep an eye on your serving size and you're likely to shave carbs and calories naturally!

- Arborio rice
- Barilla pastas: ProteinPLUS or whole wheat
- Cornflakes
- Cornmeal
- Cornstarch
- Flatout Light Original Flatbreads
- Flaxseed meal
- Fresh Gourmet lightly salted tortilla strips
- Hoagie buns
- La Tortilla Factory low-carb, high-fiber whole wheat tortillas
- Panko bread crumbs
- Pillsbury Artisan Pizza Crust with Whole Grains
- Pillsbury Grands! Jr. Golden Homestyle Buttermilk Biscuits
- Pillsbury Grands! Jr. Golden Layers Flaky Biscuits
- Pillsbury Reduced Fat Crescent Rolls
- Oyster crackers
- Quaker Quick 5-Minute Grits
- Quinoa
- Refrigerated whole wheat cheese tortellini
- Rolled oats

- Uncle Ben's Ready Rice
- White whole wheat flour
- Whole wheat egg noodles
- Whole wheat hamburger buns
- Whole wheat hot dog buns
- Whole wheat pitas
- Whole Wheat Ritz Crackers

TIP: When purchasing breads and grains, read the labels and aim to purchase items that say "100 percent whole wheat," as opposed to "made with whole wheat."

CANNED AND JARRED GOODS

Typically the name brands listed in this category are called out for their lower-sodium, lower-fat, and sugar content. If you're concerned about sodium content, when it comes to other items like beans and vegetables, feel free to rinse them or look for "reduced sodium" or "no salt added." I want to encourage you in one thing: Do not be afraid of canned and jarred foods. It wasn't canned foods that moved the scale in the wrong direction. Of course, fresh is always best. But when it's not an option, feel confident in purchasing canned and jarred.

- Black olives
- Capers
- Chickpeas
- Chipotle peppers in adobo
- Chopped green chilies
- Del Monte no-sugar-added fruit: mandarin oranges, sliced peaches
- Diced pickled jalapeños
- Dill pickle chips
- Fat-free refried beans
- Hunt's no-salt-added diced tomatoes
- Hunt's tomato paste
- Kalamata olives
- Low-sodium corn, whole kernel and cream-style
- Old El Paso Thick 'n Chunky Salsa
- Pepperoncini peppers
- Pineapple chunks and tidbits in 100% juice
- Reduced-sodium black beans
- Reduced-sodium pimento-stuffed Manzanilla olives
- Reduced-sodium pinto beans
- Reduced-sodium red kidney beans
- Ro*Tel diced tomatoes and green chiles: original and mild
- Sliced beets
- Sun-dried tomatoes
- Unsweetened applesauce

Soups and Broths

- Campbell's Healthy Request condensed soups: cream of mushroom, cream of chicken, cheddar cheese, and tomato
- Pacific Organic low-sodium broths: vegetable, beef, and chicken

Sauces and Dressings

- Bolthouse Farms Classic Balsamic vinaigrette
- Bolthouse Farms Classic Ranch yogurt dressing
- Prego Light Homestyle Alfredo sauce
- Prego Light Smart Traditional pasta sauce
- Prego Veggie Smart pizza sauce
- Thai Kitchen lite coconut milk

TIP: When purchasing canned fruits, look for items packed in water or juice, not syrup, and when purchasing canned or jarred vegetables, look for items packed in water, not oil; as always, look for lower-sodium options.

SEASONINGS AND CONDIMENTS

I love to cook with fresh herbs and spices. I even grow many of my favorites, such as rosemary, dill, basil, cilantro, and parsley, in my own herb garden in my back-yard. However, I realize that fresh herbs are not always available, so feel free to replace fresh seasonings with dried in any of the recipes. I have also denoted in every recipe throughout the cookbook when I use fresh or dried.

- Basil
- Bay leaves
- Black pepper
- Blackened seasoning
- Brown sugar
- Cajun seasoning
- Caribbean jerk seasoning
- Cayenne pepper
- Chili powder
- Chinese five-spice powder
- Chives
- Cilantro
- Creole seasoning
- Curry powder
- Dried basil
- Dried oregano
- Dried rosemary
- Dry Italian dressing mix
- Garlic powder
- Ground cumin
- Ground ginger
- Italian seasoning
- Kosher salt
- Lemon-pepper seasoning
- Less-sodium taco seasoning
- McCormick Grill Mates hamburger seasoning
- Old Bay seasoning
- Onion powder
- Paprika
- Parsley
- Poppy seeds
- Poultry seasoning
- Powdered sugar
- Ranch salad dressing and seasoning mix
- Red pepper flakes
- Rosemary
- Sesame seeds
- Stevia
- Vanilla extract

Oils, Vinegars, and Sauces

- Apple cider vinegar
- Balsamic vinegar
- Coconut oil
- Cooking red wine
- Cooking sherry
- Cooking white wine
- Dijon mustard
- Extra virgin olive oil
- Frank's RedHot Original Sauce
- Heinz reduced-sugar ketchup
- Kikkoman less-sodium teriyaki marinade
- Less-sodium soy sauce
- Light mayonnaise
- Maple Grove Farms sugar-free maple-flavor syrup
- Oyster sauce
- Rice vinegar
- Sesame oil
- Smucker's natural creamy peanut butter
- Smucker's no-sugar-added preserves
- Sriracha sauce
- Stubb's Original All-Natural Bar-B-Q Sauce
- Thai Kitchen sweet red chili sauce
- White wine vinegar
- Worcestershire sauce
- Yellow mustard

TIP: In talking about condiments, I feel it is important to share my take on sweeteners. You will see that none of my recipes use white, refined sugar. In its place, I use a variety of sweeteners, depending on the recipe. When a recipe calls for a granulated sugar, I like stevia. My advice to you is to find a sweetener that works for you and your family, remembering the closest to nature is always best.

THE MEAT AND SEAFOOD DEPARTMENTS

The person behind the counter is there to assist you, so don't be afraid to ask questions, request that fat be trimmed from the meat, or ask for assistance in choosing the leanest cuts of meat. Becoming more knowledgeable about serving sizes is likely to drastically cut the fat and calories on your supper table (not to mention save you some money). For your benefit, the serving sizes for the recipes in *Skinny Suppers* are clearly noted to take out the guesswork.

- Al Fresco Andouille chicken sausage
- Beef shoulder chuck roast
- Beef top round roast
- Boar's Head lower-sodium meats
- Boneless, center-cut pork tenderloin
- Boneless pork chops
- Boneless, skinless chicken breast
- Canned chopped clams
- Chicken drumsticks, skin removed
- Cod fillets
- Diced ham
- Eggs
- Flank steak
- Ground turkey (80/20 or leaner)
- Jumbo lump crabmeat
- Lean ground beef (90/10 or leaner)
- Lean stew meat

- Medium shrimp, peeled and deveined
- Pork baby back ribs
- Pork shoulder
- Pork tenderloin

- Salmon fillets
- Solid white albacore tuna
- Tilapia fillets
- Turkey bacon

- Turkey cutlets/ medallions
- Turkey pepperoni

> TIP: Although a scale is the most accurate way to gauge serving sizes, always remember that a 3- to 4-ounce serving is about the size of a deck of cards.

DAIRY

I like to shave off calories where I can, and the dairy section is a great place to do just that. I almost always look for reduced-fat and reduced-calorie varieties. If I ever use "the real stuff," I just remind myself that a little goes a long way. I once read that when using real butter and/or oils, you could shave off one-third of what the recipe calls for and not change the texture or flavor. I have definitely found this to be true when preparing boxed desserts like brownies and cakes. Might be a great time to play around with a trusted family recipe that calls for excessive butter or oil. You can slash hundreds of calories using this little trick!

- Daisy Low Fat Cottage Cheese
- Light sour cream
- ⅓ less fat cream cheese
- Part-skim ricotta
- Plain 0% (nonfat) Greek yogurt

- Reduced-fat blue cheese
- Reduced-fat feta cheese
- Sargento Grated Parmesan Cheese
- Sargento Natural Light String Cheese Snacks

- Sargento Reduced Fat Shredded Cheese Varieties
- Sargento Ultra Thin Sliced Cheese Varieties
- Skim milk
- Unsalted butter

> TIP: Just remember, you can always add more butter and cheese, but you can't take it away. Always start with less. You're likely to be surprised with how little you really need!

THE FROZEN SECTION

For quick, easy meal prep, the frozen section of your grocery store is your friend. Feel free to purchase frozen fruits and veggies in place of fresh when you know you will be pressed for time, or just to have on hand in a pinch. It's also impor-tant to remember that certain fruits and veggies are "in season" certain times of the year. Purchasing frozen varieties allows for their availability any time of the year.

- Blueberries
- Broccoli
- Cauliflower
- Mangos
- Mixed vegetable blends
- Pearl onions
- Spinach
- Strawberries
- Yellow corn

TIP: I love to keep frozen fruits on hand. They're great in a pinch: blended in smoothies and used for topping ice cream, oatmeal, cereals, yogurt, and more.

MISCELLANEOUS ITEMS

Below is a list of items that don't really fall into a specific category, but that I like to have on hand.

Nuts

- Pecans
- Raw cashews
- Raw unsalted sunflower seeds
- Roasted and shelled unsalted pistachios
- Slivered almonds
- Walnuts

Juice and Beverages

- Reduced-sugar apple juice
- Pomegranate juice
- Silk Unsweetened Original Almondmilk
- Tropicana Trop50 Orange Juice (reduced-calorie, stevia-sweetened)

Other

- Baking powder
- Baking soda
- Nonstick cooking spray

TIP: I like to have quarter-cup containers on hand (even in my purse). They are fantastic portion-control tools for nuts, seeds, trail mix, etc. Instead of counting nuts and seeds I simply fill my quarter-cup container. It's virtually impossible to overeat a high-calorie snack like nuts using these!

THE RIGHT KITCHEN TOOLS

If you're going to do a job right, you're going to need the right tools. You wouldn't send your son to his first football practice with a basketball or your daughter to her first day of piano with a violin, would you? Of course not. So why are you still using the same dull knives and the well-worn cutting board from your wedding shower? (If you've been married more than ten years, this message is really for you!) Here are ten tools that will make your meal prep a breeze.

1. **A set of quality sharp knives.** If a whole set is not in your budget, shop for a versatile 8-inch chef's knife, equally useful for precision dicing and heavy-duty chopping.

2. **A knife steel/honing steel.** Most knives benefit from being honed often. Honing pushes the edge of the knife back into its proper position and straightens it. Keep in mind that even the best knives need sharpening every now and then. How often you use your knives and what they're made of (carbon steel versus stainless steel) determines how often they require sharpening, but once or twice a year is likely sufficient. To sharpen your knives you can use a water stone, an electric knife sharpener, or a professional sharpening service.

3. **A worthy cutting board (or two).** Cutting boards can harbor bacteria if they're too porous and can dull your knives if they're too hard. I like a firm plastic board for meats and proteins and a wood board for my fruits and veggies. Keeping them separate relieves my concerns about bacteria infesting my fruits and vegetables. I do, however, recommend a larger one for bigger jobs and a smaller bar board for the everyday slicing and dicing of things like apples and hard-boiled eggs.

4. **A kitchen scale.** This is the best tool to ensure accurate calorie counting and monitoring of portions.

5. **A good set of pots and pans.** Seek out nonstick if saving time on cleanup is a priority for you!

6. **A high-powered blender.** Blenders are fantastic for using up fruits and vegetables that are about to go bad. Just add them to your blender with a flavored low-fat or nonfat yogurt for great-tasting, healthy smoothies! Not in the mood for a smoothie at the moment? Simply blend your fruits and veggies, place them in a freezer bag, label, and save for later!

7. **A heavy-duty mixer.** My KitchenAid mixer is one of my favorite kitchen tools of all time. Isn't it everyone's? This bad boy has been around since 1919 and is arguably

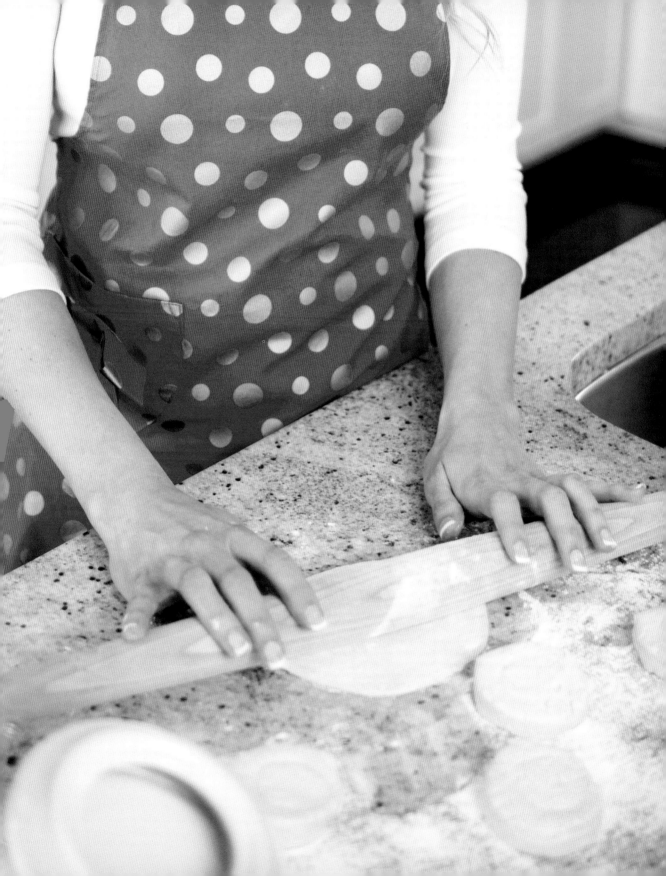

still the best. A good mixer is not just for making cakes and cookies but is also helpful for prepping and preparing dinner recipes. I use it for mixing Cauliflower Mashed Potatoes and for the creamy sweet potato topping for Creole-Style Shepherd's Pie.

8 **A set of mixing bowls.** Aim to have at least one small, one medium, and one large bowl.

9 **A set of measuring tools.** I like measuring spoons that are connected, so I'm less likely to misplace one. Nesting measuring cups are great space savers, too!

10 **A quality slow cooker.** A personal favorite, slow cookers save time, money, and are virtually mistake-proof. Just toss in the ingredients, come back in a few hours, and voilà! Supper is served!

Have fun with this, but don't break the bank. Purchase one thing at a time and spruce up your tools by buying things like measuring tools and cutting boards in your favorite colors. Your kitchen will be your new favorite place in the house!

For me, feeling organized helps to inspire and motivate me. So I want to help you organize that all-important workspace known as your kitchen. In addition to the ten tools I listed earlier, here is a list of kitchen tools I use for the preparation of all the suppers in this cookbook.

Utensils

- Tongs
- Wooden spoon
- Spatulas: metal and silicone
- Fish turner or wide slotted metal spatula
- Slotted spoon
- Whisk
- Ladle

- Meat mallet
- Silicone pastry brush
- Cutting boards with rubber grippers (or place a wet paper towel underneath to ensure nonslip cutting)

- Measuring spoons: ⅛ teaspoon, ¼ teaspoon, ½ teaspoon, 1 teaspoon, ½ tablespoon, 1 tablespoon
- Dry-ingredient measuring cups: ¼ cup, ⅓ cup, ½ cup, 1 cup
- 2-cup liquid measuring cup

Sharp Tools

- Chef's knife: 8- or 10-inch
- Paring knife
- Serrated knife
- Knife steel (to hone in between getting it sharpened professionally)
- Y-shaped peeler
- Microplane grater
- Box grater

Pots and Pans

- 13 x 9-inch baking dish
- 11 x 7-inch baking dish
- 9-inch loaf pan
- 9-inch pie pan
- Deep 2-quart baking dish
- Two rimmed baking sheets
- Cast iron skillet
- Large 12-inch skillet with lid
- Large pot with lid or soup pot with lid
- Medium saucepan with lid
- Small saucepan with lid
- Grill pan or electric indoor grill (or outdoor grill)
- Muffin tin
- Dutch oven*

*WHAT'S A DUTCH OVEN? A large, heavy pot that can be used on top of the stove as well as in the oven and includes a tight-fitting lid. For more on kitchen practices and terms I wish I had known when I started cooking, turn to page 35.

Electrics

- 6-quart slow cooker
- Digital instant-read thermometer
- Digital scale

Miscellaneous

- Spoon rest (on counter next to range)
- Butcher's twine
- Toothpicks
- Oven mitts
- Potholders
- Spiral slicer
- Plastic storage containers
- Gallon-size resealable plastic bags
- Aluminum foil
- Parchment paper
- Plastic wrap

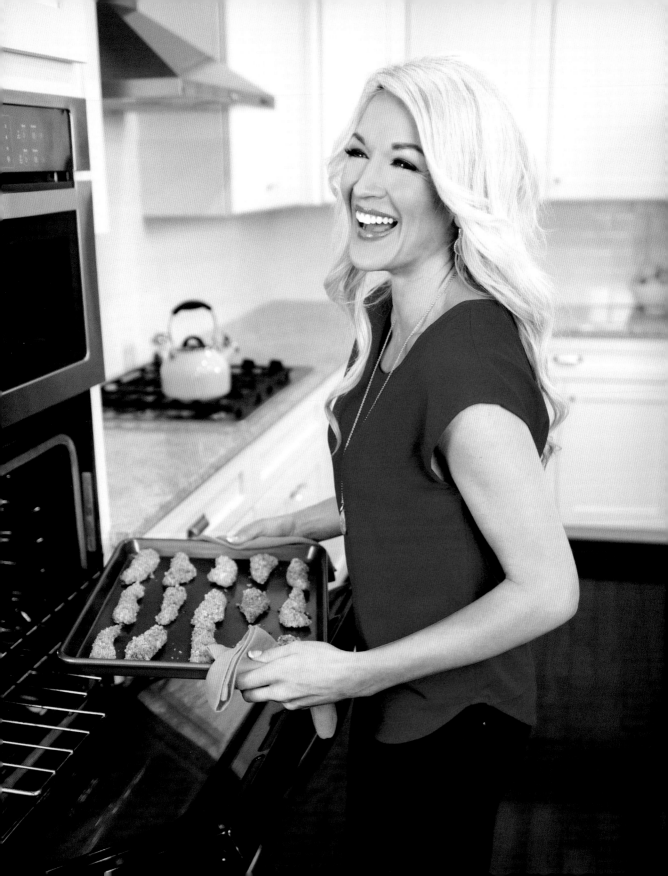

③ *meal planning for*
BALANCED, WAIST-FRIENDLY SUPPERS

I t's all in the plan. I once read a saying: "If you fail to plan, you plan to fail." The best way to ensure the success of your suppers is to plan them. Know in advance which meals you plan to cook for the week, and create your grocery list accordingly. Later in this chapter, I will share with you all you need to know about following a menu calendar for an entire month. But for now, realize this: Knowing what you're preparing for supper each night of the week is extremely empowering and an incredible stress reliever. It also helps to ensure you are aware of the calorie count and nutritional value of the foods you are consuming and feeding those you love. You can do all this in three simple steps:

1 Tailor your grocery shopping.

2 Choose a weekly prep night (it's not as scary as it sounds and is completely doable).

3 Create a supper calendar.

Let's break these components down so you can be one step closer to balanced, waist-friendly suppers!

TAILOR YOUR GROCERY SHOPPING

There's more to the grocery list than just the list. Follow these tips and your trip to the grocery store will be less stressful, more inviting, and overall a positive addition to your day and lifestyle!

Keep an ongoing grocery list in plain sight. Don't rely on your memory to remind you that you need milk or Cajun seasoning for a recipe this week. Keep a pen and paper on the counter by the stove or fridge (or on the fridge) so that you and anyone else can add to the list as necessary throughout the week. And for you techies out there, utilizing the virtual notepads on your phone or tablet is a great way to stay organized, too. It also makes it easier for you to refer back and see how often you're buying items. Recently, I've discovered apps just for grocery lists. My new favorite is the Out of Milk app (free for Android and iPhone). It keeps a running list for me and even alerts me to special sales at stores close to me!

Organize the list before you go to the grocery. I am never more frustrated than when I have crossed off everything on my list and I'm ready to check out, only to realize I forgot the romaine lettuce and the produce section is clear on the other side of the store. Organize your grocery list by section or aisle, so that you're less likely to forget an item or waste precious time crisscrossing the store for things you forgot.

Go through the fridge and pantry before heading out. This way, you can ensure that you don't already have a certain item. I remember at one point I had four bags of brown sugar in my pantry simply because I couldn't remember if I had it at home when I was at the grocery store and knew that a recipe I was preparing called for it. Save time, money, and space by giving these areas a quick once-over before heading out.

Shop when it's convenient for you. Preferably when you're not too tired or hungry. Studies indicate that when we're tired and hungry, we're more vulnerable and likely to purchase foods that aren't on our list and that are typically less nutritious. At the very least, have a nutrition bar and keep a bottle of water handy as you shop.

Make your trip to the grocery store enjoyable. To coincide with your weekly (or biweekly) trip to the grocery store, splurge on your favorite cup of coffee. But do it only when you're going to the grocery so that it seems more special. If you're shopping with the kids, use it as an educational experience by quizzing them on names of produce and asking them to find items for you like a scavenger hunt.

CHOOSE AND KEEP A WEEKLY PREP NIGHT (AKA POWER PLANNING SUNDAYS)

When I first heard about "prep days," I have to admit, I was a little skeptical. I just wasn't sure if I wanted to devote part of my weekend to chopping veggies, cooking and dicing chicken breasts, and pre-portioning everything when I wasn't even cooking a meal.

But here's what I found: Preparing food ahead of time doesn't just solve time-management issues around supper, it solves everyday situations like midday and late-night snacking, and what to pack for everyone's lunches.

On Sundays, I can do the bulk of the labor in getting my meals prepped and portioned for the week. I find that it's so much easier to set aside one and a half to two hours each week to chop veggies, cook, shred and/or dice chicken and other meats, and portion it all out as well as label items and place them in the fridge or freezer (depending on when I need certain things) than to worry about it all week long. There's a reason I now refer to these prep days as Power Planning Sundays.

If you have kiddos who come home starving every day after school, the prep day is another way to already have healthier options available for them. Having healthy snacks portioned out and readily available empowers them to make healthier choices during tempting times, like after school and after mealtimes. It can also help to relieve stress for you—if you can't be home during those times, at least you know you left them options to make healthy choices.

Power Planning Sundays give you a head start on packing lunches, too. It makes mornings a little less crazy. But hey! Don't worry if Sunday doesn't work for you. Pick any day or evening that works and mark it on the calendar just like any other appointment. Remember, if it's important to you, you'll find the time to fit it in.

Another way to make prep time more inviting is to make it about the family. Doing the prep work doesn't have to fall on your shoulders every week. Give everyone a job to do: One person can be in charge of cooking the meats; one person gets to chop veggies; another gets to label and package the portions. Even toddlers can help out by counting out the portions. This, once again, puts some control into your children's hands and naturally educates them about things like planning and healthy eating. If you have adolescents in the home, take the opportunity to educate them about which vegetables are good for their skin and hair. Athletes in that same age group love to know which lean proteins will help them build muscle and perform better in sports. Is there a techie teen in the family? Great time to instill knowledge in them about which veggies are good for focus and concentration.

CREATE A SUPPER CALENDAR

The supper calendar is a powerful tool for many reasons. Taking the guesswork out of meal planning takes the stress out of meal planning. Many women have testified, too, that knowing what they were preparing for supper every night has actually helped in their weight-loss journey. And knowing what is being prepared every night for an entire month truly simplifies grocery shopping. This tool alone is likely to transform the way you approach supper! Get ready for change!

Here's a monthlong supper calendar made up completely of Skinny Suppers. Use this sample calendar to get started right away. Just make your grocery list, take it to the grocery store, stock up, and have fun making lightened-up suppers for your family. Note: Keep in mind that many of the recipes in *Skinny Suppers* make six servings, so if you are preparing meals for a smaller crowd, be sure to incorporate leftovers into your calendar every month. More simplicity!

At some point, you are going to need to be able to create a calendar on your own. So, I want to show you how I create a month of suppers. Here are my eight simple steps to creating an entire month of guilt-free and deliciously light and balanced suppers.

1. **Start with a blank calendar.** Just Google "blank calendars" and you'll find hundreds. Print several and place in a folder marked "Supper Calendars." If you're not the pen-and-paper type, feel free to store it digitally.

2. **Add the family's schedule.** This means practices, nights you will be working late, and any other events that may interfere with the amount of time you have to cook.

3. **Pencil in meal requests.** Somewhere throughout the month, plug in what everyone is craving. This can eliminate everyone's desire for eating out. It's also

A Month of Suppers

Sunday	Monday	Tuesday	Wednesday	Thursday	Friday	Saturday
	1 Chipotle Black Bean Burgers (page 247) Southwest "Fried" Pickles (page 284)	2 Sour Cream Enchiladas (page 122) Quinoa Mexi-Lime Salad (page 289)	3 Tomato Tortellini Soup (page 232) Green salad	4 Parmesan Chicken Nuggets (page 113) Broccoli Mac 'n' Cheese (page 265)	5 Autumn Chopped Salad (page 217) Southern Sweet Beets (page 296)	6 Carnitas Veggie Bowl (page 158) Cilantro-Lime Rice (page 271)
7 Slow-Cooker Chicken and Dumplings (page 119) Easy Roasted Vegetables (page 277)	8 Veggie and Cheese Manicotti (page 138) Green salad	9 Un-Sloppy Janes (page 126) Skillet Corn (page 291)	10 Quick Shrimp and Vegetable Stir-Fry (page 202) Edamame	11 Grilled Pineapple Teriyaki Pork Chops (page 168) Sweet and Spicy Coleslaw (page 287)	12 Blackened Chicken with Avocado Cream Sauce (page 101) Parmesan-Garlic Quinoa (page 285)	13 Apple-Stuffed Pork Tenderloin with Dijon Mustard Sauce (page 156) Caramelized Brussels Sprouts with Pecans (page 298)
14 Southern "Fried" Chicken (page 110) Sun-Dried Tomato and Pesto Potato Salad (page 292)	15 Vegetarian Tikka Masala (page 257) Quick Cauliflower Couscous (page 286)	16 Deep-Dish BBQ Hawaiian Skillet Pizza (page 164) Green salad	17 Farmers' Market Garden Bake (page 82) Skinny Sweet Potato Biscuits (page 272)	18 Philly Cheesesteak Stuffed Peppers (page 52) Carrot and Raisin Salad (page 268)	19 Grilled Chicken and Fruit Salad Wraps (page 208) Old Bay Deviled Eggs (page 282)	20 Shrimp and Sausage Jambalaya (page 186) Cheesy Jalapeño Cornbread (page 270)
21 Kentucky Bourbon Fall-off-the-Bone Ribs (page 161) Skillet Corn (page 291)	22 Spinach-Artichoke Flatbread Pizza (page 253) Italian Chickpea Salad (page 278)	23 Cowgirl Casserole (page 79) Skinny Fried Apples (page 297)	24 Easy Asian Salmon with Orange Sweet Glaze (page 196) Mango Slaw (page 281)	25 Slow-Cooker Creamy Chicken and Wild Rice Soup (page 222) Rustic Rosemary Root Vegetables (page 290)	26 Cheesy Mexican Meatloaf (page 45) Cilantro-Lime Rice (page 271)	27 Supreme Pizza Pasta Casserole (page 73) Skinny Broccoli Salad (page 295)
28 Thai-Style Hot Dogs (page 65) Easy Roasted Vegetables (page 277)	29 Santa Fe Quinoa Sizzling Skillet (page 243) Southwest "Fried" Pickles (page 284)	30 Crispy Coconut Fish Sticks (page 195) Cajun-Style Sweet Potato Fries (page 267)	31 BBQ Turkey Chili (page 221) Cheesy Jalapeño Cornbread (page 270)			

another great way to encourage the kids to help out. If you're preparing their favorite meal at least once a month, they're likely to want to learn how to cook it, too!

4 **Create theme nights at least once a week.** Meatless Monday is the trend in our house. We also have Taco Tuesday (it's not always tacos, but it is always Mexican) and Clean the Fridge Friday, combining leftovers.

5 **Challenge yourself to try a new recipe often.** Plug those in accordingly. Make sure you plan those for when you have a little more time.

6 **Repeat your favorites.** Feel free to plug in the same dish more than once a month. If the whole family really loves the Jalapeño Popper Chicken Casserole (page 74), make it two or even three nights this month. (It will help to simplify your grocery shopping, too!)

7 **Schedule dining out.** Since you're not doing it several times a week, once or twice a month makes it more special.

8 **Get ready for grocery shopping.** Once the calendar is full, proceed to making your weekly grocery lists.

SAVING TIME AND MONEY

Making a change in the way you eat does not have to mean spending more on groceries. By utilizing the strategies below, you will naturally begin to spend less on your grocery bill without even thinking about it. I also want to encourage you to look at the money you *do* spend at the supermarket as an investment in the future of your family. Eating healthier now is likely to save you on doctor bills and prescriptions later.

Even though we've made leaps and bounds in terms of creating a new perspective on the grocery store, you still don't want to live there. For additional help in maximizing your savings, here are a few general rules that I use when I grocery-shop:

Buy in bulk when you can. Megastores like Sam's Club and Costco often offer lower prices for buying in bulk. For staples like chicken breasts and lean ground beef or turkey, you can save big-time. I portion them out into individual freezer bags labeled with the date and contents and can often scratch these items off my weekly grocery list!

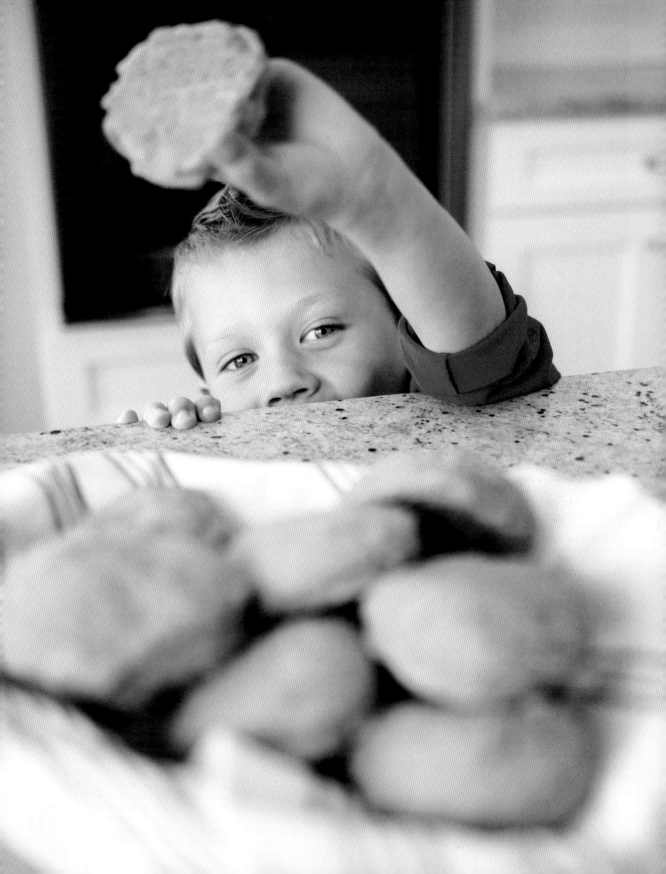

Take inventory. It's always a good idea to go through the pantry, fridge, and freezer once a month to get an idea of what's there. I often freeze leftovers, so if I'm not taking stock every now and then, I quickly forget what's there.

Know the floor plan of the stores you frequent. If you frequent the same stores, learn the layout and plan your route so you don't derail to the cookie aisle.

Plan your suppers by the sales. I like to look over the grocery ads once a week and see what's on sale. Once I determine the items I plan to purchase, I peruse my recipes and plan accordingly. Having a calendar of meals planned ahead of time allows me to easily swap suppers from one week to another based on specific items that might be on sale.

The less you frequent the store, the less you buy. I used to be an "I'm just going to run in and get one thing" kind of girl. I quickly realized the time and extra money I was spending could be cut drastically with a little planning. Did you know that we're more likely to impulse-buy when our trips to the grocery are unplanned or we go without a list?

Freeze or feast on what is soon to be expired. Americans typically toss about 25 percent of the groceries they buy, according to the National Resources Defense Council. To prevent your food from turning into wasted money, sort through your fridge and pantry about once a week for items that are about to expire and place those in a designated space so that you remember to eat them before they go bad. If you're struggling to use up all the leftovers, remember this: Most of them can be frozen until you're ready to eat them.

TOP FIVE STRATEGIES FOR BALANCED MEALS

In addition to knowing what you are planning, below are my top five strategies for ensuring the suppers you plan are balanced and waist-friendly. As we move closer to cooking I wanted to share a few tips with you regarding how to plan for light and balanced eating. Keeping these five strategies in mind as you embark on this fun, new way of eating and living will empower and naturally train your mind to make more informed decisions about what you purchase and how you fill your plate. Which all translates into lighter and more balanced eating for you and the ones you love.

1 **Be "in the know."** Pay attention to food labels and know the fat and calorie content. Typically, suppers should be about 500 calories.

2 **Portion control is key.** Consider eating off smaller plates, like salad plates, so you can fill your plate and trick your mind into thinking you're actually eating more. Seriously, it works!

3 **Fill your plate with fruits and veggies.** I find myself serving the fruits and veggies first, covering half my plate. That way, I am less likely to fill my plate with higher-fat and -calorie items.

4 **Water! Water! Water! Really, no one can argue with water.** It serves so many important jobs: great for hair, skin, and nails, and it's a natural diuretic. I usually drink 12 to 20 ounces right before I'm getting ready to eat. Studies indicate that just this trick alone promotes a calorie-consumption drop of 100 to 200 calories when sitting down to eat!

5 **Remake your favorite Skinny Suppers regularly.** Remember how I told you that I'm a creature of habit? Well, most of us are. Chances are you have a spaghetti recipe you know like the back of your hand, and when all else fails, you can whip it up in no time. That's the idea behind the staples and recipes in this cookbook. I want you to be able to "whip up" five to ten of them without thinking about it. So as you begin to explore the suppers in *Skinny Suppers*, listen to the feedback from the family. And when they say, "Mom, this is the bomb!" be sure to take note. You just found a light and balanced supper to feed your family for a lifetime!

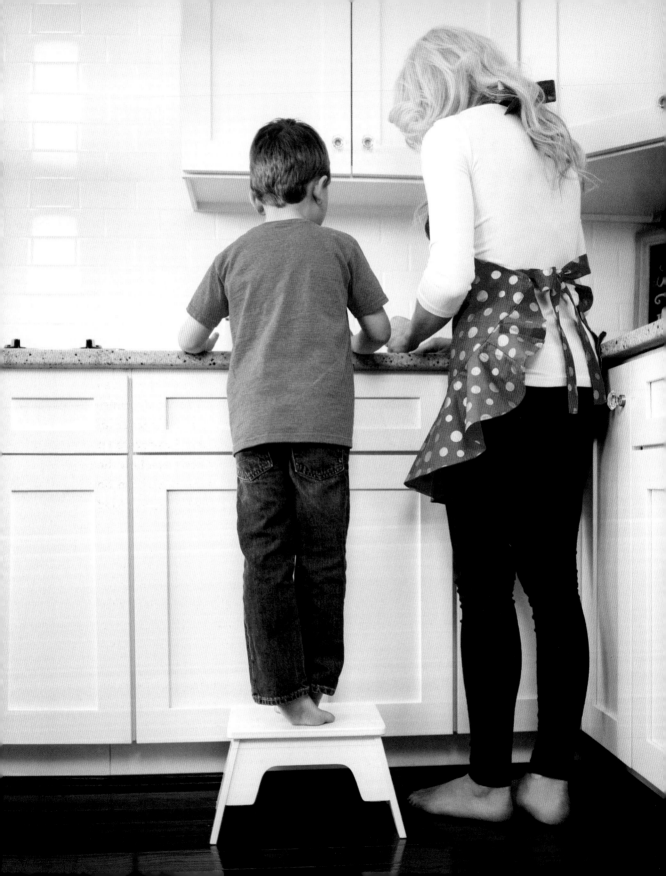

4 *let's get* COOKING

N ow it's time to get cooking. You are about to dig into more than one hundred of my favorite skinny suppers and side dishes, all of which you can feel confident about serving up to your loved ones. To simplify things even more, look for the following icons and sidebars that will provide more information regarding the recipes. Inspiration, simplicity, leftovers. I've covered it all. And to add some fun along the way, for those of you who aren't sure how the conversation will flow after the food is on the table, I've got that covered, too. So tie your apron on and get out your skillet, you're about to make some great food and memories!

READING THE RECIPES

Throughout this book, I have included **Skinny Sense** ideas, which were designed to provide you with insightful tips and facts about specific ingredients, techniques, or health benefits that relate to the recipes. I love learning new information about the food that I prepare, and I hope you take away a new piece of knowledge from these ideas.

You will also find **Suppertime Inspirations.** These are messages of encouragement and inspiration—my way of cheering you on throughout your journey. I know it's not easy to find balance, fulfill your responsibilities within your career, raise a family, *and* eat healthy. I'm on the journey with you. Sprinkled in the pages of this book are quotes that have carried me through some of the toughest times and inspired me to keep going, even when I didn't want to. It's my hope that they will do the same for you!

I have also included **Suppertime Chat** ideas designed to guide you in how to lighten up the conversation, bring out some laughs, and genuinely learn how to enjoy one another while getting to know each other just a little more.

Be on the lookout for tips called **Quick and Easy,** which are interesting ideas and suggestions that will help you make preparation as quick as possible, cue you in on recipes that are easy to double up or freeze, or offer easy ingredient swaps.

If you spot **Make It Homemade** in the ingredients lists, it's a reference to easy seasoning and sauce recipes that you can make in advance and substitute for packaged seasonings and prepared sauces that are called for in some of the recipes. Most of the homemade recipes can be made using pantry staples that you will likely have on hand, and the homemade version not only adds wonderful flavor but also cuts down on sodium.

Many of the dinner recipes will feature a **Suggested Side Dish** that calls attention to a side dish recipe along with the page on which it is located. I handpicked the side dishes based on flavors that pair well with the main entrées and tried to be mindful of nutritional values to create a well-balanced supper for you and your family.

For all recipes that use a slow cooker, **No Slow Cooker, No Problem** offers instructions for how to prepare the recipe without one.

🕐 Even though all the recipes in this cookbook take right around 30 minutes, I call attention to my **Weeknight Wonders.** These are recipes that take 30 minutes or less from prep to the table and have fewer overall ingredients. You'll definitely want to plug a few Weeknight Wonders into your supper calendar every month!

⊟ If you see a recipe with the **Waist-Friendly** icon, that means that the supper contains fewer than 350 calories per serving or the side dish contains fewer than 150 calories per serving.

(2x) Finally, I have marked several recipes in this cookbook that taste just as good (if not better) the second time around. Look for recipes labeled **Twice as Nice** sprinkled throughout, and you no longer have to feel guilty about serving up leftovers!

⭐ Twenty-five of the 125 recipes in *Skinny Suppers* are recipes I lovingly refer to as **Fan Favorites.** These are the recipes readers rave about on the Skinny Mom website month after month. They have been taste-tested by you—the busy cook with no time to spare—and have passed the test of being simple, balanced, waist-friendly, and delicious! They are skinny and likely to become "favorites" in your home, too! I absolutely recommend adding a few Fan Favorites to your calendar every month!

PRACTICES AND TERMS I WISH I'D KNOWN ABOUT WHEN I STARTED COOKING

Because I'm not a chef, when I first started flipping through cookbooks, the cooking terms began to frustrate me. Between words like "slurry" and "roux," I found myself becoming discouraged before I even got started. Knowledge gives you power and confidence in the kitchen, and I want to make sure you know the basics. Here are a list of terms and definitions that you'll see in the recipes

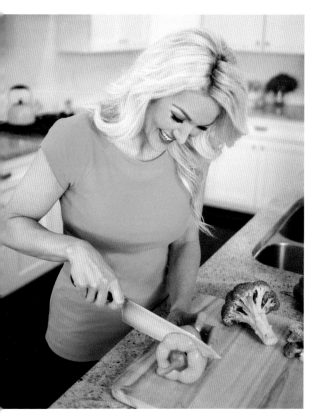

that follow. They're important to know because they do have an impact on the outcome of your recipes.

al dente: Some people translate this Italian phrase as cooked "just right." It refers to pasta, vegetables, rice, or beans that are cooked to be firm to the bite.

broil: Cooking food directly under high, intense heat. This is good for finishing a dish with cheese, so you can get a nice bubbling brown top.

butterfly: A technique used when you want to cut down on cooking time by making the boneless protein you are working with thinner, or when you are stuffing a protein. You cut the protein lengthwise but not all the way through, leaving it attached on one side so it can be opened up like a book.

chop: To cut something into uniform size, but where the shape of the pieces does not matter.

deglaze: A fancy way of saying that I'm about to use my pan drippings to make gravy (that's what my granny would have said) or other sauce. You can deglaze a pan with water, or a flavorful liquid, like cooking wine or stock.

dice: To cut something into uniform cubes; dice can be small, medium, or large.

glaze: Thinner than gravies and often brushed on food several times during preparation, glazes adhere to the surface, often becoming part of the food.

julienne: Sometimes referred to as a "matchstick" cut, this is a knife cut that is a long, thin strip. Technically, the dimensions are 1/8 inch x 1/8 inch x 2 inches. This cut is most often used with vegetables.

mince: Cutting something down very small, where the shape of the cuts do not matter (for example, garlic).

roux: A cooked thickening agent used as the base of many soups and sauces. It is equal parts flour and fat (typically butter). You'll melt the butter first, then mix in the flour and cook for 1 to 2 minutes until it releases a nutty aroma. Be sure to cook the roux long enough to cook out the flour taste before adding the liquid. Next you will gradually whisk in the liquid, and continue whisking until the roux is smooth and has thickened.

rub: A spice and/or herb mixture rubbed on foods before cooking. Typically rubs are used on meats/poultry and seafood. Rubs can be wet (paste) or dry.

sauté: To fry something quickly in a little fat.

sear: Cooking meat or fish at a very high temperature for a brief period of time. On contact, the hot cooking surface caramelizes the sugars and the sugars brown the protein, producing incredible flavor.

simmer: To heat a liquid just below the boiling point. You know your liquid is at a simmer when you start seeing tiny bubbles coming up from the bottom of the pot and breaking at the surface.

slurry: An uncooked thickening agent that is typically added at the end of cooking to thicken a sauce. It is equal parts starch (usually cornstarch) and liquid (water, stock, or juice).

COOKING TIMES

Food safety is always important. It's vital to make sure foods are cooked to the correct and safe temperature to avoid growth of bacteria and other food poisoning organisms. Below is the most recent guide put forth by the USDA for safe cooking temperatures. (Along with accurate cooking temperatures, I also like to be sure that I frequently wash my hands and the surfaces on which I am preparing food.)

Internal Temperatures

Product	Minimal Internal Temperature
Beef, Pork, Veal, and Lamb (steaks, chops, roasts)	**145°F** (62.8°C) and allow to rest for at least 3 minutes
Ground meats	**160°F** (71.1°C)
Ham, fresh or smoked (uncooked)	**145°F** (62.8°C) and allow to rest for at least 3 minutes
Ham, fully cooked (to reheat)	Reheat cooked hams packaged in USDA-inspected plants to **140°F** (60°C) and all others to **165°F** (73.9°C)
Poultry (breasts, whole bird, legs, thighs, wings, ground poultry, and stuffing)	**165°F** (73.9°C)
Eggs	**160°F** (71.1°C)
Fish and Shellfish	**145°F** (62.8°C)
Leftovers	**165°F** (73.9°C)
Casseroles	**165°F** (73.9°C)

This chart lists the USDA's recommended safe internal temperatures as of January 2015.
http://www.fsis.usda.gov/wps/portal/fsis/topics/food-safety-education/get-answers/food-safety-fact-sheets/safe-food-handling/safe-minimum-internal-temperature-chart/ct_index

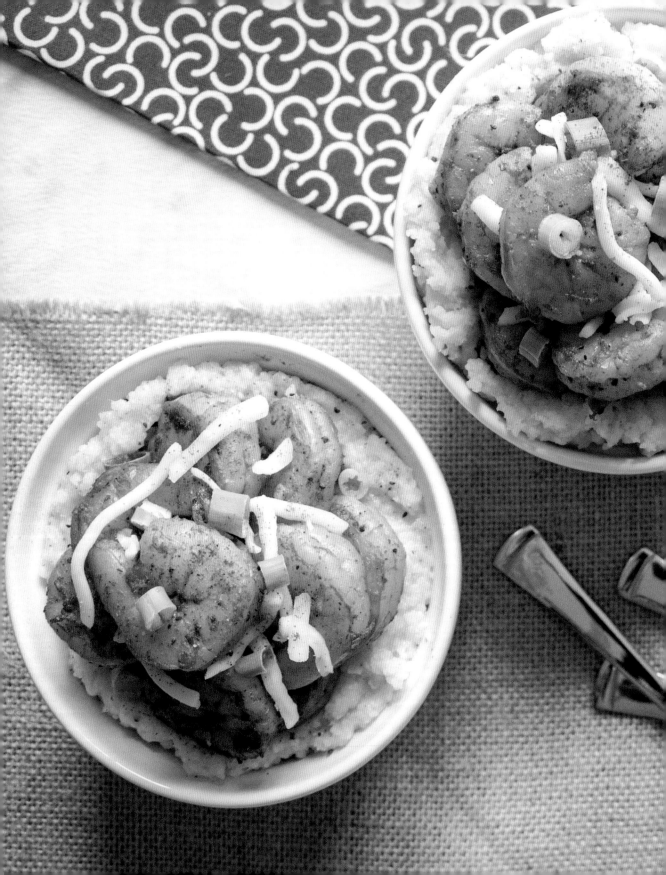

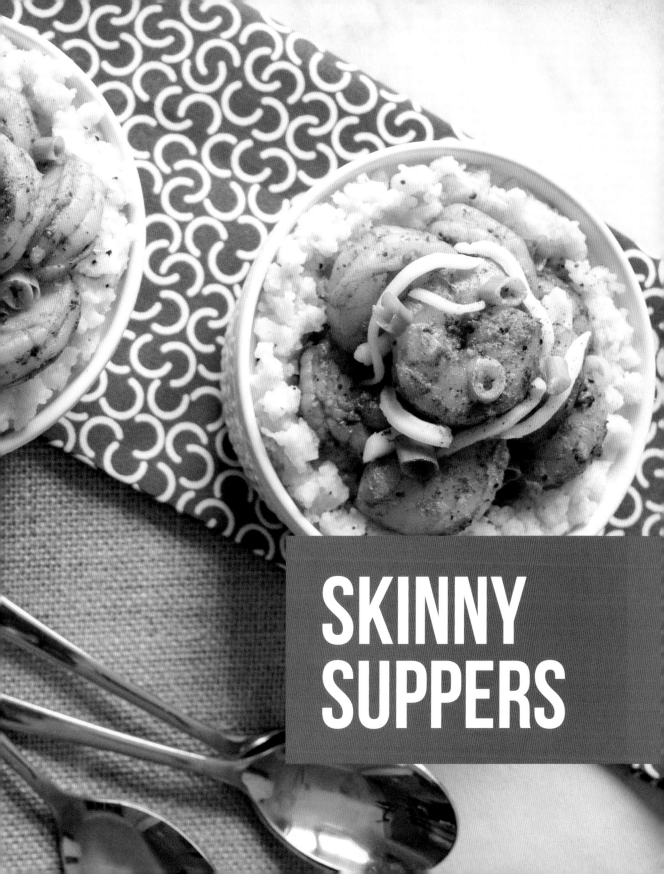

SKINNY SUPPERS

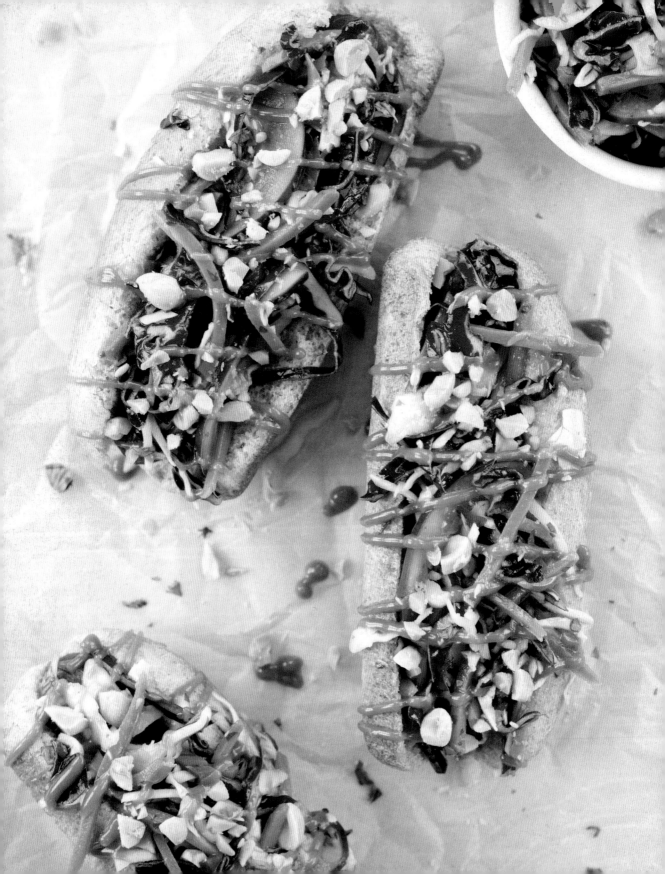

⑤ HOME COOKING ON THE RANGE
BEEF SUPPERS

Cheeseburger Lettuce Wraps

These lettuce wraps have all the yummy cheeseburger flavor, but the guilt is left at the door! By eliminating one of the highest-carb and -calorie features—the bun—and replacing it with vegetables, you can get this new and improved all-American tradition on your monthly meal calendar many times a month!

Prep Time: 10 minutes | **Cook Time:** 12 minutes
Serves: 6 | **Serving Size:** 2 stuffed lettuce leaves

Beef Filling:

1½ pounds lean ground beef

1 large onion, diced

1 tablespoon minced garlic

1 (10.5-ounce) can Campbell's Healthy Request condensed cheddar cheese soup

½ tablespoon McCormick Grill Mates hamburger seasoning

Sauce:

2 tablespoons light mayonnaise

1 tablespoon Heinz reduced-sugar ketchup

½ tablespoon yellow mustard

For Serving:

12 large romaine lettuce leaves

¾ cup shredded reduced-fat sharp cheddar cheese (I like Sargento)

4 dill pickle spears, chopped

1 cup diced tomato

1. To make the beef filling: In a large skillet over medium-high heat, cook the ground beef, 1 cup of the diced onion, and the garlic until the beef is no longer pink, 7 to 8 minutes. Use a wooden spoon to break the beef up as it cooks. Drain any excess fat and return the skillet to the stovetop, turning the heat down to low.

2. Add the cheddar soup and hamburger seasoning to the ground beef, mix well to combine, and simmer for 2 to 3 minutes.

3. Meanwhile, to make the sauce: In a small bowl, whisk together the mayonnaise, ketchup, and mustard.

4. To assemble the lettuce wraps: Spoon a heaping ¼ cup of the ground beef mixture into the bottom of a lettuce leaf. Top with 1 tablespoon cheddar, 1 heaping tablespoon each chopped pickles and diced tomatoes, and 1 teaspoon of the remaining diced onion. Drizzle with 1 teaspoon of the sauce. Repeat for a total of 12 wraps.

Suggested Side Dish: Cajun-Style Sweet Potato Fries (page 267)

quick and easy: Make this dish even more fun for your family by setting it up as a "serve yourself bar." Once cooked, set out the hamburger mixture along with a platter of lettuce leaves, cheese, pickles, tomatoes, onions, etc., and let everyone dress their wrap to their liking!

Calories 268 • Fat 14g • Carbohydrate 12g • Fiber 2g • Sugar 4g • Protein 26g

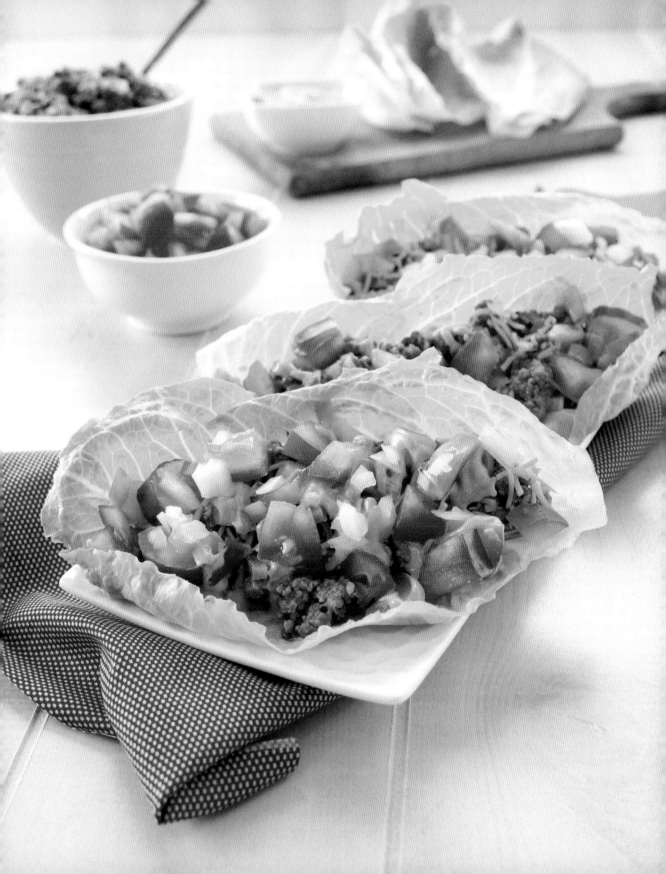

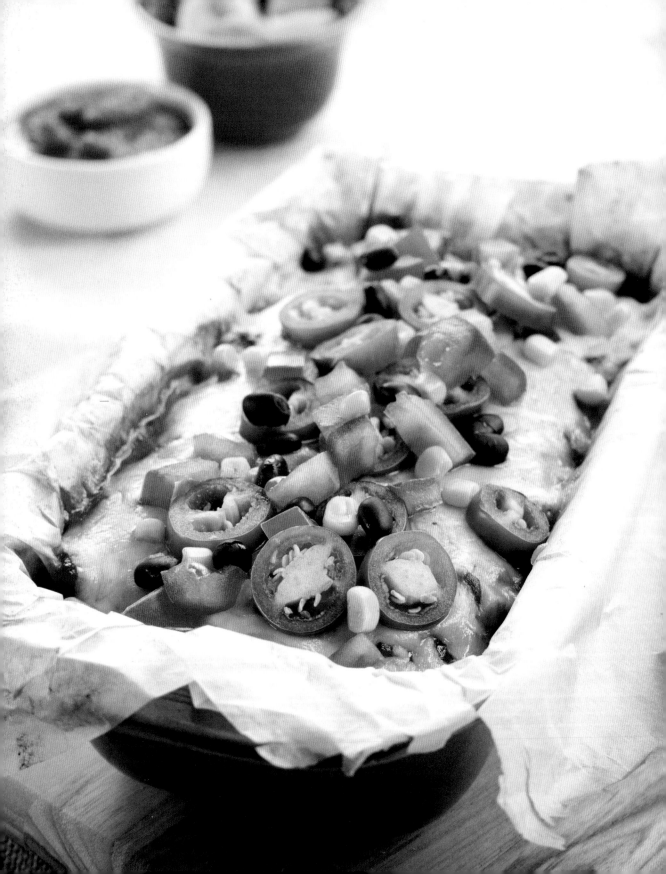

Cheesy Mexican Meatloaf

I'm a Southern girl, so meatloaf is near and dear to my heart. However, I realize not everyone shares my love for this dish. But just you wait! With the right blend of cheese and Mexican flare, the meatloaf doubters in your house will be singing a new tune!

Prep Time: 10 minutes | **Cook Time:** 1 hour 10 minutes
Serves: 6 | **Serving Size:** 1½-inch-thick slice of meatloaf

1½ pounds lean ground beef

1 cup reduced-sodium black beans, drained and rinsed

1 (7-ounce) can Del Monte Fiesta Corn, drained

1 (4.5-ounce) can chopped green chilies

1 (1-ounce) packet less-sodium taco seasoning or Make It Homemade (page 299)

2 egg whites, beaten

½ cup plain bread crumbs

1 cup shredded reduced-fat four-cheese Mexican blend (I like Sargento)

½ cup medium tomato salsa

1 tablespoon brown sugar

1 medium tomato, diced

2 jalapeño peppers, sliced

quick and easy: Have a little extra time over the weekend? Prepare this dish in advance. Prepared unbaked meatloaf can be refrigerated overnight, or you can freeze it baked or unbaked for future dinners.

1. Preheat the oven to 375°F. Coat a 9-inch loaf pan with cooking spray or line with parchment paper.

2. In a large bowl, combine the ground beef, black beans, corn, green chilies, taco seasoning, egg whites, and bread crumbs. Using clean hands, mix all the ingredients until well combined.

3. Divide the ground beef mixture in half and place one portion in the bottom of the loaf pan. Cover the beef with ½ cup of the shredded Mexican cheese. Layer the second portion of the ground beef mixture on top of the cheese. Bake for 1 hour.

4. While the meatloaf is baking, in a small bowl, mix together the salsa and brown sugar and set aside for a glaze.

5. After the meatloaf has baked for 1 hour, spoon the glaze over the top of the meatloaf and sprinkle with the remaining ½ cup cheese. Bake for an additional 10 minutes to melt the cheese.

6. Let the meatloaf rest for 5 minutes before cutting into 6 slices.

7. Serve garnished with the diced tomato and jalapeños.

Suggested Side Dish: Cilantro-Lime Rice (page 271)

Calories 357 • Fat 14g • Carbohydrate 31g • Fiber 3g • Sugar 6g • Protein 32g

Creole-Style Shepherd's Pie

Shepherd's pie (also known as cottage pie) has roots going back to England and Ireland in the eighteenth century. A pie-shaped casserole dish, it features meat and vegetables as its foundation, topped with a mashed potato crust. Here, I transform the traditional dish and give it a Southern makeover by infusing it with Creole seasoning, okra, and sweet potato!

Prep Time: 10 minutes | **Cook Time:** 35 minutes
Serves: 6 | **Serving Size:** ⅙ of the pie

2 large sweet potatoes, peeled and cut into 1-inch cubes

1 pound lean ground beef

1 small onion, diced

⅛ teaspoon salt

¼ teaspoon black pepper

1 tablespoon white whole wheat flour

⅓ cup low-sodium beef broth (I like Pacific Organic)

1 (12-ounce) bag frozen sliced okra

1 cup frozen yellow corn kernels

1 green bell pepper, diced

1 yellow bell pepper, diced

1 (14.5-ounce) can no-salt-added diced tomatoes (I like Hunt's), drained

1 tablespoon plus 1 teaspoon Creole seasoning

2 tablespoons light sour cream

1. In a large pot, combine the sweet potatoes with water to cover. Bring to a boil over medium-high heat and boil until the potatoes are soft, 15 to 18 minutes. Drain the potatoes, transfer to a large bowl, and set aside.

2. Meanwhile, in a large skillet over medium-high heat, cook the ground beef and onion until the beef is no longer pink, 7 to 8 minutes. Use a wooden spoon to break the beef up as it cooks. Season with the salt and pepper. Add the flour and stir an additional minute.

3. Preheat the oven to 400°F. Coat a 9-inch pie pan with cooking spray.

4. Add the beef broth to the skillet and stir in the okra, corn, bell peppers, tomatoes, and 1 tablespoon of the Creole seasoning. Reduce the heat to low, cover, and simmer until the vegetables are softened, about 10 minutes.

5. Add the remaining 1 teaspoon Creole seasoning and the sour cream to the cooked sweet potatoes. Use a mixer to blend until creamy.

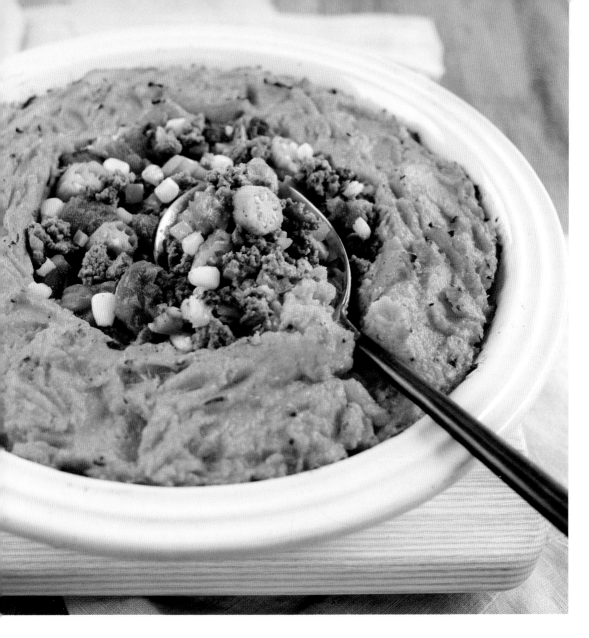

6. Transfer the meat mixture to the prepared pie dish. Evenly spread the sweet potatoes over the meat mixture. Bake until heated through, 15 to 20 minutes.

Suggested Side Dish: Easy Creamed Spinach (page 275)

quick and easy: Make this dish into "mini pies" (great for portion control) by using ramekins in place of the 9-inch pie dish.

Calories 180 • Fat 6g • Carbohydrate 20g • Fiber 4g • Sugar 7g • Protein 14g

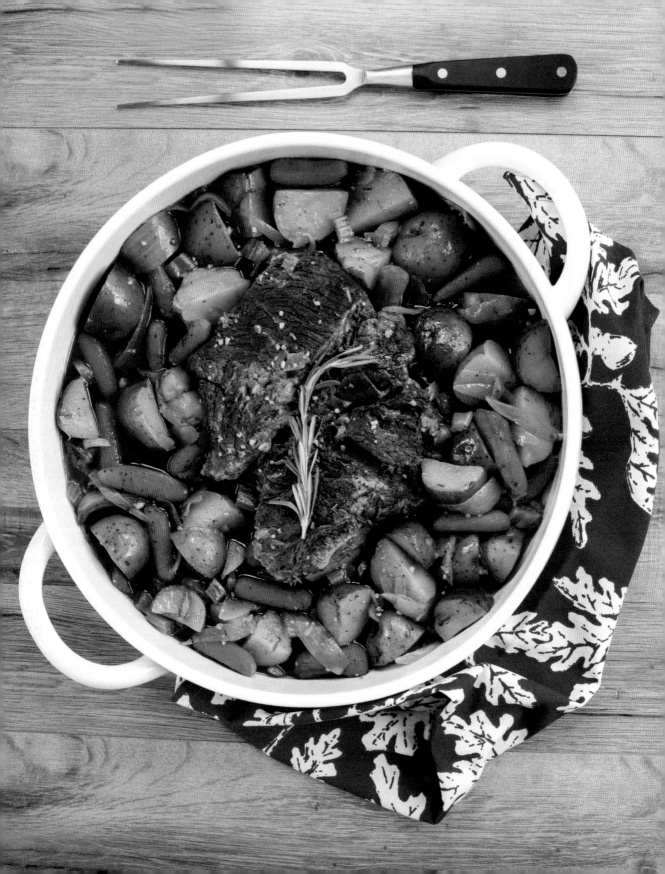

Easy Slow-Cooker Pot Roast

I used to shy away from making pot roasts for my family because choosing the right cut of beef among all the various cuts seemed overwhelming. Take it from me, picking up a relatively inexpensive chuck roast (like the one I use here) provides a moist, juicy, and tender roast every time.

Prep Time: 10 minutes | **Cook Time:** 4 hours on high or 8 hours on low
Serves: 6 | **Serving Size:** About 3 ounces beef, 1 cup vegetables plus ¼ cup broth

---

Rub:

½ tablespoon paprika

1 tablespoon chopped fresh
   rosemary

2 teaspoons garlic powder

1 teaspoon kosher salt

1 teaspoon black pepper

Roast and Vegetables:

2 pounds boneless chuck roast,
   trimmed

1 tablespoon extra virgin olive oil

2 cups whole baby carrots

1 medium onion, cut into large dice

3 stalks celery, chopped

8 red new potatoes, quartered

2½ cups low-sodium beef broth
   (I like Pacific Organic)

2 tablespoons balsamic vinegar

1 tablespoon minced garlic

2 bay leaves

1. To make the rub: In a small bowl, combine the paprika, rosemary, garlic powder, salt, and pepper.

2. To make the beef: Pat the chuck roast dry with a paper towel to remove excess moisture. Evenly pat the rub on all sides of the roast.

3. In a large skillet, heat the olive oil over high heat. Add the seasoned roast and sear on each side for 2 to 3 minutes.

4. Transfer the roast to a slow cooker. Place the carrots, onion, celery, and potatoes around the roast.

5. In a small bowl, whisk together the beef broth, vinegar, and garlic.

6. Add the beef broth mixture and the bay leaves to the slow cooker. Cover and cook for 4 hours on high or 8 hours on low. Remove the bay leaves before serving.

Suggested Side Dish: The Creamiest Mac 'n' Cheese Dish You Will Ever Make (page 264)

no slow cooker, no problem: Preheat the oven to 325˚F. Follow the recipe as directed but instead of placing the seared roast, vegetables, and broth mixture in a slow cooker, place them in a large roasting pan. Cover the roasting pan with aluminum foil and bake until the meat is fork-tender, 2 to 3 hours.

Calories 441 · Fat 12g · Carbohydrate 47g · Fiber 6g · Sugar 7g · Protein 38g

Open-Faced Aloha Sliders

Sliders have found their place in the restaurant world, from fine dining to fast takeout. So I decided it was time to create the ultimate mini burger, with a tropical twist! It has the ideal combination of sweet and tangy created by the melt-in-your-mouth Hawaiian roll coupled with the pineapple and a perfectly piquant marinade and slaw.

Prep Time: 10 minutes, plus 30 minutes marinating time | **Cook Time:** 15 minutes
Serves: 4 | **Serving Size:** 2 sliders

Sliders and Marinade:

1 pound lean ground beef

2 teaspoons minced garlic

1 teaspoon ground ginger

¼ teaspoon salt

½ teaspoon black pepper

½ cup less-sodium teriyaki marinade (I like Kikkoman)

Red Cabbage Slaw:

1 (8-ounce) can juice-packed crushed pineapple (I like Del Monte)

3 tablespoons light mayonnaise

1 tablespoon rice vinegar

1 teaspoon grated lime zest

⅛ teaspoon salt

10 ounces shredded red cabbage (about 4½ cups)

½ small red onion, thinly sliced

2 tablespoons chopped fresh cilantro

2 teaspoons sesame seeds

For Serving:

4 King's Hawaiian sweet dinner rolls

1. To make the sliders: In a medium bowl, mix together the lean ground beef, minced garlic, ginger, salt, and black pepper.

2. Using clean hands, form the beef into 8 slider-size patties using about ¼ cup of the beef for each.

3. Place the sliders in a single layer in a baking dish and pour the teriyaki marinade over them to cover. Cover with foil and refrigerate for 30 minutes to 1 hour, making sure the sliders are evenly covered in the marinade.

4. Meanwhile, to make the slaw: Reserving the juice, drain the crushed pineapple. Set the pineapple aside for serving. Measure out 3 tablespoons of the juice and transfer to a small bowl (discard the remaining juice). Whisk the mayonnaise, vinegar, lime zest, and salt into the pineapple juice.

5. In a medium bowl, toss the cabbage, red onion, cilantro, and sesame seeds together. Pour the dressing mixture over the cabbage mixture and toss to evenly cover.

6. Heat an indoor or outdoor grill to medium-high heat or heat a grill pan over medium-high heat. Coat the grill rack or grill pan with cooking

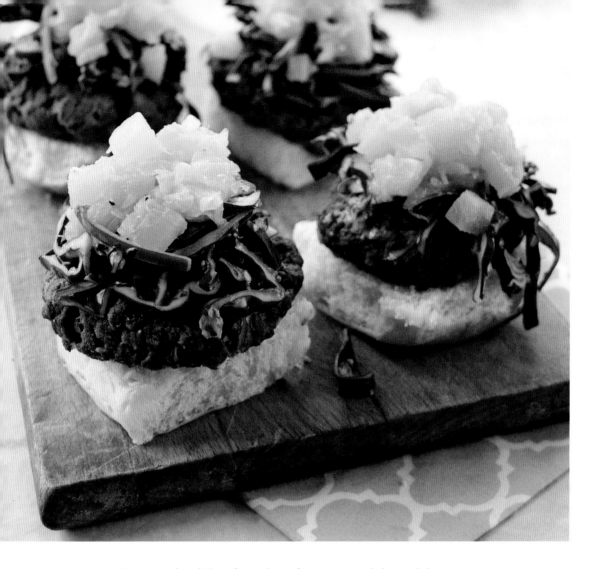

spray. Remove the sliders from the refrigerator and discard the
marinade. Grill the sliders for 2 to 3 minutes on both sides, or until
desired doneness.

7. In a small skillet over low heat, warm the crushed pineapple for
about 2 minutes.

8. To serve, split the Hawaiian rolls in half and top each half with
1 slider, followed by 1 heaping tablespoon of the slaw and
1 tablespoon of the warm crushed pineapple.

Suggested Side Dish: Asparagus Fries with Garlic Lemon Aioli (page 262)

Calories 390 · **Fat** 15g · **Carbohydrate** 39g · **Fiber** 3g · **Sugar** 20g · **Protein** 26g

Philly Cheesesteak Stuffed Peppers

"Colorful," "fun," and "flavorful" are just a few words that come to mind when I prepare this tasty treat at home. So much goodness in one little pepper. Boiling the peppers softens them so that they're easier to eat—and what's more fun than eating with your hands? No utensils for this fun supper. These stuffed peppers are mild enough for the most sensitive of taste buds, yet packed with vitamins and nutrients.

Prep Time: 10 minutes | **Cook Time:** 10 minutes
Serves: 6 | **Serving Size:** 1 stuffed pepper half

3 green bell peppers

2 teaspoons extra virgin olive oil

1 (8-ounce) container baby bella (cremini) mushrooms, sliced

1 red bell pepper, diced

1 small onion, diced

1 tablespoon minced garlic

¼ teaspoon salt

¼ teaspoon black pepper

8 ounces flank steak, trimmed of fat and thinly sliced against the grain into bite-size strips

2 tablespoons Worcestershire sauce

6 slices Sargento Ultra Thin sliced provolone cheese, halved

1. In a large pot, bring 4 cups of water to a boil over high heat.

2. Halve the green bell peppers lengthwise and remove the ribs and seeds. Place the pepper halves, 2 at a time, in the boiling water for 2 to 4 minutes. (The pepper skin will lose a little brightness after cooking in boiling water.) Use tongs to carefully remove the peppers from the pot and place open side down on paper towels to drain.

3. In a large skillet over medium-high heat, heat the olive oil . Add the mushrooms, red bell pepper, onion, garlic, salt, and black pepper. Sauté until the onion and pepper have softened, 2 to 3 minutes.

4. Preheat the oven to 400°F. Coat an 11 x 7-inch baking dish with cooking spray.

5. Add the flank steak to the skillet. Stir in the Worcestershire sauce and cook for 2 to 4 minutes. The steak should still be slightly pink in the middle for medium or cook until no longer pink for medium well.

6. Place the green bell pepper halves open side up in the baking dish. Line the inside of each pepper half with 1/2 slice of provolone cheese.

7. Using a slotted spoon, transfer 1/2 cup of the flank steak mixture to each bell pepper half. Top each pepper with a 1/2 slice of the remaining provolone cheese.

8. Bake the peppers for 10 minutes in the preheated oven until the cheese is melted.

Suggested Side Dish: Carrot and Raisin Salad (page 268)

quick and easy: Use your "prep day" to dice the red pepper and onion for this Skinny Supper.

suppertime inspiration: Managing the ups and downs and demands of life requires extreme focus. Becoming sidetracked or distracted can really set me back. So finding a scripture or quote that inspires me is very powerful. This verse has been a constant reminder for me that although life doesn't always make sense, God is in control: "And we know that all things work together for the good of those who love him, who have been called according to his purpose." Romans 8:28 NIV.

suppertime chat: What qualities are important in a person? Why? This is a great way to understand character traits that other family members deem important, and what they might be seeking from you!

Calories 155 • Fat 14g • Carbohydrate 10g • Fiber 3g • Sugar 4g • Protein 18g

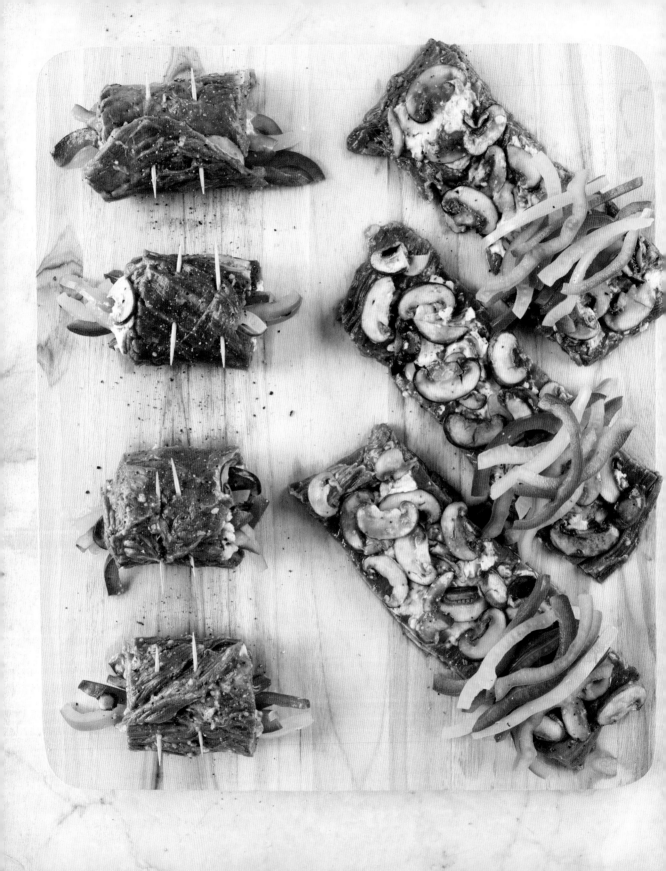

Grilled Red Wine and Balsamic Flank Steak Roll-Ups

It doesn't have to be a special occasion to enjoy a good steak! Bring the steakhouse to your house with these flavorful and budget-friendly roll-ups.

Prep Time: 25 minutes, plus 4 hours marinating time │ **Cook Time:** 10 minutes
Serves: 8 │ **Serving Size:** 1 roll-up

---

2 pounds flank steak, trimmed of fat

½ teaspoon salt

½ teaspoon black pepper

½ cup cooking red wine or low-sodium beef broth

½ cup balsamic vinaigrette

1 tablespoon minced garlic

½ tablespoon Dijon mustard

1 teaspoon extra virgin olive oil

1 green bell pepper, julienned

1 red bell pepper, julienned

1 yellow bell pepper, julienned

1 (8-ounce) container baby bella (cremini) mushrooms, sliced

4 wedges Laughing Cow Creamy Swiss Light cheese

1. Butterfly the flank steak: Start with the meat grain running up and down in front of you. Carefully work a knife (preferably a filleting knife) through the middle, from one side to the other, leaving the back (long) edge still connected by about ½ inch, like the spine of a book. Open the flank steak halves like butterfly wings and lay flat—doubling the size.

2. Place the flank steak between two pieces of wax paper and gently pound with the flat side of a meat mallet or a rolling pin until the flank steak is about ¼ inch thick. Sprinkle the steak on both sides with the salt and black pepper.

3. In a small bowl, whisk together the red wine, balsamic vinaigrette, minced garlic, and mustard to make the marinade.

4. Place the steak in a 13 x 9-inch baking dish and cover with the marinade. Marinate in the refrigerator anywhere from 4 hours to overnight—depending on how much time you have—flipping the flank steak from time to time if possible.

5. To make the vegetables: In a medium skillet, heat the olive oil over medium-high heat. Add the bell peppers and mushrooms and sauté for 2 to 3 minutes. Set aside.

(recipe continues)

(continued from page 55)

suppertime inspiration:

There's an old English proverb that says, "A smooth sea never made a skilled sailor." Life is full of rough waves and unexpected storms. Through the waves and the storms we emerge as stronger and more courageous women. Embrace the storms—the sunshine always follows the rain!

6. Preheat an indoor or outdoor grill to medium-high heat or heat a grill pan over medium-high heat. Lightly coat the grill rack or grill pan with cooking spray.

7. Remove the flank steak from the dish and place on a large plate. Pour the marinade into a small bowl and set aside.

8. Slice the flank steak across the grain (perpendicular to the grain) into 8 rectangular strips. Spread the cheese wedges evenly on one side of each strip of flank steak.

9. Divide the peppers and mushrooms over the cheese-covered flank steak strips. Roll each flank steak up tight and pierce each end with a toothpick to secure.

10. Place the steak rolls on the grill or grill pan and brush often with the reserved marinade while cooking. Grill the steak rolls for 6 minutes, or until desired doneness (120°F for medium-rare, 130°F for medium). Transfer to a clean plate and allow to rest for 3 to 4 minutes before serving.

Suggested Side Dish: Easy Creamed Spinach (page 275)

Calories 245 • Fat 11g • Carbohydrate 8g • Fiber 1g • Sugar 5g • Protein 24g

Slow-Cooker Beef Stroganoff

Fork-tender beef, mixed into a warm, flavorful sauce, atop whole grain egg noodles. Need I say more? I assure you this dish will find a permanent home on your monthly supper rotation.

Prep Time: 10 minutes │ **Cook Time:** 3 hours on high or 6 hours on low
Serves: 8 │ **Serving Size:** Heaping 1½ cups

1½ pounds lean stew beef, cut into 1-inch cubes

2 (8-ounce) containers baby bella (cremini) mushrooms, thinly sliced

1 (10.5-ounce) can Campbell's Healthy Request condensed cream of mushroom soup

1 small onion, diced

¾ cup low-sodium beef broth (I like Pacific Organic)

2 tablespoons cooking sherry or low-sodium beef broth

2 tablespoons Worcestershire sauce

2 tablespoons minced garlic

1 teaspoon salt

1 teaspoon black pepper

12 ounces whole grain egg noodles

1 cup plain 0% Greek yogurt

2 tablespoons chopped fresh parsley

1. Place the meat, mushrooms, mushroom soup, onion, beef broth, sherry, Worcestershire sauce, garlic, salt, and pepper in the slow cooker and stir together.

2. Cook on high heat for 3 hours or low heat for 6 hours. About 30 minutes before the cooking time is up, bring a large pot of salted water to a boil over high heat. Cook the noodles to al dente according to the package directions.

3. Drain the noodles and add to the slow cooker along with the yogurt. Stir to combine and heat through on low heat before serving.

4. Serve garnished with the parsley.

Suggested Side Dish: Rustic Rosemary Root Vegetables (page 290)

suppertime chat: What is your all-time favorite movie? Who starred in it? Why is it your favorite? Is there a movie coming out that you would like to see? Plan and commit to that date night or family night that is long overdue!

no slow cooker, no problem: Place all the ingredients into a large pot or Dutch oven and cook over low heat for 2 to 3 hours until the meat is cooked through. Cook the noodles separately as directed and add to the stew.

Calories 323 • Fat 8g • Carbohydrate 40g • Fiber 6g • Sugar 4g • Protein 29g

Spicy Szechuan Beef with Zoodles

"We're having zoodles for supper!" Just the word "zoodles" gets everyone's attention. This is one of those recipes my little guy loves to help out with. Just watching a giant zucchini be transformed into noodles mesmerizes him. But for me, it's the addition of the blended sweet, nutty spice in the sauce that makes this supper so special.

Prep Time: 15 minutes | **Cook Time:** 15 minutes
Serves: 6 | **Serving Size:** 1½ cups zoodles, ¾ cup meat sauce, 1 tablespoon green onion, and 1 teaspoon sesame seeds

5 large zucchini

½ tablespoon sesame oil

1 pound lean ground beef

1 red bell pepper, julienned

1 small onion, thinly sliced

2 tablespoons minced garlic

1 teaspoon red pepper flakes

1 teaspoon Chinese five-spice powder

½ teaspoon ground ginger

¼ teaspoon salt

Sauce:

1 tablespoon cornstarch

1½ cups low-sodium beef broth (I like Pacific Organic)

2 tablespoons less-sodium soy sauce

1 tablespoon creamy natural peanut butter (I like Smucker's)

1 tablespoon sugar-free maple-flavor syrup (I like Maple Grove Farms)

2 teaspoons rice vinegar

1 teaspoon sriracha sauce

For Serving:

4 green onions, thinly sliced

4 teaspoons sesame seeds

1. Use a spiral slicer or a vegetable peeler to make noodles (zoodles) from your zucchini.

2. In a large skillet, heat the sesame oil over medium-high heat. Add the zucchini noodles and cook until slightly tender, about 2 minutes (make certain not to overcook). Remove from the heat and let sit in the pan—allowing the moisture to release. Remove the zoodles from the pan and drain the excess water. Place the zoodles in a covered dish to keep warm.

3. Carefully wipe the same skillet clean, then reheat over medium-high heat. Add the ground beef, bell pepper, onion, and garlic and cook until the beef is no longer pink, 7 to 8 minutes. Use a wooden spoon to break the beef up as it cooks. Drain any excess fat and return the skillet to the stovetop, turning the heat down to low. Season with the pepper flakes, five-spice powder, ginger, and salt.

4. Meanwhile, to make the sauce: Place the cornstarch in a small bowl. Whisk in the broth. Then whisk in the soy sauce, peanut butter, syrup, vinegar, and sriracha.

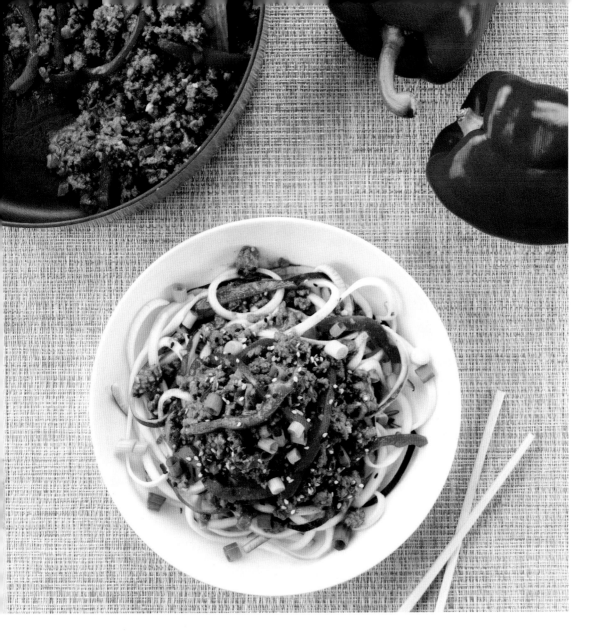

5. Pour the sauce over the meat mixture in the skillet and simmer for 2 to 3 minutes, constantly stirring to evenly cover the meat.

6. To serve, place 1¹/₂ cups of the zoodles in each bowl and top with ³/₄ cup of the meat mixture. Garnish each with 1 tablespoon green onion and 1 teaspoon sesame seeds.

Suggested Side Dish: Mango Slaw (page 281)

Calories 346 · **Fat** 16g · **Carbohydrate** 26g · **Fiber** 6g · **Sugar** 14g · **Protein** 31g

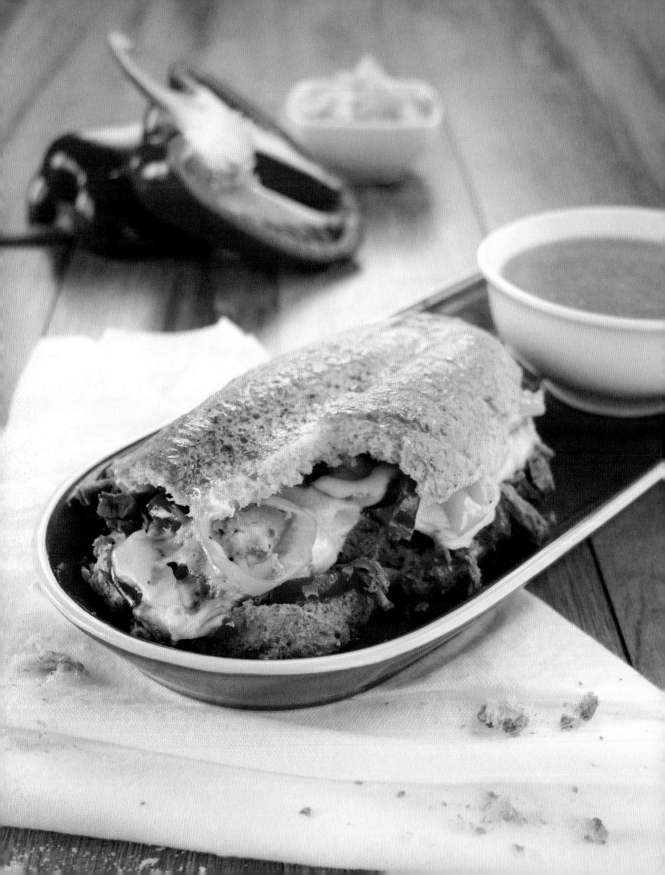

Slow-Cooker Italian Beef Hoagies

I love a good hoagie, but restaurant buns are often loaded with added butter and salt. This recipe preserves the big Italian flavor, but not the big Italian calories.

Prep Time: 10 minutes | **Cook Time:** 4½ hours on high or 9 hours on low
Serves: 8 | **Serving Size:** 1 prepared sandwich

3 pounds beef top round roast, trimmed of fat

½ teaspoon onion powder

½ teaspoon black pepper

½ teaspoon kosher salt

1 (.06-ounce) packet Italian salad dressing mix or Make It Homemade (page 299)

3 cups low-sodium beef broth (I like Pacific Organic)

1 tablespoon minced garlic

1 bay leaf

2 cups pepperoncini slices

2 red bell peppers, julienned

8 whole wheat hoagie buns (see Quick and Easy)

8 slices Sargento Ultra Thin sliced provolone cheese

no slow cooker, no problem: Coat the roast with the rub as directed and place the roast and broth mixture into a large pot or Dutch oven and cook over low heat until the meat is fork-tender, 2 to 3 hours. Shred the meat and remove the bay leaves. Add the pepperoncinis, bell peppers, and shredded meat to the pot and cook for an additional 30 minutes over low heat.

1. Pat the roast dry with a paper towel to remove excess moisture.

2. In a small bowl, make a rub by mixing together the onion powder, black pepper, and salt. Generously rub the roast with the seasoning and place the roast in a slow cooker.

3. Add the salad dressing mix, broth, garlic, and bay leaf to the slow cooker. Cover and cook on high heat for 4 hours or on low heat for 8 hours; the meat should be very tender.

4. After cooking, remove the roast from the slow cooker and shred the roast. Remove the bay leaf and return the shredded roast to the slow cooker.

5. Add 1 cup of the pepperoncinis and the bell peppers to the slow cooker. Cover and continue cooking on high heat for 30 minutes or on low heat for 1 hour.

6. To serve, top each whole wheat hoagie bun with 3 ounces of the meat mixture. Top the meat with 1 slice of provolone and some of the remaining pepperoncinis. Serve the liquid remaining in the slow cooker as a dip for the sandwiches.

quick and easy: Toast the hoagie buns before preparing the sandwiches. Place the prepared hoagie under the broiler for 2 to 3 minutes to melt the provolone cheese.

Calories 430 • Fat 16g • Carbohydrate 33g • Fiber 5g • Sugar 6g • Protein 56g

Salisbury Steak Meatballs

Say hello to this hearty supper with a skinny twist. Hearty for its rich, beefy flavor, but the twist is that the smart combination of ingredients also yields a light and balanced nutrition panel. Plus, transforming a traditional dish into a meatball entrée is just fun.

Prep Time: 10 minutes | **Cook Time:** 25 minutes
Serves: 8 | **Serving Size:** ¾ cup noodles, 4 meatballs, and ⅓ cup sauce

Meatballs:

1½ pounds lean ground beef

½ cup plain bread crumbs

3 tablespoons Heinz reduced-sugar ketchup

2 tablespoons Dijon mustard

1 tablespoon Worcestershire sauce

1 egg, beaten

1 tablespoon minced garlic

¼ teaspoon onion powder

¼ teaspoon black pepper

½ teaspoon salt

1 tablespoon extra virgin olive oil

Mushroom Gravy:

1 teaspoon extra virgin olive oil

1 medium onion, thinly sliced

1 (8-ounce) container baby bella (cremini) mushrooms, sliced

¾ cup low-sodium beef broth (I like Pacific Organic)

1 (10.5-ounce) can Campbell's Healthy Request condensed cream of mushroom soup

1 tablespoon Worcestershire sauce

1 tablespoon white whole wheat flour

(ingredients continue)

1. To make the meatballs: In a large bowl, combine the ground beef, bread crumbs, ketchup, mustard, Worcestershire sauce, egg, garlic, onion powder, pepper, and salt. Using clean hands, mix together. Using a tablespoon, form into 32 meatballs.

2. In a large skillet, heat the olive oil over medium heat. Add the meatballs to the skillet and brown all over (they do not have to be cooked in the center, as they will continue cooking in the gravy), using a spatula to turn them to cook evenly on all sides. Transfer to a plate and set aside.

3. To make the gravy: In the same large skillet, heat the olive oil. Add the onion and mushrooms and cook until the onion and mushrooms have softened, 5 to 6 minutes. Reduce the heat to low.

4. In a medium bowl, whisk together the beef broth, mushroom soup, and Worcestershire sauce.

5. Lightly sprinkle the flour into the skillet and stir gently to combine. Pour the soup mixture into the skillet, ¼ cup at a time, and stir to evenly combine.

6. Return the meatballs to the skillet and simmer until the meatballs have cooked through and the gravy has thickened, about 15 minutes.

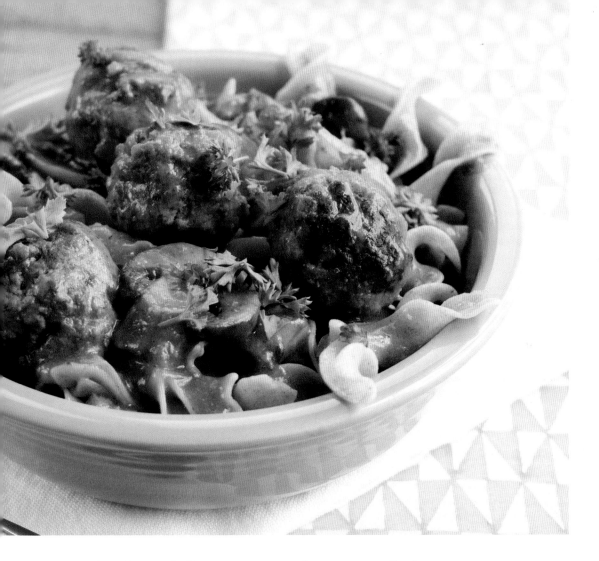

7. While the meatballs simmer, prepare the egg noodles. Bring a large pot of salted water to a boil over high heat. Cook the egg noodles to al dente according to the package directions. Drain.

8. To serve, place ³/₄ cup of the noodles onto a plate with 4 meatballs and ¹/₃ cup of the mushroom gravy, and garnish with a sprinkle of the parsley.

Suggested Side Dish: Cauliflower Mashed Potatoes (page 269)

For Serving

8 ounces whole grain wide egg noodles

¼ cup chopped fresh parsley

suppertime chat: Encourage those around your supper table to make someone else's day special by asking, "What did you do today to help someone? Hold a door open? Stand up for someone who was being bullied?"

Calories 308 · Fat 11g · Carbohydrate 33g · Fiber 5g · Sugar 4g · Protein 23g

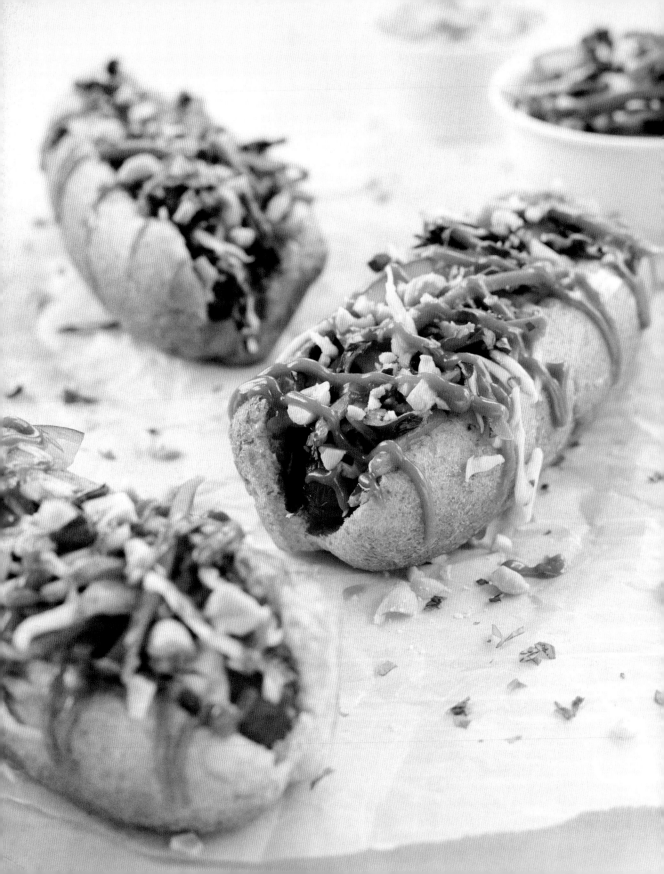

Thai-Style Hot Dogs

This unique dish gets its inspiration from one of my favorite restaurants in Cincinnati, Ohio: Senate. It is actually famous for hot dogs! There's nothing basic about these gourmet dogs. I know, it sounds like an oxymoron, but trust me. Try one and you'll be convinced. Here, I infuse some of my favorite Thai flavors on top of an all-beef dog with a fresh slaw drizzled with an impeccable peanut sauce. This supper redeems the notoriously unhealthy all-American tradition.

Prep Time: Less than 5 minutes | **Cook Time:** 5 minutes
Serves: 6 | **Serving Size:** 1 prepared hot dog, 2 tablespoons slaw, and 1 teaspoon sesame seeds

Thai-Style Slaw:

½ cucumber, halved lengthwise and sliced crosswise

½ cup shredded carrots

½ (10-ounce) bag shredded red cabbage

3 tablespoons fresh cilantro, chopped

1 tablespoon sesame oil

2 teaspoons less-sodium soy sauce

1 tablespoon rice vinegar

2 tablespoons Thai red chili sauce

Peanut Sauce

2 tablespoons creamy natural peanut butter (I like Smucker's)

2 tablespoons sesame oil

1 tablespoon sugar-free maple-flavor syrup (I like Maple Grove Farms)

1½ teaspoons less-sodium soy sauce

For Serving:

6 all-beef kosher hot dogs

6 whole wheat hot dog buns

¼ cup raw unsalted peanuts, coarsely chopped

6 teaspoons sesame seeds

1. To make the slaw: In a large bowl, combine the cucumber, carrots, red cabbage, and cilantro. In a small bowl, whisk together the sesame oil, soy sauce, vinegar, and Thai red chili sauce. Pour this over the vegetables and toss to evenly cover. Refrigerate until ready to serve.

2. To make the peanut sauce: In a small bowl, whisk together the peanut butter, sesame oil, syrup, and soy sauce. Set aside until ready to serve.

3. To assemble: Preheat an indoor grill, grill pan, or outdoor grill to medium-high heat. Coat the indoor grill or grill pan with cooking spray. Grill the hot dogs for 2 to 3 minutes on all sides.

4. Place one grilled hot dog in a bun, top with 2 tablespoons slaw, 3/4 tablespoon peanut sauce, a heaping 1/2 tablespoon peanuts, and 1 teaspoon sesame seeds.

5. Refrigerate any leftover slaw or serve it as a side dish.

Suggested Side Dish: Easy Roasted Vegetables (page 277)

Calories 312 · Fat 16g · Carbohydrate 31g · Fiber 4g · Sugar 7g · Protein 14g

Zucchini Taco Boats

Zucchini boats are such a natural fit for taco fixin's that your family can easily say *adios!* to traditional shells (which are high in carbs and notorious for breaking midcrunch). Have some fun and turn the dining table into a taco bar!

Prep Time: 10 minutes | **Cook Time:** 40 minutes
Serves: 4 | **Serving Size:** 2 taco boats

¾ cup mild low-sodium tomato salsa (I like Frog Ranch)

4 large zucchini, halved lengthwise

1 pound lean ground beef

1 (1-ounce) packet less-sodium taco seasoning or Make It Homemade (page 299)

1 (4.5-ounce) can chopped green chilies

1 (8.8-ounce) pouch Uncle Ben's Ready Rice Spanish-style rice

½ cup shredded reduced-fat four-cheese Mexican blend (I like Sargento)

Toppings:

2 cups shredded iceberg lettuce

1 jalapeño pepper, sliced

1 tomato, diced

¼ cup black olives, sliced (optional)

4 tablespoons light sour cream (optional)

1. Preheat the oven to 350°F. Lightly coat a 13 x 9-inch baking dish with cooking spray.

2. Evenly spread the salsa in the bottom of the baking dish and set aside.

3. Bring a large pot of salted water to a boil over high heat. Add the zucchini halves and boil for 1 to 2 minutes. Remove and set aside to cool. Once cooled, use a melon baller or a teaspoon to hollow out the zucchini halves so that they resemble boats. Chop the scooped-out flesh into bite-size pieces and set aside.

4. In a large skillet over medium-high heat, cook the ground beef until the beef is no longer pink, 7 to 8 minutes. Use a wooden spoon to break the beef up as it cooks. Drain any excess fat and return the skillet to the stovetop, turning the heat down to low.

5. Stir the taco seasoning and ¼ cup water into the beef in the skillet and bring to a boil. Reduce the heat to low, add the reserved zucchini flesh, green chilies, and rice, and simmer for 5 minutes, stirring occasionally.

6. Place the zucchini halves in the prepared baking dish and stuff each half with a heaping ½ cup of the meat filling. Top the zucchini boats with the Mexican cheese.

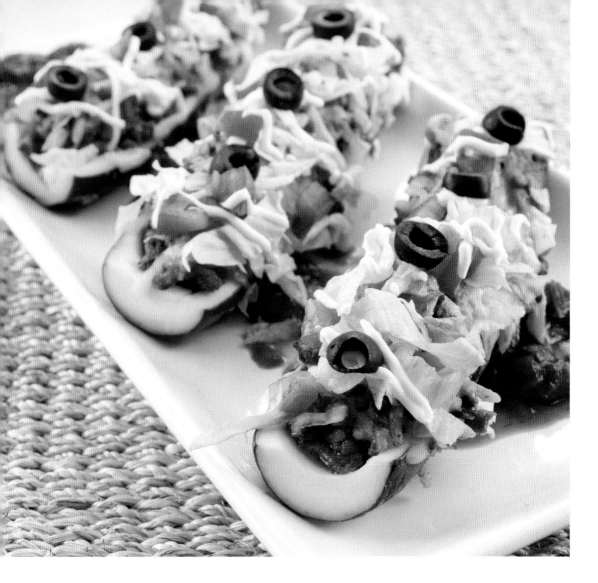

7. Cover the baking dish with foil and bake for 30 minutes, until the cheese is melted and the zucchinis are cooked through.

8. Garnish the taco boats evenly with toppings before serving.

Suggested Side Dish: Quinoa Mexi-Lime Salad (page 289)

skinny sense: Make this supper vegetarian by swapping out the ground beef for two cans of black beans. The dish will still have a good amount of protein, but it will be lower in fat and calories and much higher in fiber!

Calories 401 · **Fat** 13g · **Carbohydrate** 39g · **Fiber** 4g · **Sugar** 13g · **Protein** 30g
Nutrition does not include optional toppings.

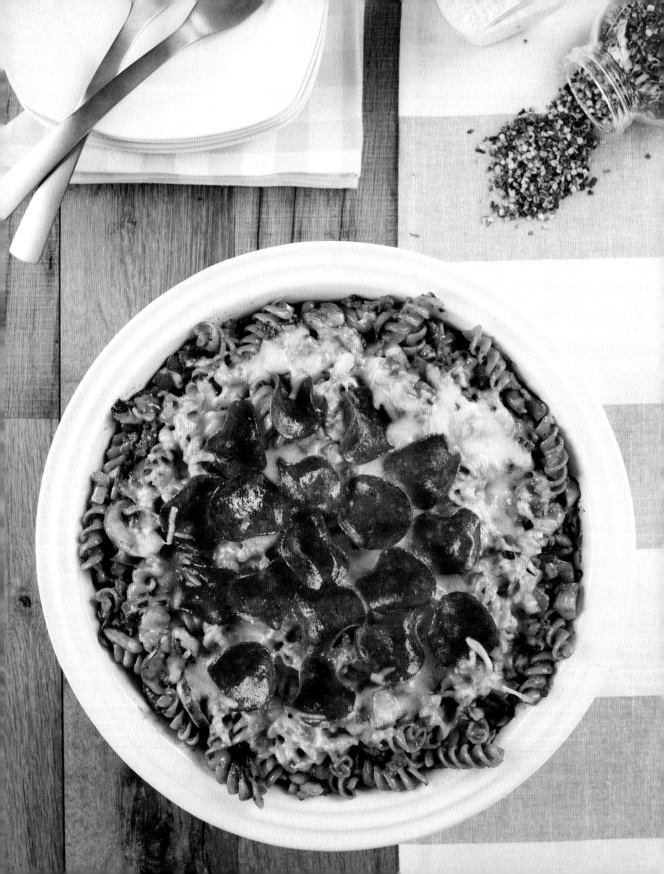

6 SERVE UP SOME COMFORT
CASSEROLE SUPPERS

A Casserole to Be Thankful For

This casserole was born out of my love for Thanksgiving. The flavorful foods served around the Thanksgiving table are so warm and gratifying. I hate that it only comes once a year. So I was determined to capture the essence of Thanksgiving staples, like turkey and stuffing, in a dish that could be prepared year-round. The addition of creamy mushroom soup with rice provides a whole new texture. Plus, the nutty aroma of butternut squash fills the house, creating a warm and comforting feeling.

Prep Time: 10 minutes | **Cook Time:** 30 minutes
Serves: 6 | **Serving Size:** Heaping 1 cup

2 tablespoons unsalted butter

1 cup peeled, cubed (1-inch) butternut squash

1 small onion, diced

2 stalks celery, diced

1½ cups Stovetop Stuffing Mix for Turkey, seasoning packet discarded

2 cups cubed (1-inch) cooked turkey breast (see Quick and Easy)

1 (10.5-ounce) can Campbell's Healthy Request condensed cream of mushroom soup

1 (10.5-ounce) can Campbell's Healthy Request condensed cream of celery soup

½ cup plain 0% Greek yogurt

⅛ teaspoon salt

⅛ teaspoon black pepper

1 (8.8-ounce) pouch Uncle Ben's brown and wild rice medley

¼ cup pecans, coarsely chopped

2 tablespoons Reduced Sugar Craisins Dried Cranberries

1. Preheat the oven to 350°F. Coat an 11 x 7-inch baking dish with cooking spray.

2. In a large skillet, melt 1 tablespoon of the butter over medium heat. Add the squash, onion, and celery and cook until soft, 10 to 12 minutes.

3. Meanwhile, prepare the stuffing: In a medium saucepan, combine 1½ cups water and the remaining 1 tablespoon butter and bring to a boil. Add the stuffing mix, stir, and remove from the heat. Fluff the stuffing with a fork and set aside.

4. Stir the turkey, mushroom soup, celery soup, yogurt, salt, and pepper into the skillet with the vegetables. Add the rice and carefully stir until mixed. Pour into the prepared baking dish. Evenly spoon the prepared stuffing over the top of the turkey mixture.

5. Bake for 15 minutes. Sprinkle with the pecans and Craisins and bake for 5 minutes longer. Serve warm.

quick and easy: No worries if it's not the day after Thanksgiving and you're craving this comforting dish (but there's no leftover turkey). You can purchase lean turkey medallions at your local grocery store any time of year.

Calories 366 • **Fat** 11g • **Carbohydrate** 42g • **Fiber** 4g • **Sugar** 7g • **Protein** 25g

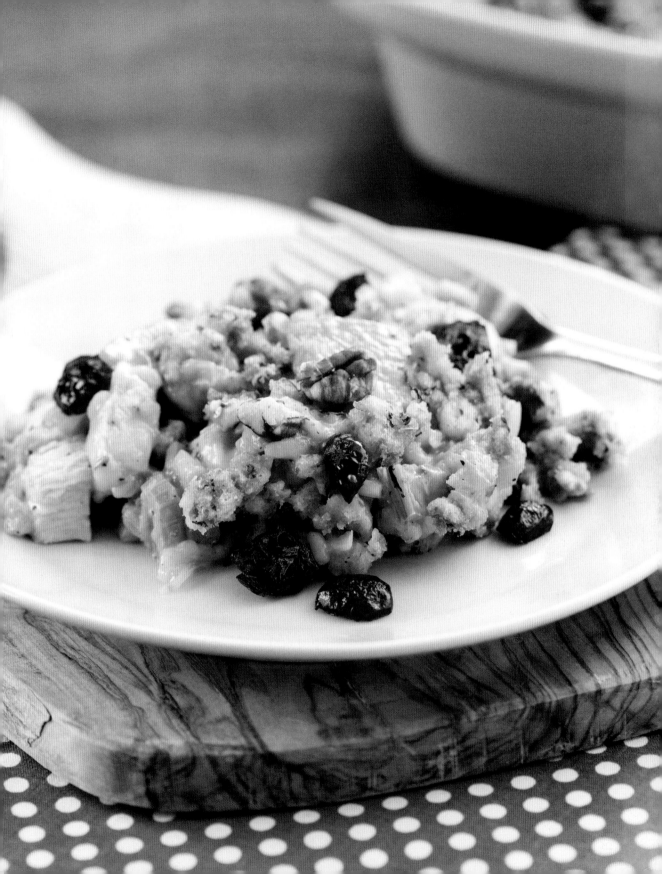

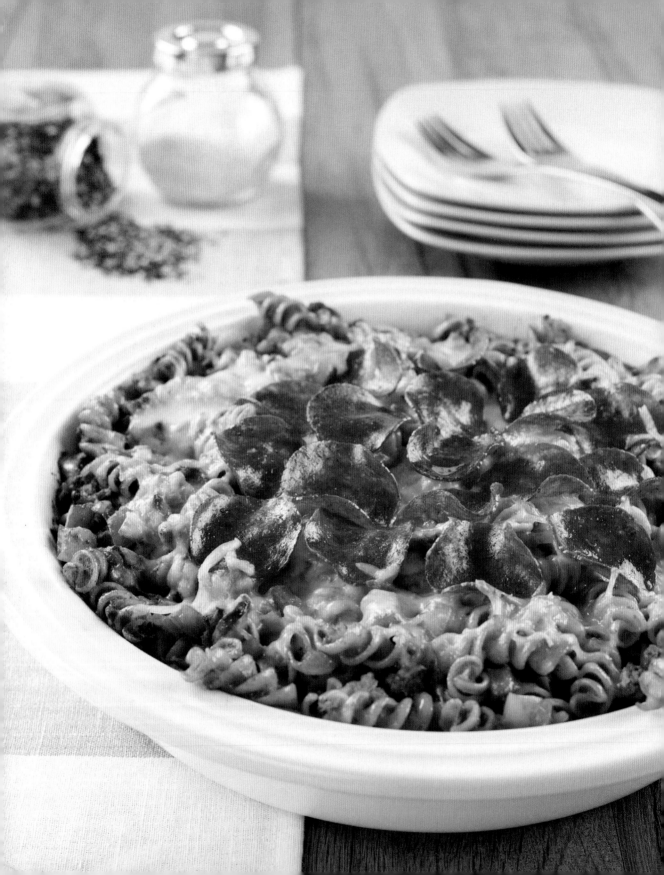

Supreme Pizza Pasta Casserole

It's the best of Italy—pizza and pasta in one! It's fun for your toddlers, has a grown-up taste, and is surprisingly low in calories. This casserole will have everyone at the supper table saying, "That's *amore!*"

Prep Time: 10 minutes | **Cook Time:** 30 minutes
Serves: 6 | **Serving Size:** 1⅓ cups

8 ounces whole wheat rotini pasta (I like Barilla)

½ pound lean ground beef

1 teaspoon extra virgin olive oil

1 teaspoon minced garlic

1 small onion, diced

2 green bell peppers, diced

1 (8-ounce) container baby bella (cremini) mushrooms, sliced

1 (23.25-ounce) jar Prego Light Smart Traditional Pasta Sauce

1 teaspoon Italian seasoning

1 cup shredded reduced-fat mozzarella cheese (I like Sargento)

17 slices turkey pepperoni

quick and easy: Cut prep time in half by preparing this casserole the night before and refrigerating. Or double the recipe and freeze half for a future dinner or to share with family and friends.

1. Bring a large pot of salted water to a boil over high heat. Cook the pasta to al dente according to the package directions. Drain and set aside.

2. In a large skillet over medium-high heat, cook the ground beef until no longer pink, 7 to 8 minutes. Use a wooden spoon to break the beef up as it cooks. Transfer the beef to a plate and drain any excess fat from the skillet.

3. Add the olive oil to the skillet over medium-high heat. Add the garlic, onion, bell peppers, and mushrooms and cook until the vegetables are softened, 4 to 6 minutes.

4. Preheat the oven to 350°F. Coat a 13 x 9-inch baking dish or a 14-inch round baking dish with cooking spray.

5. Return the cooked ground beef to the skillet and mix with the vegetables. Reduce the heat to low. Pour the pasta sauce into the skillet. Add the Italian seasoning and mix well. Stir the cooked pasta into the skillet, making sure to evenly coat the pasta.

6. Transfer the mixture to the prepared baking dish. Top with the mozzarella and pepperoni. Bake uncovered until the cheese is melted, 20 to 25 minutes.

Suggested Side Dish: Skinny Broccoli Salad (page 295)

Calories 314 • Fat 9g • Carbohydrate 42g • Fiber 8g • Sugar 10g • Protein 22g

Jalapeño Popper Chicken Casserole

Every now and then I like to kick it up a notch with the spices in my recipes. But the star in this casserole is definitely the quinoa. Incredibly easy to work with, quinoa has a nutty, smoky flavor and is an excellent source of protein. In the last few years it has become much easier to find and purchase and is a staple in my pantry.

Prep Time: 5 minutes | **Cook Time:** 40 minutes
Serves: 6 | **Serving Size:** Heaping 1 cup

1 pound boneless, skinless chicken breasts

1 (4-ounce) can diced pickled jalapeños, drained

3 cups low-sodium chicken broth (I like Pacific Organic)

1 cup quinoa, rinsed

4 ounces ⅓-less-fat cream cheese, softened

¾ cup plain 0% Greek yogurt

2 tablespoons Frank's RedHot Sauce

1 cup shredded reduced-fat sharp cheddar cheese (I like Sargento)

2 fresh jalapeño peppers, sliced

¼ cup panko bread crumbs

1. In a large pot over high heat, combine the chicken, 2 tablespoons of the diced jalapeños, and enough water to cover the chicken. Bring to a boil and cook until the chicken reaches an internal temperature of 145°F, 12 to 15 minutes. Remove the chicken from the water and set on a plate to cool. Discard the water and the jalapeños. Once cool enough to handle, shred the chicken breasts.

2. Meanwhile, in a medium saucepan, combine 2 cups of the chicken broth and the quinoa. Bring to a boil, reduce to a simmer, cover, and cook until the seeds are translucent and have "spiraled out," 12 to 15 minutes. Uncover and fluff with a fork.

3. Preheat the oven to 350°F. Coat a 13 x 9-inch baking dish with cooking spray.

4. In a large bowl, combine the cream cheese, yogurt, hot sauce, remaining 1 cup chicken broth, and remaining diced jalapeños from the can. Stir to mix well.

5. Add ½ cup of the cheddar, the cooked quinoa, and the shredded chicken to the cream cheese mixture. Combine until the chicken and quinoa are evenly covered.

6. Pour the mixture into the prepared baking dish. Top with the remaining ½ cup cheddar and the fresh jalapeño slices. Sprinkle with the panko.

7. Coat the top of the casserole generously with cooking spray and bake for 20 minutes, until the cheese is melted and bubbly.

suppertime chat: If you have kids at the table, tell them about the day they were born. Describe your excitement at meeting them for the first time. Mention what you remember best about seeing them and hearing their sounds in those first few moments. Kids love to hear stories about themselves!

skinny sense: Try quinoa for breakfast! If you're already cooking it up for dinner, make a little extra, refrigerate, and reheat in the morning. Drizzle with your favorite liquid sweetener and top with fresh fruit. It's a super quick and nutrient-dense way to start off anyone's day!

Calories 320 • **Fat** 10g • **Carbohydrate** 25g • **Fiber** 3g • **Sugar** 2g • **Protein** 30g

Chicken Noodle Soup Casserole

Growing up in the South, we always (and I do mean always) brought chicken noodle soup to sick family members and friends. This casserole is simple and quick to make, and it's the perfect way to say "I care," with ease.

Prep Time: 10 minutes | **Cook Time:** 30 minutes
Serves: 6 | **Serving Size:** 1½ cups

1 tablespoon extra virgin olive oil

3 stalks celery, diced

2 cups crinkle-cut carrots

1 small onion, diced

1½ pounds boneless, skinless chicken breasts, cut into 1-inch cubes

1 teaspoon salt

½ teaspoon black pepper

1 cup low-sodium chicken broth (I like Pacific Organic)

6 ounces whole wheat egg noodles

1 (10.5-ounce) can Campbell's Healthy Request condensed cream of mushroom soup

1 (10.5-ounce) can Campbell's Healthy Request condensed cream of chicken soup

½ cup light sour cream

1 teaspoon garlic powder

½ teaspoon poultry seasoning

½ cup oyster crackers

quick and easy: Consider doubling up the ingredients and making two casseroles at once. Freeze one to surprise an unexpected neighbor or family member one evening or to have on hand when someone you love is going through a time of need (surgery, new baby, etc.).

1. In a large pot, heat the oil over medium-high heat. Add the celery, carrots, and onion and cook until they start to soften, 5 to 6 minutes.

2. Sprinkle the chicken with ¼ teaspoon of the salt and ¼ teaspoon of the pepper and add to the pan with the vegetables. Cook the chicken on all sides for 3 to 4 minutes.

3. Add the broth to the pan, cover, and simmer for 8 to 10 minutes, stirring and turning the chicken occasionally, until the chicken is cooked through.

4. While the chicken is simmering, bring a pot of salted water to a boil over high heat. Cook the noodles to al dente according to the package directions. Drain and set aside.

5. Preheat the oven to 350°F. Coat a 13 x 9-inch baking dish with cooking spray.

6. In a small bowl, combine the mushroom soup, chicken soup, sour cream, garlic powder, poultry seasoning, and remaining ¾ teaspoon salt and ¼ teaspoon pepper. Add to the pan with the chicken and vegetables and stir to evenly combine.

7. Mix the cooked noodles into the chicken mixture, then transfer the mixture to the prepared baking dish.

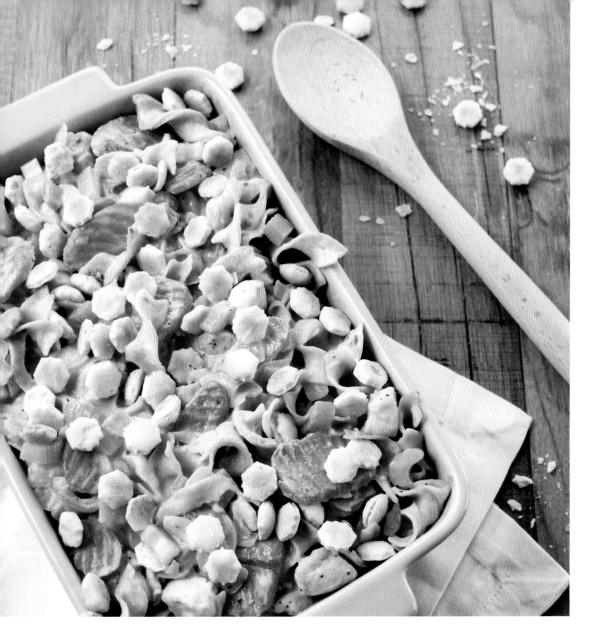

8. Cover with the oyster crackers and bake until the casserole is heated through and bubbly, 12 to 15 minutes.

suppertime inspiration: Sometimes the best way to boost my own mood is simply to help someone else. I often find myself busy or preoccupied when a loved one is going through a tough time. Follow the Quick and Easy tip on page 76 and you'll always be ready to reach out when someone is in need!

Calories 358 • **Fat** 11g • **Carbohydrate** 40g • **Fiber** 5g • **Sugar** 6g • **Protein** 30g

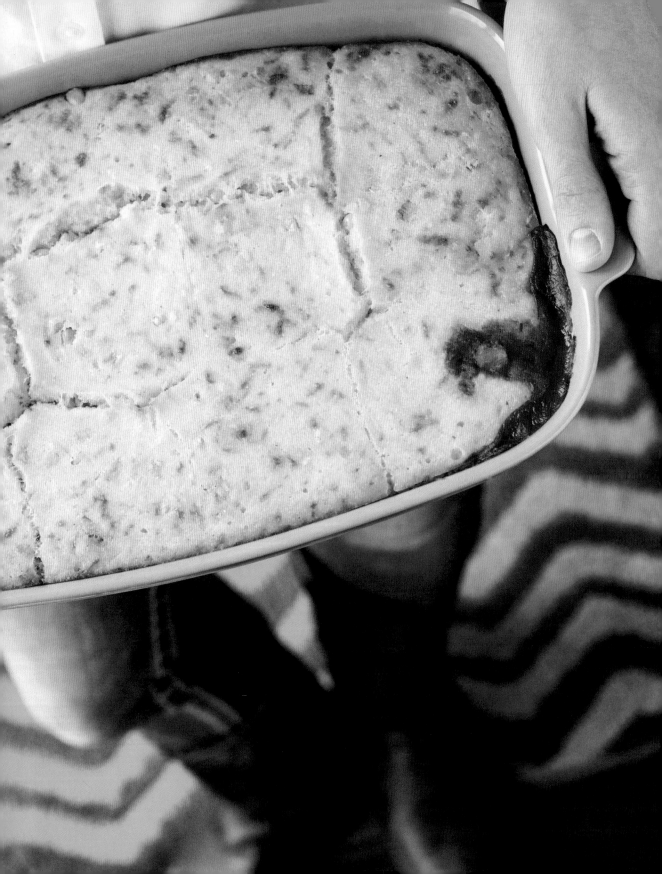

Cowgirl Casserole

Every Southern girl needs a hearty cowgirl casserole recipe, and this is mine. It's also one of my favorite ways to get solid, wholesome sources of protein into my diet. Getting enough protein helps to control both blood sugar and weight, since protein is a fat-burning, muscle-building macronutrient. Between the lean ground beef and the great source of protein found in the three beans here, this cowgirl creation is a low-calorie and low-fat powerhouse!

Prep Time: 15 minutes | **Cook Time:** 40 minutes
Serves: 6 | **Serving Size:** 1/6 of the casserole

½ pound lean ground beef

1 small onion, diced

1 (8-ounce) container baby bella (cremini) mushrooms, sliced

1 red bell pepper, diced

1 teaspoon chili powder

½ teaspoon ground cumin

¼ teaspoon salt

¼ teaspoon black pepper

1 (15-ounce) can reduced-sodium pinto beans, drained and rinsed

1 (15-ounce) can reduced-sodium dark red kidney beans, drained and rinsed

1 (15-ounce) can reduced-sodium black beans, drained and rinsed

½ cup Stubb's Original All-Natural Bar-B-Q Sauce

2 tablespoons Heinz reduced-sugar ketchup

1 tablespoon sugar-free maple-flavor syrup (I like Maple Grove Farms)

1 tablespoon Worcestershire sauce

½ tablespoon apple cider vinegar

Cheesy Cornbread Topping:

⅔ cup white whole wheat flour

½ cup cornmeal

1 tablespoon stevia

1½ teaspoons baking powder

¼ teaspoon salt

1 cup canned cream-style corn

2 egg whites, beaten

¼ cup light sour cream

½ cup shredded reduced-fat sharp cheddar cheese (I like Sargento)

1½ tablespoons sugar-free maple-flavor syrup (I like Maple Grove Farms)

3 green onions, thinly sliced

(recipe continues)

(continued from page 79)

suppertime inspiration:

It's no secret that there are just not enough hours in the day. Making the most of the time you have is vital. Never underestimate the power of 10: 10 minutes playing with your toddler, 10 minutes listening to your teen tell you about her day, 10 minutes praying about something on your mind. The old cliché is true: It's not quantity, it's quality. Give someone in your family "10" today.

1. Preheat the oven to 350°F. Coat a 13 x 9-inch baking dish with cooking spray.

2. In a large skillet over medium-high heat, cook the ground beef, onion, mushrooms, and bell pepper until the beef is no longer pink, 7 to 8 minutes. Use a wooden spoon to break up the beef as it cooks. Drain any excess fat and return the skillet to the stovetop, turning the heat down to low.

3. Set the skillet over low heat. Add the chili powder, cumin, salt, and black pepper to the meat mixture and stir to evenly combine. Add the pinto beans, kidney beans, and black beans and stir to combine.

4. In a small bowl, whisk together the barbecue sauce, ketchup, syrup, Worcestershire sauce, and vinegar. Add the sauce mixture to the skillet and stir to combine. Transfer the mixture to the prepared baking dish.

5. To make the cheesy cornbread topping: In a large bowl, whisk together the flour, cornmeal, stevia, baking powder, and salt.

6. In a small bowl, mix together the creamed corn, egg whites, sour cream, cheddar, and syrup.

7. Add the corn mixture to the flour mixture and use a spoon to mix well. Gently fold in the green onions.

8. Drop the cornbread mixture in even spoonfuls on top of the bean mixture.

9. Cover the baking dish with foil and bake for 30 minutes. Uncover and bake until the cornbread is golden brown and the casserole is heated through, about 10 minutes longer.

Suggested Side Dish: Skinny Fried Apples (page 297)

Calories 341 • Fat 16g • Carbohydrate 32g • Fiber 2g • Sugar 8g • Protein 19g

Easy Chicken and Rice Casserole

There are some nights when easy isn't even easy enough! This recipe is for those nights. I designed this recipe for the days when I have so much to do, it's a wonder I get anything accomplished. If you can relate, this one's for you!

Prep Time: 5 minutes | **Cook Time:** 40 minutes
Serves: 6 | **Serving Size:** 1½ cups

4 cups broccoli florets

1 pound boneless, skinless chicken breasts (see Quick and Easy)

1 (10.5-ounce) can Campbell's Healthy Request condensed cream of chicken soup

⅓ cup plain 0% Greek yogurt

¾ cup fat-free milk

½ teaspoon salt

½ teaspoon black pepper

1 (8.8-ounce) pouch Uncle Ben's Ready Rice brown rice

1 cup shredded reduced-fat sharp cheddar cheese (I like Sargento)

¼ cup panko bread crumbs

quick and easy: Save time by picking up an already prepared rotisserie chicken. That way most of the cooking is done ahead of time!

1. Preheat the oven to 350°F. Coat a 13 x 9-inch baking dish with cooking spray.

2. Bring a large pot of water to a boil over high heat. Add the broccoli and blanch for 1 to 2 minutes, until it is bright green. Remove the broccoli with a slotted spoon and set aside.

3. Add the chicken to the water and bring back up to a boil. Cook until the chicken is cooked through, 15 to 20 minutes. Remove the chicken breasts and set on a plate to cool. When cool enough to handle, shred the chicken breasts with a fork.

4. In a large bowl, mix together the soup, yogurt, milk, salt, and pepper. Add the chicken, broccoli, rice, and ½ cup of the cheddar. Use a large spoon to stir and combine, making sure the soup mixture evenly coats all of the ingredients.

5. Transfer the chicken and rice mixture to the prepared baking dish. Top with the remaining ½ cup cheddar and the panko.

6. Bake uncovered until the cheese is melted and the casserole is heated through, about 20 minutes.

Calories 260 · Fat 8g · Carbohydrate 24g · Fiber 1g · Sugar 3g · Protein 27g

Farmers' Market Garden Bake

This is truly a garden of goodness. The variety of colors, tastes, and textures in this refreshing dish captures what light and balanced eating is all about. If in season, consider taking a trip to your local farmers' market to pick up the wonderful veggies that go into making this supper. It's a great way to invest in the local agriculture and express appreciation to your local farmers. Feel free to use any vegetables that you choose in this dish.

Prep Time: 10 minutes | **Cook Time:** 20 minutes
Serves: 6 | **Serving Size:** 2 cups

8 ounces high-protein farfalle pasta
(I like Barilla ProteinPLUS)

1 tablespoon extra virgin olive oil

1 tablespoon minced garlic

1 small yellow squash, diced

1 small zucchini, diced

1 orange bell pepper, diced

1 pound asparagus, cut into 1-inch
pieces

½ cup frozen pearl onions

1 tomato, diced

Sauce:

¼ cup cooking sherry or low-
sodium vegetable broth

1 cup part-skim ricotta cheese

1 teaspoon grated lemon zest

1 teaspoon dried basil

½ teaspoon dried oregano

¼ teaspoon salt

¼ teaspoon black pepper

1 cup shredded reduced-fat
mozzarella (I like Sargento)

1. Preheat the oven to 350°F. Coat a 13 x 9-inch baking dish with cooking spray.

2. Bring a large pot of salted water to a boil over high heat. Cook the pasta to al dente according to the package directions. Reserving ½ cup of the pasta water, drain the pasta and set aside.

3. In a large skillet, heat the olive oil over medium-high heat. Add the garlic, squash, zucchini, bell pepper, asparagus, and onions and sauté for 5 minutes. Add the tomato and sauté for an additional 2 minutes, until the vegetables have softened.

4. Remove the vegetables from the heat and fold in the cooked pasta.

5. To make the sauce: In a small saucepan, bring the sherry to a simmer over medium heat. Add the reserved ½ cup pasta water and the ricotta and whisk for 2 minutes to incorporate. Season with the lemon zest, basil, oregano, salt, and black pepper. Add ½ cup of the mozzarella and stir until melted, about 2 minutes. Carefully transfer the sauce to a blender (or use an immersion blender) and blend for 1 to 2 minutes until smooth.

(recipe continues)

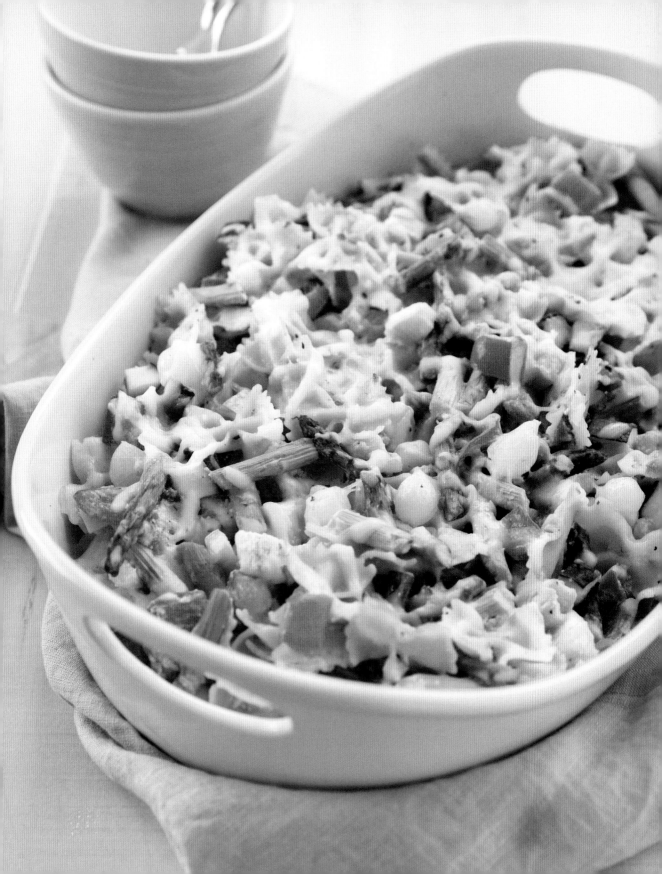

(continued from page 82)

suppertime inspiration:
Your body craves what it is
consistently fed. So, if you feed it
"good food," eventually it will crave
"good food."

6. Pour the sauce over the pasta and vegetables.
   Mix until everything is evenly covered.

7. Transfer the mixture to the prepared baking dish
   and top with the remaining 1/2 cup cheese. Bake
   until the cheese is melted, 15 to 20 minutes.

*Suggested Side Dish: Skinny Sweet Potato Biscuits
(page 272)*

suppertime chat: Infuse some gratitude into your
family tonight by going around the table and expressing to
each person why you are grateful for them today.

Calories 311 • **Fat** 10g • **Carbohydrate** 42g • **Fiber** 5g • **Sugar** 8g • **Protein** 17g

Stuffed Pepper Casserole

Why do I love casseroles so much? One dish makes for easy cleanup! Yet, when you see the words "stuffed" and "casserole" in the title of the recipe you might not expect it to be good for you. Think again! This skinny yet satisfying supper packs vitamins and nutrients onto everyone's dinner plate, with fewer calories than most dishes of its kind.

Prep Time: 10 minutes │ **Cook Time:** 30 minutes
Serves: 6 │ **Serving Size:** 1 1/3 cups

- 1 pound lean ground beef
- 2 green bell peppers, diced
- 2 red bell peppers, diced
- 1 small onion, diced
- 1 tablespoon minced garlic
- 2 (8.8-ounce) pouches Uncle Ben's Ready Rice brown rice
- 1 (23.25-ounce) jar Prego Light Smart Traditional pasta sauce
- ½ tablespoon dried basil
- ½ tablespoon dried oregano
- 1 teaspoon salt
- 1 teaspoon black pepper
- 1 cup shredded reduced-fat four-cheese Italian blend (I like Sargento)

1. Preheat the oven to 350°F. Coat a 13 x 9-inch baking dish with cooking spray.

2. In a large skillet over medium-high heat, cook the ground beef, bell peppers, onion, and garlic until the vegetables soften and the beef is no longer pink, 10 to 12 minutes. Use a wooden spoon to break the beef up as it cooks. Drain any excess fat and return the skillet to the stovetop, turning the heat down to low.

3. Microwave the rice according to the package directions.

4. Add the cooked rice, pasta sauce, basil, oregano, salt, and pepper to the beef in the skillet and mix well. Transfer the skillet ingredients to the prepared baking dish.

5. Sprinkle the Italian cheese on top of the casserole.

6. Bake uncovered until the cheese is melted, 18 to 20 minutes.

Calories 359 • **Fat** 11g • **Carbohydrate** 43g • **Fiber** 7g • **Sugar** 10g • **Protein** 25g

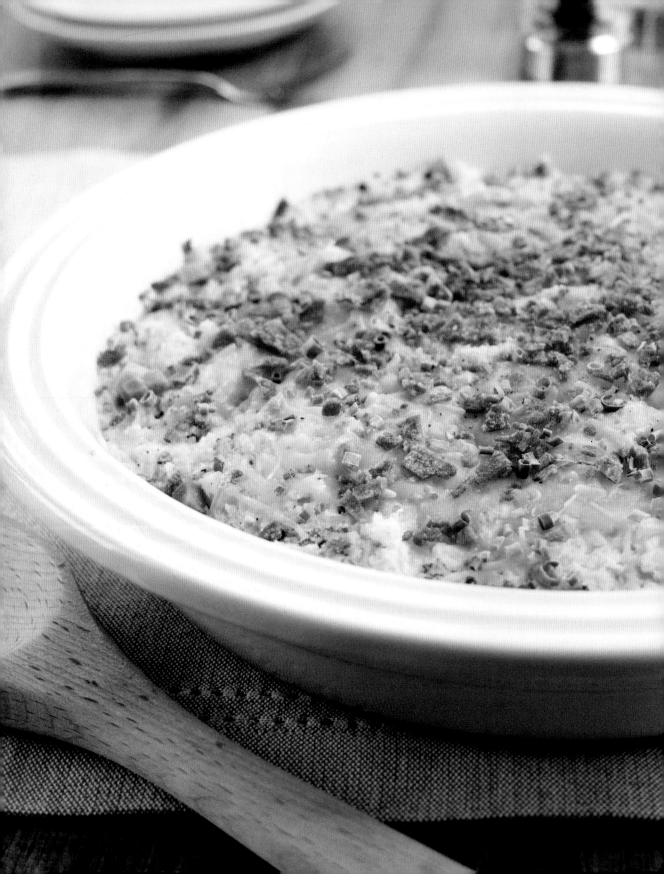

Loaded "Baked Potato" Casserole

This dish is loaded with everything except the potato. Cauliflower is celebrated for its ability to effortlessly impersonate the famous spud, and this dish further substantiates the notion by allowing you to trim the carbs and calories but keep the tried-and-true taste.

Prep Time: 10 minutes | **Cook Time:** 20 minutes
Serves: 4 | **Serving Size:** Heaping 1⅓ cups

2 (12-ounce) bags frozen cauliflower florets

⅓ cup low-sodium chicken broth (I like Pacific Organic)

¼ cup light sour cream

1 (1-ounce) packet ranch salad dressing and seasoning mix

¼ teaspoon salt

¼ teaspoon black pepper

1 (12-ounce) bag frozen broccoli florets

1 cup diced ham

1 cup shredded reduced-fat sharp cheddar cheese (I like Sargento)

½ cup fresh chives, chopped

5 slices lower-sodium turkey bacon

quick and easy: If you haven't reached your desired crispiness in the turkey bacon after 2½ minutes, continue cooking in 30-second increments.

1. Preheat the oven to 350°F. Coat a 13 x 9-inch baking dish with cooking spray.

2. Microwave both of the bags of cauliflower according to the package directions. Drain the cauliflower and place in a large bowl.

3. Add the chicken broth, sour cream, ranch dressing mix, salt, and pepper to the cauliflower. Using an immersion blender or a potato masher, blend or mash until almost smooth (or leave it a little chunky, if you desire).

4. Microwave the broccoli according to the package directions. Drain.

5. Fold the broccoli, ham, ½ cup of the cheddar, and ¼ cup of the chives into the cauliflower mixture.

6. Pour the mixture into the prepared baking dish and spread evenly. Bake for 20 minutes.

7. Meanwhile, arrange the turkey bacon slices in a single layer on a microwave-safe plate lined with paper towels. Microwave on high for 1½ to 2½ minutes (see Quick and Easy). Once cool enough to handle, crumble the bacon into pieces.

8. Top the casserole with the bacon and the remaining ½ cup cheddar and ¼ cup chives. Bake until the cheese is melted, 7 to 8 minutes longer.

Calories 258 · Fat 11g · Carbohydrate 16g · Fiber 4g · Sugar 7g · Protein 19g

PB&J "Brinner" Casserole

At least once a month, I love to surprise my little guy with "brinner," i.e., breakfast for dinner. It can be such a welcome break in our daily routine. But I don't like to always serve up your typical eggs and bacon kind of brinner. That's why this one-of-a-kind casserole has become a favorite in our house. It combines the classic breakfast of French toast with everyone's favorite afternoon snack—peanut butter and jelly. It's an unusual mix for sure, but definitely worth trying out on your family, as it's super kid-friendly. My little man never frowns when he hears that it's peanut butter and jelly time.

Prep Time: 10 minutes, plus 2 hours chilling time | **Cook Time:** 1 hour
Serves: 8 | **Serving Size:** ⅛ of the casserole (a 3 x 4¼-inch square)

---

6 tablespoons creamy natural peanut butter (I like Smucker's)

6 whole wheat hamburger buns

⅓ cup reduced-sugar raspberry preserves (I like Smucker's Low Sugar)

4 ounces ⅓-less-fat cream cheese, softened

2 teaspoons stevia

2 eggs

4 egg whites

2½ cups Silk Unsweetened Original Almondmilk

3 tablespoons sugar-free maple-flavor syrup (I like Maple Grove Farms)

2 teaspoons vanilla extract

¼ cup old-fashioned rolled oats

½ cup fresh raspberries

1. Coat a 13 x 9-inch baking dish with cooking spray.

2. Spread 1 tablespoon of the peanut butter onto the bottom of each of the bun halves. Put the top and bottom halves back together and cut the buns into 1-inch cubes. Spread the bread cubes evenly in the baking dish. Using a teaspoon, drop mounds of raspberry jam evenly over the bread cubes.

3. In a medium bowl, fold the cream cheese and stevia together until mixed well. Use the teaspoon again to drop the cream cheese evenly over the bread cubes.

4. In a separate medium bowl, whisk together the whole eggs, egg whites, almond milk, syrup, and vanilla. Pour the egg mixture over the bread cubes. Cover with foil and refrigerate for at least 2 hours or up to overnight.

5. Remove the baking dish from the refrigerator and let stand at room temperature for 20 minutes.

(recipe continues)

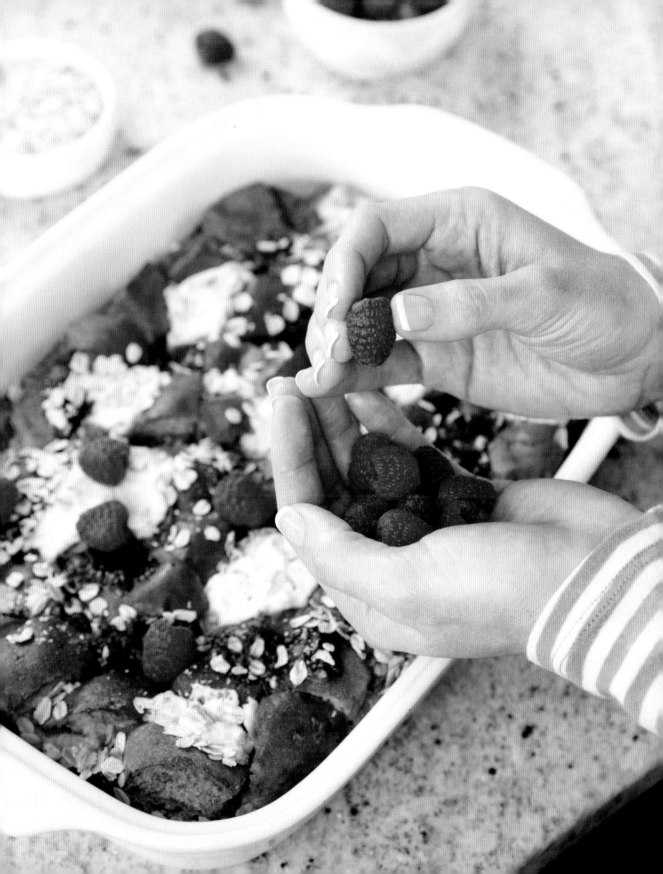

(continued from page 88)

skinny sense: If you're like me, you still love to serve up a classic peanut butter and jelly sandwich for lunch every now and then. Here's a tip to help keep the complaints down regarding soggy bread (from the jelly) in the lunch boxes: Try smoothing a thin layer of peanut butter on both slices of the bread (to create a seal) before spreading the jelly on top. This will eliminate the soggy bread, but keep the smiles!

6. Preheat the oven to 350°F.

7. Uncover the baking dish and sprinkle the oats evenly over the top of the casserole.

8. Re-cover with the foil and bake for 40 minutes, rotating the baking dish front to back after 20 minutes. Uncover and bake until a knife inserted into the center comes out clean, about 20 minutes longer, rotating the baking dish front to back halfway through the cooking.

9. Remove from the oven. Cool on a wire rack for 10 minutes before serving. Cut into squares and serve sprinkled with the fresh raspberries.

Calories 225 · Fat 11g · Carbohydrate 23g · Fiber 7g · Sugar 3g · Protein 11g

Tuna Rice Casserole

The benefits of adding fish to your family's diet are endless. The main reason I like to keep it on the weekly menu in our house is that the omega-3 fats found in fish (like the albacore tuna I use in this dish) help reduce my family's overall risk for heart disease, work as a great anti-inflammatory, and assist in brain function—perfect for helping my little man do well in school.

Prep Time: 10 minutes | **Cook Time:** 30 minutes
Serves: 6 | **Serving Size:** 1 1/3 cups

½ teaspoon extra virgin olive oil

1 tablespoon minced garlic

1 onion, diced

1 red bell pepper, diced

1 (8-ounce) container baby bella (cremini) mushrooms, sliced

1 (10.5-ounce) can Campbell's Healthy Request condensed cream of mushroom soup

1 cup Prego Light Homestyle Alfredo sauce or Make It Homemade (page 132)

¼ teaspoon salt

½ teaspoon black pepper

1 (12-ounce) bag frozen peas, thawed

2 (5-ounce) cans solid white albacore tuna, drained and flaked

1 (8.8-ounce) pouch Uncle Ben's Ready Rice brown rice

¼ cup shredded Parmesan cheese (I like Sargento Artisan Blends)

½ cup whole wheat Ritz cracker crumbs (about 13 crackers)

1. Preheat the oven to 350°F. Coat a 13 x 9-inch baking dish with cooking spray.

2. In a large skillet, heat the olive oil over medium-high heat. Add the garlic, onion, and bell pepper and cook until softened, 4 to 5 minutes. Add the mushrooms and cook until they have softened, 4 to 5 minutes longer.

3. Stir in the mushroom soup and Alfredo sauce. Season with the salt and black pepper. Add the peas and tuna and stir for another 1 to 2 minutes to evenly combine.

4. Remove from the heat and add the rice. Transfer the tuna mixture to the baking dish and sprinkle with the Parmesan and cracker crumbs and bake until heated through and the sauce is bubbly, about 20 minutes.

suppertime chat: What's the funniest thing that happened to you today? Sometimes it's easier for all of us to focus on the stressors, like homework and to-do lists. Encouraging your family to reminisce about the humorous parts of their day will help them to develop a "glass is half full" kind of attitude. Bonus: You might realize your day wasn't all that bad either!

Calories 286 • Fat 8g • Carbohydrate 37g • Fiber 5g • Sugar 7g • Protein 18g

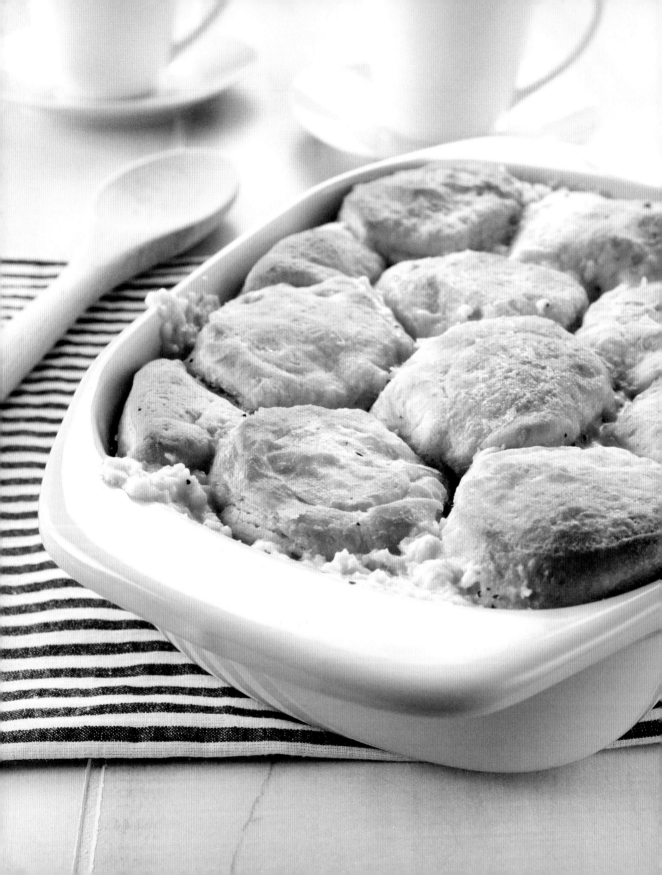

Southern Biscuits and Gravy Casserole

I'm from the South, so I couldn't write a cookbook without including a recipe with biscuits and gravy. This Southern specialty combines the best of all things breakfast, but when it's lightened up, it makes one delicious suppertime casserole. And, like most casseroles, it's one dish in the oven—and done! Easy cleanup means more time for me to enjoy the little free time I have with the ones who mean the most—family!

Prep Time: 10 minutes | **Cook Time:** 40 minutes
Serves: 6 | **Serving Size:** 1/6 of the casserole

2 eggs

4 egg whites

1/2 cup shredded reduced-fat sharp cheddar cheese (I like Sargento)

1/2 cup fat-free milk

8 fully cooked turkey sausage links, cut into 1/2-inch pieces

Gravy:

2 tablespoons unsalted butter

2 tablespoons white whole wheat flour

1 1/2 cups fat-free milk

1/2 teaspoon salt

1/2 teaspoon black pepper

1 (12-ounce) can Pillsbury Grands! Jr. Golden Layers Flaky Biscuits

skinny sense: Leave baking dishes in the kitchen and serve from there. You're less likely to go for seconds if you have to get up from the table to get a second helping!

1. Preheat the oven to 350°F. Coat an 11 x 7-inch baking dish with cooking spray.

2. In a medium bowl, whisk together the eggs, egg whites, cheddar, and milk.

3. Pour the egg mixture into the baking dish. Top with the turkey sausage. Cover with foil and bake for 20 to 25 minutes.

4. While the eggs and sausage are baking, prepare the gravy: In a small saucepan, melt the butter over low heat. Whisk the flour into the butter for about 30 seconds, until smooth and the mixture smells nutty, making a roux. Whisk in the milk and bring to a boil over medium heat, making sure to stir constantly. Season with the salt and pepper. Reduce the heat to low and continue to stir until the gravy is thickened, 5 to 8 minutes.

5. Remove the baking dish from the oven. Pour the gravy over the eggs and sausage to cover. Carefully arrange the biscuits evenly on top of the gravy mixture, leaving space in between each biscuit.

6. Bake uncovered until the biscuits are golden brown, 14 to 16 minutes.

Calories 341 · Fat 16g · Carbohydrate 32g · Fiber 2g · Sugar 8g · Protein 19g

Tex-Mex Casserole

Tex-Mex is a fusion of American and Mexican cuisine, characterized by the use of cheese, beef, beans, and various spices. In this creamy casserole you'll get big Tex-Mex flavor, with quick, easy, and inexpensive ingredients. Adding whole wheat pasta makes it a nutritionally balanced supper.

Prep Time: 10 minutes | **Cook Time:** 30 minutes
Serves: 8 | **Serving Size:** Heaping 1½ cups

8 ounces whole wheat penne pasta
(I like Barilla)

1 pound lean ground beef

1 small onion, diced

1 teaspoon minced garlic

1 (10.5-ounce) can Campbell's
Healthy Request condensed
tomato soup

1 (15-ounce) can reduced-sodium
black beans, drained and rinsed

1 (15.25-ounce) can low-sodium
whole kernel corn, drained

1 (10-ounce) can Ro*Tel "Original"
diced tomatoes and green chilies

1 (4.5-ounce) can chopped green
chilies

2 teaspoons chili powder

1½ teaspoons ground cumin

½ teaspoon salt

½ teaspoon black pepper

½ cup shredded reduced-fat
four-cheese Mexican blend
(I like Sargento)

1 tomato, diced

1. Preheat the oven to 350°F. Coat a 13 x 9-inch baking dish with cooking spray.

2. Bring a large pot of salted water to a boil over high heat. Cook the pasta to al dente according to the package directions. Drain and set aside.

3. In a large skillet over medium-high heat, cook the ground beef, onion, and garlic until the beef is no longer pink, 7 to 8 minutes. Use a wooden spoon to break the beef up as it cooks. Drain any excess fat and return the skillet to the stovetop, turning the heat down to low.

4. Add the cooked pasta, soup, beans, corn, diced tomatoes, green chilies, chili powder, cumin, salt, and black pepper to the skillet and stir until well combined.

5. Transfer the pasta mixture to the prepared baking dish. Sprinkle the Mexican cheese evenly over the top. Bake uncovered until the cheese is melted and the casserole is heated through, 18 to 20 minutes.

6. Top with the diced tomato before serving.

suppertime inspiration: All too often, the goals I want to achieve in life seem far away. It's in these moments that I hang on to a quote I heard many years ago: "Believe you can and you are halfway there!" A powerful reminder that the mind plays a vital role in our ability to succeed.

Calories 319 • **Fat** 8g • **Carbohydrate** 48g • **Fiber** 7g • **Sugar** 11g • **Protein** 21g

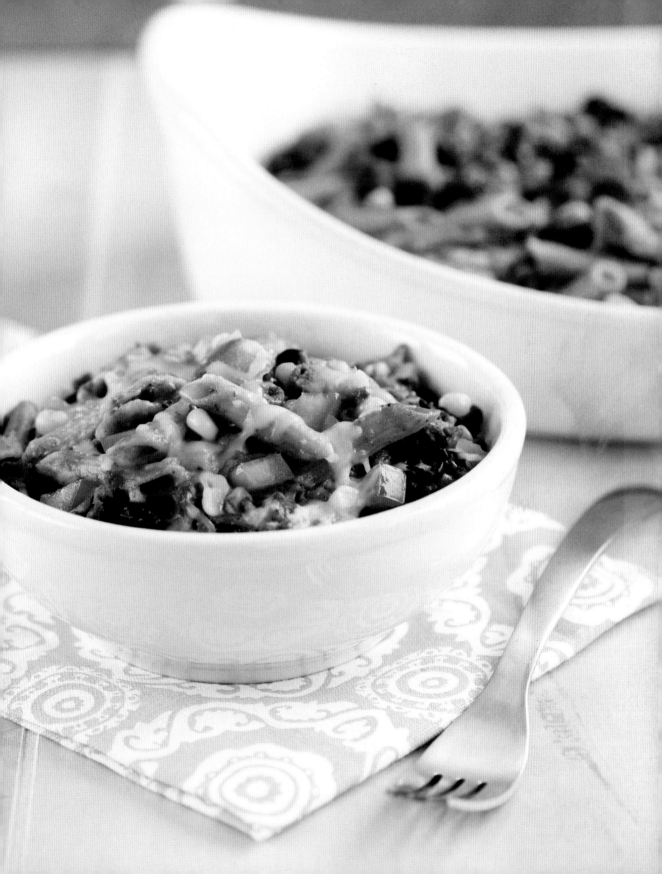

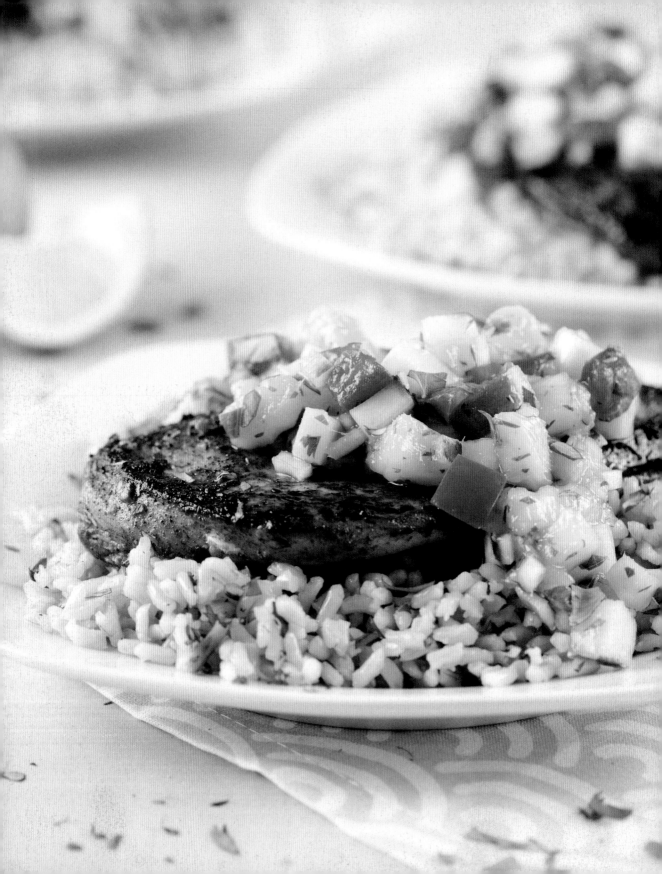

7 BAKED, SHAKED, AND UNFRIED
CHICKEN AND TURKEY SUPPERS

Baked Sweet and Sour Chicken

My version of sweet and sour chicken is tender, juicy, and full of flavor. With only 10 minutes of prep and less than 1 hour of cook time, you'll be able to serve up this tasty dish whenever someone in the house says, "I feel like Chinese food tonight!"

Prep Time: 10 minutes | **Cook Time:** 50 minutes
Serves: 4 | **Serving Size:** 1¾ cups

1 pound boneless, skinless chicken breasts, cut into 1-inch cubes

⅓ cup plus 2 teaspoons cornstarch

2 tablespoons extra virgin olive oil

1 (8-ounce) can juice-packed pineapple chunks (I like Del Monte)

¼ cup Heinz reduced-sugar ketchup

2 tablespoons rice vinegar

1 tablespoon less-sodium soy sauce

1 teaspoon minced garlic

1 teaspoon stevia

⅛ teaspoon red pepper flakes

1 small onion, chopped

1 red bell pepper, chopped

1 yellow bell pepper, chopped

3 green onions, thinly sliced

suppertime chat: Who's your favorite superhero and why? If you could have a superhero power, what would it be and why? Get ready to reminisce about the days when you wanted to grow up and be Wonder Woman or Superwoman!

1. Preheat the oven to 350°F. Coat an 11 x 7-inch baking dish with cooking spray.

2. Place the chicken and ⅓ cup of the cornstarch in a large resealable bag. Seal and shake the bag a few times to evenly coat the chicken.

3. In a wok or large skillet, heat the olive oil over medium-high heat. Add the chicken in a single layer and cook the chicken until browned all over but not cooked through, 1 to 2 minutes, turning the chicken occasionally. Remove from the heat.

4. Drain the pineapple and reserve the juice for the sauce.

5. In a small bowl, whisk together the reserved pineapple juice, ketchup, rice vinegar, soy sauce, garlic, stevia, red pepper flakes, and remaining 2 teaspoons cornstarch.

6. Place the browned chicken pieces in the bottom of the prepared baking dish. Add the pineapple chunks, onion, and red and yellow bell peppers. Pour the sauce evenly over the chicken and vegetables.

7. Cover the baking dish loosely with foil and bake until the sauce is bubbling and the chicken is

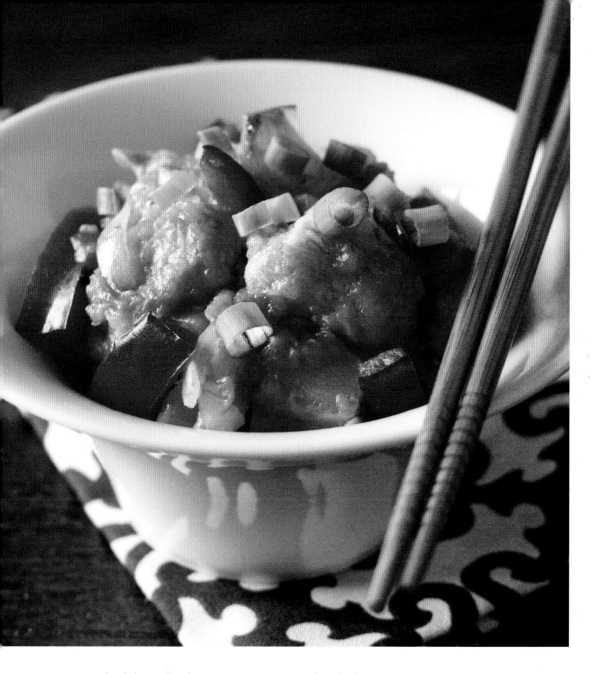

cooked through, about 45 minutes. Stir the chicken mixture and rotate the pan front to back halfway through the baking time to ensure that it cooks evenly.

8. Serve garnished with the green onions.

Calories 294 • **Fat** 10g • **Carbohydrate** 29g • **Fiber** 3g • **Sugar** 13g • **Protein** 24g

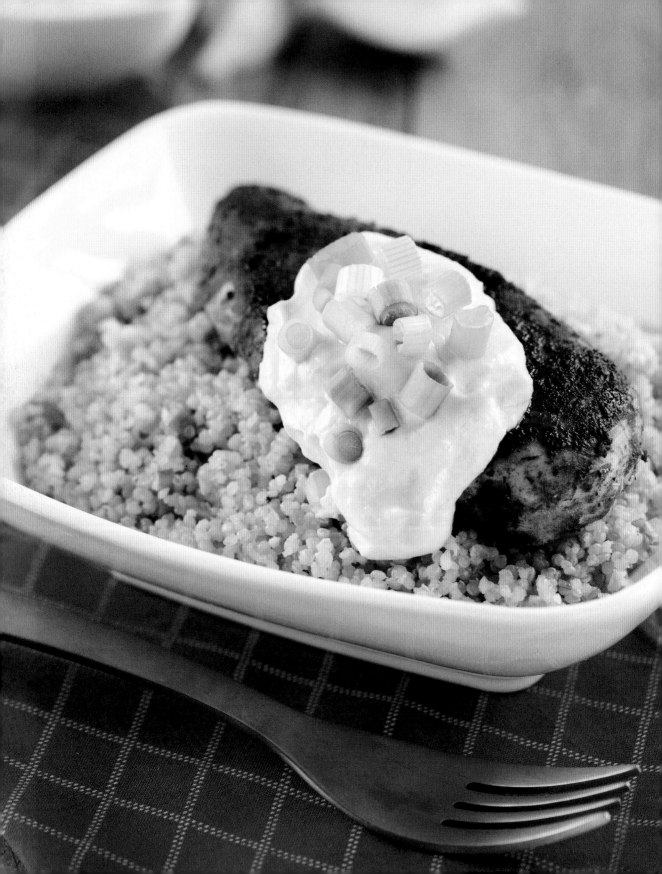

Blackened Chicken with Avocado Cream Sauce

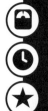

If you're trying to eat light and balanced, chicken almost always becomes part of your supper repertoire, but it can get boring fast. Diminish the boredom by offering this succulent dish to your household. With just 10 minutes of prep and less than 10 ingredients, I give it a "10"!

Prep Time: 10 minutes | **Cook Time:** 15 minutes
Serves: 4 | **Serving Size:** One 4-ounce chicken breast, 2 tablespoons avocado cream sauce

4 (4-ounce) boneless, skinless chicken breasts (see Quick and Easy)

2 tablespoons blackened seasoning

Avocado Cream Sauce:

⅓ cup plain 0% Greek yogurt

½ avocado

1 teaspoon lemon juice

½ teaspoon garlic powder

⅛ teaspoon salt

For Serving:

2 tablespoons green onions, thinly sliced

quick and easy: Cut larger chicken breasts (more than 4 ounces) in half lengthwise to make 4-ounce breast servings. This also cuts down on the cook time and helps the chicken cook more evenly.

1. Place the chicken breasts and blackened seasoning in a large resealable bag. Seal and shake a few times to evenly coat the chicken.

2. Lightly coat a large skillet with cooking spray and heat over medium-high heat. Add the chicken and cook until cooked through, 4 to 6 minutes per side.

3. Meanwhile, prepare the avocado cream sauce: In a food processor, combine the yogurt, avocado, lemon juice, garlic powder, and salt and pulse until smooth and creamy.

4. To serve, top each chicken breast with 2 tablespoons of the creamy avocado sauce and garnish with ½ tablespoon green onions.

Suggested Side Dish: Parmesan-Garlic Quinoa (page 285)

Calories 162 · Fat 6g · Carbohydrate 4g · Fiber 2g · Sugar 1g · Protein 25g

2x

Blueberry Rosemary Chicken

Who would think to pair a blueberry sauce with chicken? Trust me, it's phenomenal! Sweet and just a little tart, it's the perfect way to welcome spring and summer. I also like to make a little extra blueberry sauce to serve for dessert over low-fat vanilla ice cream or over whole grain waffles the next morning for breakfast.

Prep Time: 5 minutes, plus 30 minutes marinating time | **Cook Time:** 15 minutes
Serves: 4 | **Serving Size:** One 4-ounce chicken breast, 2 tablespoons sauce

4 (4-ounce) boneless, skinless chicken breasts

⅓ cup balsamic vinegar

1 teaspoon minced garlic

½ teaspoon kosher salt

¼ teaspoon black pepper

1 teaspoon dried rosemary (see Quick and Easy)

2 teaspoons extra virgin olive oil

Blueberry Sauce:

1 tablespoon cornstarch

⅓ cup balsamic vinegar

1 (10-ounce) bag frozen blueberries

2 tablespoons light brown sugar

1 teaspoon grated lemon zest

2 tablespoons lemon juice

Pinch of salt

quick and easy: Fresh rosemary is one of my favorite herbs to grow in the summer. Feel free to use fresh rosemary in place of the dried.

1. Place the chicken breasts, balsamic vinegar, and minced garlic in a large resealable bag. Marinate in the refrigerator for 30 minutes.

2. Remove the chicken from the marinade and set aside on a plate (discard any remaining marinade). Season the chicken with the kosher salt, pepper, and rosemary.

3. In a large skillet, heat the olive oil over medium-high heat. Add the chicken breasts and cook until the chicken is no longer pink in the center but still juicy, 4 to 6 minutes per side. Set aside to rest.

4. Meanwhile, to make the blueberry sauce: In a small bowl, dissolve the cornstarch in the balsamic vinegar to make a slurry.

5. In a medium saucepan, combine the slurry, blueberries, brown sugar, lemon zest, lemon juice, and salt. Stir together over medium heat until the blueberries release their juices and start to break apart and the sauce thickens, 4 to 6 minutes.

6. To serve, spoon the blueberry sauce over the chicken.

Suggested Side Dish: Caramelized Brussels Sprouts with Pecans (page 298)

Calories 230 · Fat 5g · Carbohydrate 24g · Fiber 2g · Sugar 18g · Protein 24g

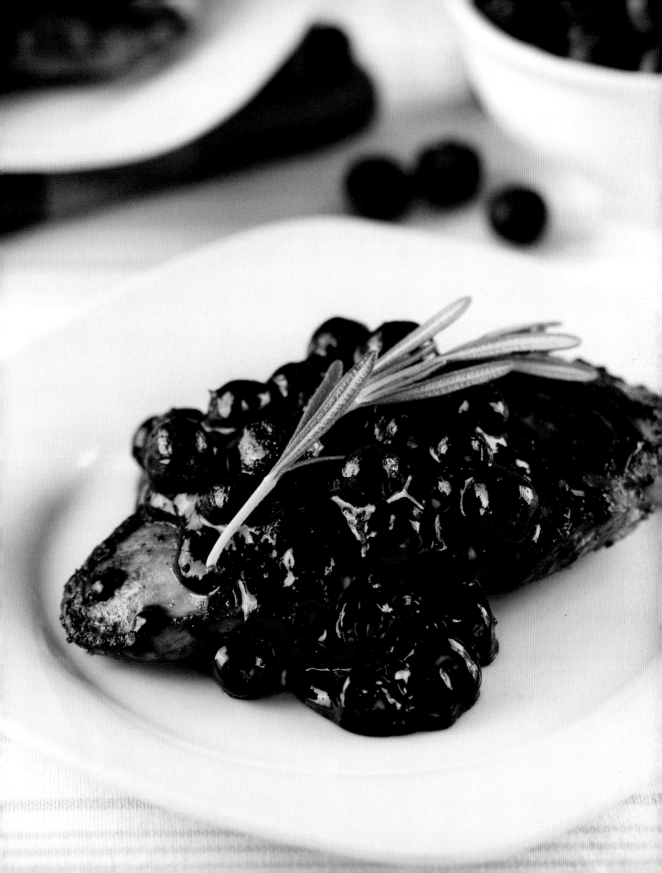

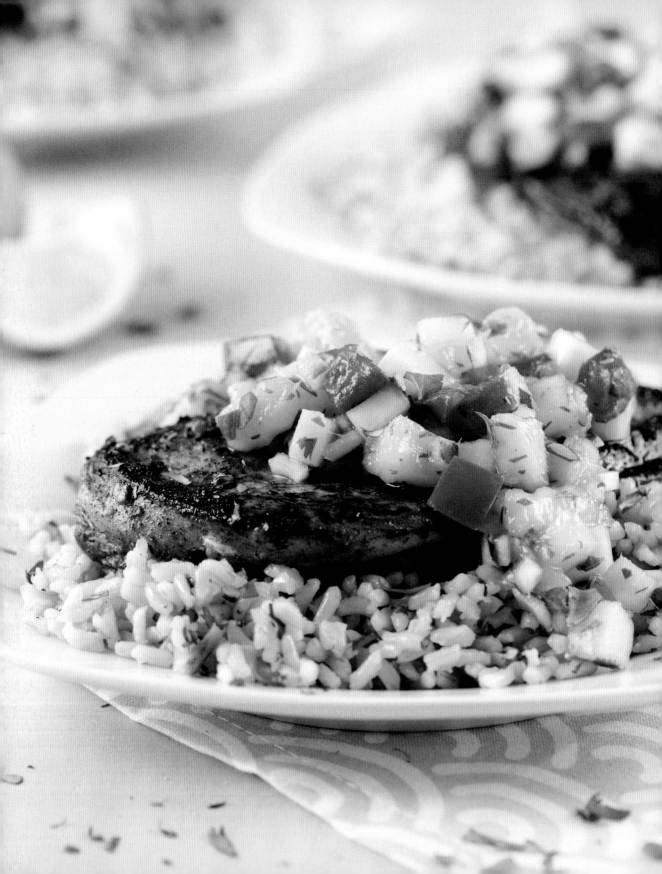

Caribbean Jerk Chicken with Mango Salsa

The mango salsa in this dish really adds a Caribbean flair. I love to serve this meal when having guests over for an outdoor party. It presents like it would take hours to prepare, but really takes around 30 minutes!

Prep Time: 10 minutes | **Cook Time:** 15 minutes
Serves: 4 | **Serving Size:** One 4-ounce chicken breast, ¼ cup mango salsa

Mango Salsa:

1 mango, peeled and diced
   (see Quick and Easy)

1 Roma (plum) tomato, diced

½ cup diced red onion

2 tablespoons finely chopped fresh
   cilantro

1 teaspoon grated lime zest

2 teaspoons lime juice

¼ teaspoon salt

Jerk Chicken:

4 (4-ounce) boneless, skinless
   chicken breasts

2 tablespoons Caribbean jerk
   seasoning or Make It Homemade
   (page 299)

2 teaspoons extra virgin olive oil

1. To make the salsa: In a medium bowl, stir together the mango, tomato, onion, cilantro, lime zest, lime juice, and salt to combine. Refrigerate until ready to serve.

2. To make the jerk chicken: Place the chicken breasts and jerk seasoning in a large resealable bag. Seal and shake a few times to evenly coat the chicken.

3. In a large skillet, heat the olive oil over medium heat. Add the chicken and cook until done, 4 to 6 minutes per side.

4. Serve the chicken warm topped with the mango salsa.

Suggested Side Dish: Cilantro-Lime Rice (page 271)

quick and easy: Feel free to purchase frozen mango for this recipe. To thaw the mango, place 1 cup frozen mango in a bowl and refrigerate for at least 5 hours before ready to use. Try to stir or turn the fruit a few times while in the refrigerator for an even thaw and drain any juice or water from the mango before using.

Calories 210 • Fat 5g • Carbohydrate 21g • Fiber 2g • Sugar 13g • Protein 24g

Greek Turkey Meatballs with Tzatziki Sauce

Easier to prepare than pronounce (*tsat-ZEE-kee*), this Greek sauce has delicious fresh cucumber and dill flavor and smooth, creamy texture. Here I pair it with turkey meatballs atop pita quarters as a fun way for me to serve up goodness to my little guy.

Prep Time: 15 minutes │ **Cook Time:** 30 minutes
Serves: 6 │ **Serving Size:** 4 meatballs, 1 pita, ¼ cup tzatziki sauce, and 4 Kalamata olives

1 pound lean ground turkey

1 (12-ounce) bag frozen spinach, thawed and drained

½ cup plain bread crumbs

½ cup reduced-fat feta cheese crumbles

½ small onion, finely diced

1 egg, beaten

1 tablespoon minced garlic

1 tablespoon lemon juice

1 teaspoon dried oregano

¼ teaspoon salt

¼ teaspoon black pepper

Tzatziki Sauce:

1 medium cucumber, peeled

1 cup plain 0% Greek yogurt

2 tablespoons chopped fresh dill

2 tablespoons minced garlic

1 tablespoon lemon juice

¼ teaspoon salt

½ teaspoon black pepper

For Serving:

2 medium cucumbers, cut into 24 (¼-inch) slices

6 whole wheat pitas, quartered

24 Kalamata olives

1. Preheat the oven to 400°F. Lightly coat a 13 x 9-inch baking dish with cooking spray.

2. In a large bowl, with clean hands, combine the ground turkey, spinach, bread crumbs, feta, onion, egg, garlic, lemon juice, oregano, salt, and pepper. Using a heaping tablespoon for a measure, form the mixture into 24 meatballs.

3. Place the meatballs in the prepared baking dish and bake for 20 minutes. Turn the meatballs and bake for 10 minutes longer, until browned.

4. Meanwhile, to make the tzatziki sauce: Halve the cucumber lengthwise and scrape out the seeds with a spoon. Mince the cucumber and place in a medium bowl. Add the yogurt, dill, garlic, lemon juice, salt, and pepper. Stir well and set aside.

5. To assemble, place one cucumber slice on each pita quarter. Top with a meatball and 1 tablespoon of tzatziki sauce. Finish by securing a Kalamata olive to the top with a toothpick. Serve 4 pita quarters per person.

Suggested Side Dish: Quick Cauliflower Couscous (page 286)

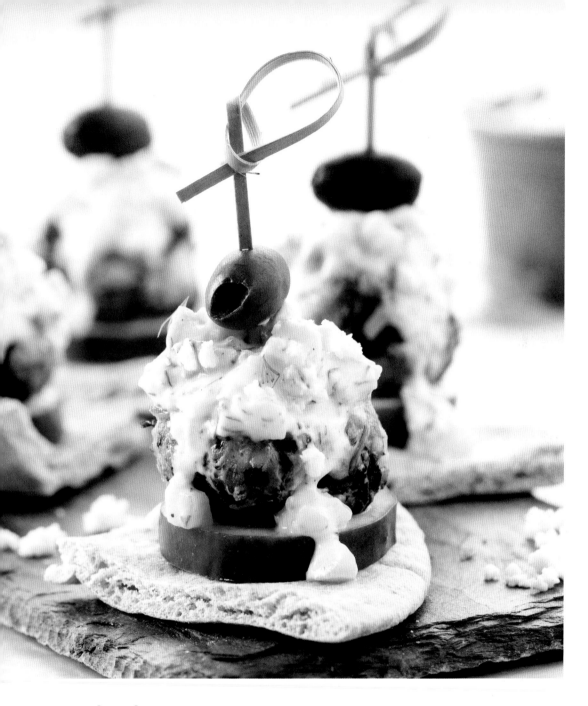

quick and easy: I like to make two or even three batches
of these delicious meatballs at a time and freeze any extras in
a resealable bag. (I usually freeze 24 to 30 per bag.)

Calories 449 · Fat 14g · Carbohydrate 47g · Fiber 5g · Sugar 6g · Protein 31g

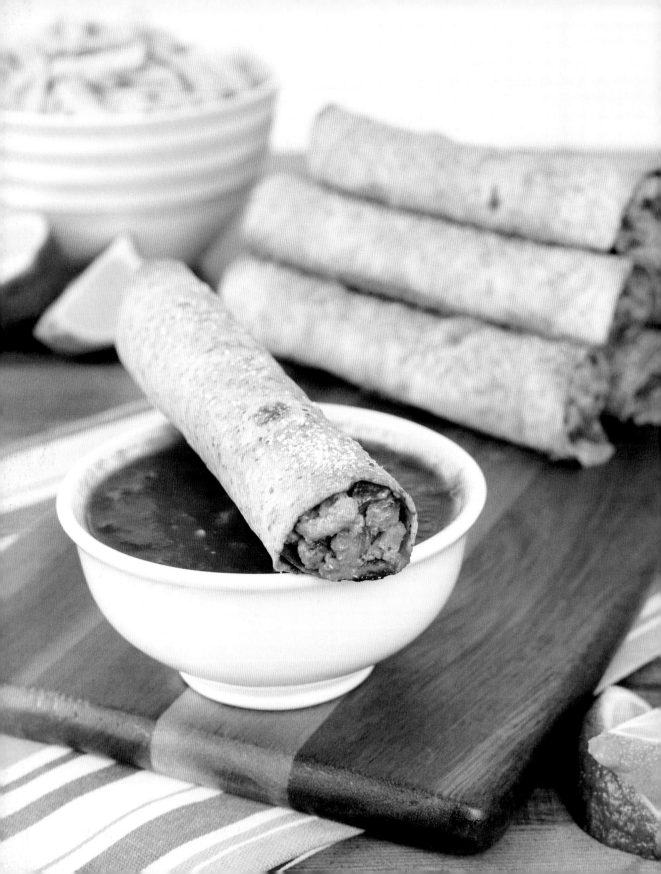

Turkey Taquitos

We love Mexican food at our house, and in this recipe I've found a way to preserve the golden, crispy goodness of the taquito without the deep fryer. The smart blend of the cream cheese and Greek yogurt provides the ultimate creamy base for this Mexican favorite.

Prep Time: 5 minutes | **Cook Time:** 30 minutes
Serves: 8 | **Serving Size:** 2 taquitos

1 pound lean ground turkey

1 small onion, diced

1 red bell pepper, diced

1 (1-ounce) packet less-sodium taco seasoning or Make It Homemade (page 299)

4 ounces ⅓-less-fat cream cheese, softened

⅓ cup plain 0% Greek yogurt

1 tablespoon lime juice

1 (4.5-ounce) can chopped green chilies

16 low-carb, high-fiber whole wheat tortillas (I like La Tortilla Factory original size)

½ cup shredded reduced-fat four-cheese Mexican blend (I like Sargento)

1 cup mild low-sodium tomato salsa (optional; I like Frog Ranch)

quick and easy: If a recipe calls for softened cream cheese and you forgot to set it out in advance, put the cream cheese in a microwave-safe bowl and heat it in the microwave for 10 to 15 seconds.

1. Preheat the oven to 350°F. Coat a baking sheet with cooking spray.

2. In a large skillet over medium-high heat, cook the ground turkey, onion, and bell pepper until the ground turkey is browned, 7 to 8 minutes. Use a wooden spoon to break the turkey up as it cooks. Reduce the heat to low and add the taco seasoning and 1 tablespoon water, stirring to mix well. Simmer for 2 to 3 minutes, then remove from the heat.

3. While the ground turkey is cooking, in a bowl, stir together the cream cheese, yogurt, lime juice, and chopped green chilies. Mix until well combined.

4. Add the cream cheese mixture to the ground turkey mixture and stir to mix well.

5. To assemble, spoon 3 tablespoons of the turkey mixture along the edge of each tortilla, top with ½ tablespoon of the shredded cheese, and roll up.

6. Place the rolls seam side down on the greased baking sheet. Coat the tops of the rolls with cooking spray.

7. Bake until the rolls are golden brown, 25 to 30 minutes.

8. Serve warm, with salsa for dipping, if desired.

Suggested Side Dish: Cilantro-Lime Rice (page 271)

Calories 334 • Fat 14g • Carbohydrate 43g • Fiber 25g • Sugar 5g • Protein 55g
Nutrition does not include optional ingredient.

Southern "Fried" Chicken

My hometown of Corbin, Kentucky, is also hometown to the original Colonel Sanders and the very first Kentucky Fried Chicken. But the fried chicken I grew up on was homemade by my granny. Here, I've preserved the spicy Southern flavors of my family's secret recipe, but not the Southern fat and calories!

Prep Time: 10 minutes, plus 4 hours marinating time | **Cook Time:** 30 minutes
Serves: 4 | **Serving Size:** 3 pieces of chicken

4 (4-ounce) boneless, skinless
   chicken breasts

¾ cup fat-free milk

1 tablespoon Frank's RedHot Sauce

1 cup cornflakes

1 teaspoon paprika

1 teaspoon salt

2 teaspoons black pepper

½ cup panko bread crumbs

skinny sense: Did you know that allowing your children to help prepare meals encourages their desire to eat healthy? The next time your little one asks to help out, hand him a serving spoon and a bowl, and whip up a yummy memory!

1. Place the chicken breasts between 2 pieces of wax paper and gently pound with the flat side of a meat mallet or rolling pin until the breasts are about ½ inch thick. Cut each breast into 3 equal pieces.

2. In a small bowl, whisk together the milk and hot sauce.

3. Place the chicken pieces in a large resealable bag and pour in the milk mixture. Squeeze out any excess air, seal the bag, and marinate in the refrigerator for at least 4 hours and up to overnight (depending on how much time you have).

4. When you're ready to cook, preheat the oven to 400°F. Coat a baking sheet with cooking spray.

5. In a food processor, combine ½ cup of the cornflakes, the paprika, salt, and pepper. Pulse until the cornflakes become crumbs. Pour them into a shallow baking dish and stir in the panko.

6. In a small resealable bag, gently crush the remaining ½ cup cornflakes by hand into small pieces. Transfer the hand-crushed cornflakes to the panko-crumb mixture.

7. Remove the chicken pieces one at a time from the marinade and place in the cornflake mixture. Evenly cover each piece of chicken.

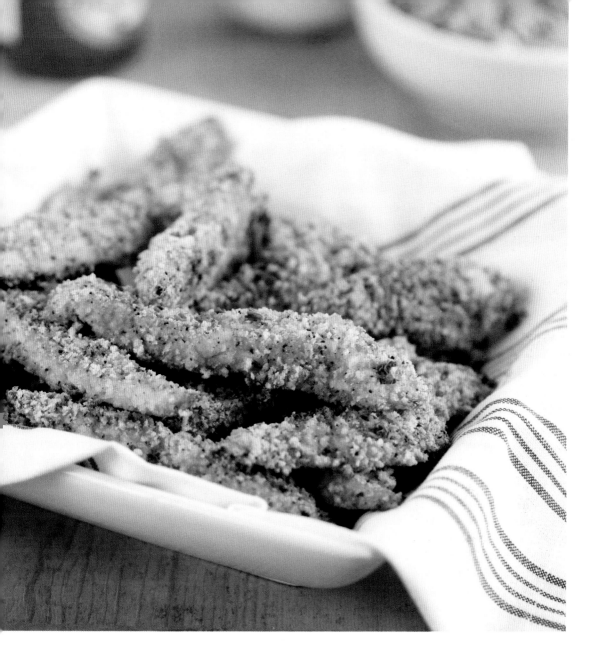

8. Arrange the chicken in a single layer on the baking sheet. Bake for 15 minutes at 400°F, then reduce the oven temperature to 350°F and bake until the chicken is cooked through and crispy, 5 to 10 minutes longer.

Suggested Side Dish: Sun-Dried Tomato and Pesto Potato Salad (page 292)

Calories 177 · **Fat** 3g · **Carbohydrate** 14g · **Fiber** 0g · **Sugar** 3g · **Protein** 26g

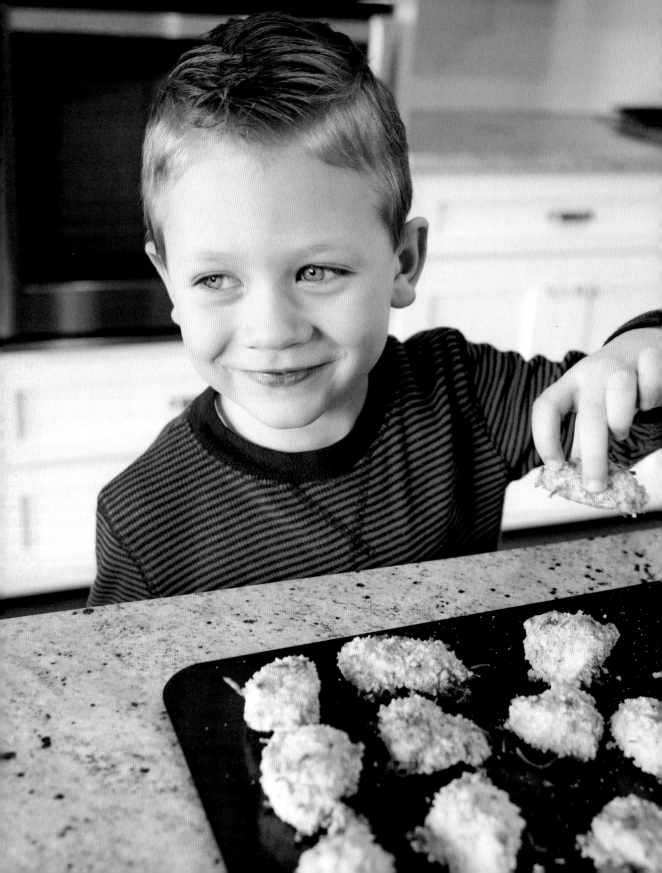

Parmesan Chicken Nuggets

My little guy (pictured here) is five, so we live and die by chicken nuggets in my house. You can understand how painstakingly I worked to come up with a (more natural) chicken nugget recipe he'd be happy to eat. Here it is, for all you moms out there battling Drive-Thru Guilt Syndrome. Be free! And, to relieve yourself of another guilty compromise (packaged macaroni and cheese), pair these yummy nuggets with my Broccoli Mac 'n' Cheese (page 265).

Prep Time: 10 minutes | **Cook Time:** 20 minutes
Serves: 6 | **Serving Size:** 6 nuggets

3 egg whites

¼ cup white whole wheat flour

⅓ cup panko bread crumbs

⅓ cup plain bread crumbs

⅓ cup shredded Parmesan cheese (I like Sargento Artisan Blends)

1 teaspoon garlic powder

1 teaspoon black pepper

1 teaspoon salt

1½ pounds boneless, skinless chicken breasts, cut into 1-inch cubes

2 tablespoons chopped fresh parsley

½ cup marinara sauce, for dipping (optional)

1. Preheat the oven to 400°F. Coat a baking sheet with cooking spray.

2. In a small shallow dish, lightly beat the egg whites. Place the flour in a separate small shallow dish. In a medium shallow dish, mix together the panko and plain bread crumbs, Parmesan, garlic powder, pepper, and salt.

3. Working in batches, dredge the chicken pieces in the flour, followed by the egg whites, and then the Parmesan mixture. Make sure to coat each chicken piece evenly.

4. Arrange the coated chicken pieces in a single layer on the baking sheet.

5. Bake until the chicken is cooked through, 15 to 18 minutes, turning the chicken at least once.

6. Serve garnished with the parsley. If desired, put out marinara sauce for dipping.

Suggested Side Dish: Broccoli Mac 'n' Cheese (page 265)

Calories 192 • Fat 5g • Carbohydrate 11g • Fiber 1g • Sugar 1g • Protein 27g
Nutrition does not include optional ingredient.

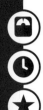

Skinny Cheeseburger Pie

You can't have family suppers without cheeseburgers, but you can have cheeseburgers without excessive fat and calories. No one will be craving the golden arches after diving into this skinny sensation!

Prep Time: 10 minutes | **Cook Time:** 20 minutes
Serves: 6 | **Serving Size:** 1/6 of the pie

1 pound lean ground turkey

1 small onion, diced

1 tablespoon minced garlic

2 teaspoons McCormick Grill Mates hamburger seasoning

2 tablespoons Worcestershire sauce

2 tablespoons Heinz reduced-sugar ketchup

1 cup low-fat cottage cheese

¼ teaspoon black pepper

1 (8-ounce) can Pillsbury Reduced Fat Crescent Rolls

1 cup shredded reduced-fat sharp cheddar cheese (I like Sargento)

4 tomato slices

1. Preheat the oven to 350°F. Coat a 9-inch round baking dish with cooking spray.

2. Heat a large skillet over medium-high heat. Add the ground turkey, onion, and garlic and sprinkle with the hamburger seasoning. Cook until the ground turkey is browned, 7 to 8 minutes. Use a wooden spoon to break the turkey up as it cooks. Remove from the heat.

3. Add the Worcestershire sauce and ketchup to the turkey mixture and stir to combine. Stir in the cottage cheese, season with the pepper, and stir to combine.

4. Line the baking dish with the crescent rolls. To do this, start by separating each individual triangle. Then align the long side of the triangles around the edge of the baking dish. Slightly overlap the triangles as you make your way around them and fill in the bottom of the dish using the remaining triangles. Pinch the seams together. Gently poke a few holes in the dough triangles with a fork.

5. Prebake the crust for 6 to 7 minutes.

6. Remove the crust from the oven and add the ground turkey mixture. Sprinkle the cheddar evenly over the pie. Place the tomato slices on top of the cheese. Cover just the crust with a thin strip of foil to avoid charring the edges.

suppertime inspiration:
Albert Einstein was quoted as saying, "Life is like riding a bicycle. To keep your balance, you must keep moving." That's good to know for those of us who can't seem to slow down!

7. Return to the oven and bake until the cheese is melted, about 20 minutes.

8. To serve, cut into 6 wedges.

Suggested Side Dish: Cauliflower Mashed Potatoes (page 269)

suppertime chat: Which season (winter, spring, summer, or fall) is your favorite and why? (And if you have toddlers, preface the conversation with a fun little lesson about the four seasons!) Discussing the seasons prompts reminiscing about "the time we went to Disney World," or the fact that "it's time to plan that canoeing trip we've been talking about." Just a few minutes chatting together every day can spur dreams and provoke precious memories of the past.

Calories 335 • **Fat** 14g • **Carbohydrate** 23g • **Fiber** 0g • **Sugar** 7g • **Protein** 28g

Slow-Cooker Asian Drumsticks

This saucy little number is a healthier alternative to the traditional way most Americans eat drumsticks—fried! These drumsticks make for an easy, delicious Sunday supper. Paired with my Mango Slaw (page 281), it feels like an indulgent supper without overindulging. And the thick stickiness of the saucy drumsticks is finger-licking good.

Prep Time: 10 minutes | **Cook Time:** 2 hours on high or 4 hours on low
Serves: 4 | **Serving Size:** 3 drumsticks, 3 tablespoons sauce

Sauce:

⅓ cup balsamic vinegar

¼ cup less-sodium soy sauce

1 tablespoon light brown sugar

3 tablespoons sugar-free maple-flavor syrup (I like Maple Grove Farms)

1 tablespoon Heinz reduced-sugar ketchup

1 tablespoon sriracha sauce

½ tablespoon minced garlic

½ teaspoon ground ginger

½ teaspoon onion powder

½ teaspoon black pepper

Drumsticks:

12 chicken drumsticks (about 3 pounds)

¼ teaspoon salt

¼ teaspoon black pepper

2 tablespoons cornstarch

2 tablespoons sesame seeds

2 green onions, thinly sliced

1. To make the sauce: In a medium bowl, whisk together the vinegar, soy sauce, brown sugar, syrup, ketchup, sriracha, garlic, ginger, onion powder, and pepper.

2. To make the drumsticks: Remove the skin from the drumsticks. To do this, hold a paper towel in each hand, grip the base of the chicken drumstick, and pull the skin off.

3. Season the drumsticks with the salt and pepper. Place the drumsticks in a slow cooker and pour the sauce over them. Cook on high heat for 2 hours or on low heat for 4 hours.

4. Just before serving, remove the drumsticks from the sauce. Pour the sauce into a small saucepan, then return the drumsticks to the slow cooker to keep warm until serving.

5. In a small bowl, dissolve the cornstarch in 2 tablespoons of cold water to make a slurry. Whisk the slurry into the sauce. Simmer over low heat, stirring frequently, until thick, 5 to 10 minutes.

6. To serve, brush the thickened sauce over the drumsticks and garnish with the sesame seeds and green onions.

Suggested Side Dish: Mango Slaw (page 281)

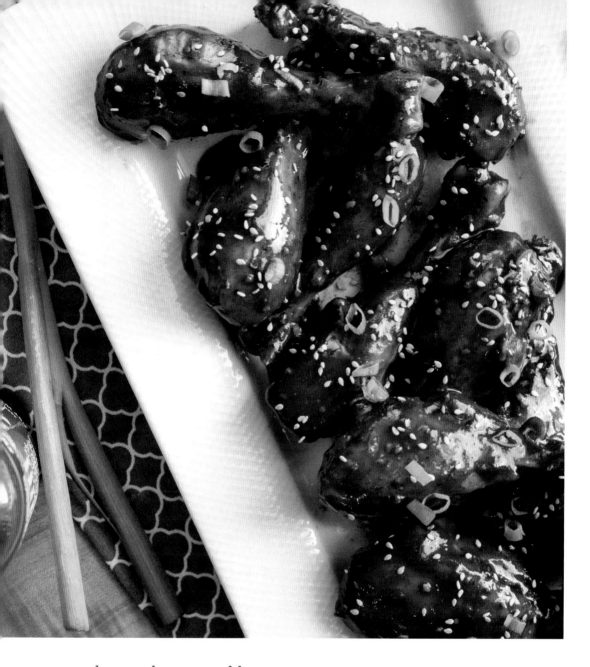

no slow cooker, no problem: Preheat the oven to 375°F. Place the seasoned drumsticks in a single layer in the bottom of a 13 x 9-inch baking dish. Prepare and pour the sauce over the drumsticks. Bake for 25 to 30 minutes, until the chicken is cooked through. Remove the chicken from the baking dish and cover with aluminum foil to keep warm, and thicken the sauce as directed.

Calories 481 · Fat 15g · Carbohydrate 14g · Fiber 1g · Sugar 7g · Protein 69g

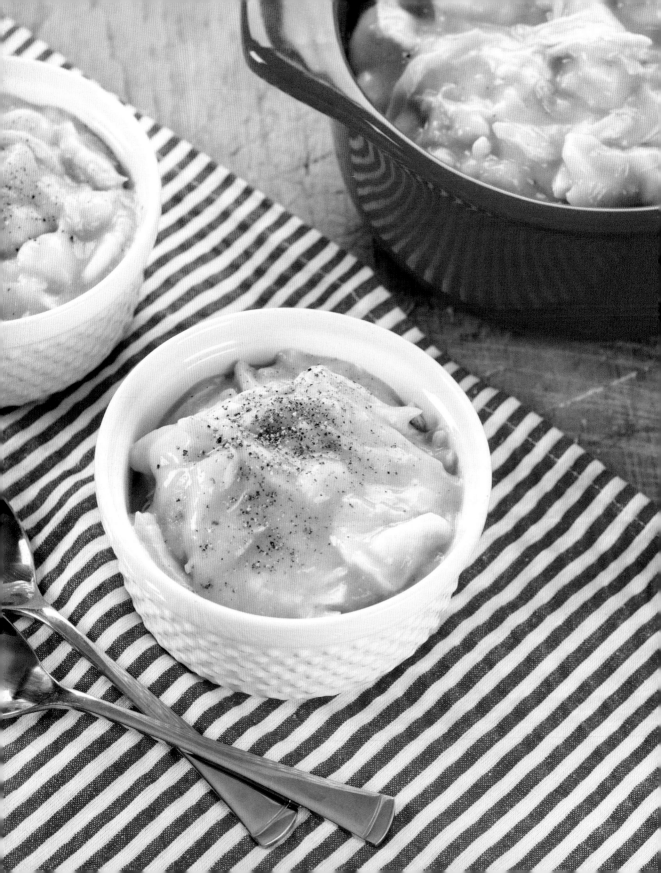

Slow-Cooker Chicken and Dumplings

Cook up an old Southern favorite with very little effort! I used to love it when my granny would make chicken and dumplings, but it seemed like she was in the kitchen all day (actually, she was). I don't have that kind of time, and I'm guessing you don't either. So I've modified this classic supper with the simplicity of prepackaged biscuits and a slow cooker. Voilà! You're cooking up Southern suppers like my granny in no time!

Prep Time: 20 minutes | **Cook Time:** 4 hours on high
Serves: 6 | **Serving Size:** Heaping 1 cup

1½ pounds boneless, skinless chicken breasts

¼ teaspoon salt

¼ teaspoon black pepper

¼ teaspoon poultry seasoning

2 (10.5-ounce) cans Campbell's Healthy Request condensed cream of chicken soup

5 cups low-sodium chicken broth (I like Pacific Organic)

1 can Pillsbury Grands! Jr. Golden Homestyle buttermilk biscuits

¼ cup white whole wheat flour

1. Coat the bottom of a slow-cooker liner with cooking spray.

2. Season both sides of the chicken breasts with the salt, pepper, and poultry seasoning.

3. Transfer the chicken to the slow cooker. Cover the chicken with both cans of the chicken soup and the chicken broth. Cook on high heat for 1½ hours.

4. When the chicken has been cooking for 1½ hours, prepare the dumplings. On a clean surface and with clean hands, sprinkle the surface with half the flour. Remove the biscuits from the can and, using a rolling pin, gently roll out each biscuit onto the flour-coated surface until about ½ inch thick. Using a knife, slice each rolled biscuit into 1-inch strips. Each biscuit should yield about 5 strips. Add additional flour to the surface as needed.

5. Adding a few at a time, drop the biscuit-strip "dumplings" into the slow cooker. Stir and

(recipe continues)

(continued from page 119)

suppertime chat: It's always fun to play a little game called "Best" and "Worst." Each person at the table gets to share the best thing that happened to them that day, along with the worst. (In our house, we like to end with the best!)

repeat. The goal is to not drop the dumplings on top of one another, otherwise they will stick together. Cover and cook the dumplings and the chicken an additional 2½ hours, stirring occasionally.

6. Remove and shred the chicken and return the chicken to the slow cooker before serving.

7. Serve the chicken and dumplings immediately after cooking.

Suggested Side Dish: Easy Roasted Vegetables (page 277)

no slow cooker, no problem: Combine the chicken, both cans of the soup, and the chicken broth in a large pot or Dutch oven and cook over medium heat until the chicken reaches an internal temperature of 145°F, 20 to 30 minutes. Remove the chicken, shred, and set aside. Roll out and cut the biscuits as directed. Bring the broth mixture to a high simmer over medium-high heat. Drop the biscuit strips one by one into the broth and stir occasionally, making sure that the biscuit strips do not stick together. Once the dumplings have cooked (they will cook quickly), reduce the heat to low and return the shredded chicken to the pot before serving.

Calories 352 • Fat 11g • Carbohydrate 37g • Fiber 1g • Sugar 4g • Protein 30g

Chicken Fried Rice

There's a Chinese take-out restaurant in every town and in nearly every mall in America. That proves two things: We love Chinese food and we desperately need a makeover for one of the most popular Chinese dishes, chicken fried rice. Look no further! I've tweaked, twisted, and fine-tuned this recipe until I got it just right.

Prep Time: 10 minutes | **Cook Time:** 15 minutes
Serves: 6 | **Serving Size:** Heaping 1 cup

2 teaspoons sesame oil

1 tablespoon minced garlic

¼ teaspoon red pepper flakes

1 pound boneless, skinless chicken breast, cut into 1-inch cubes

1 (8.8-ounce) pouch Uncle Ben's Ready Rice brown rice

1 small onion, diced

2 cups frozen peas and carrots mix

6 green onions, thinly sliced

2 eggs

¼ cup less-sodium soy sauce

2 teaspoons oyster sauce

quick and easy: There is an abundance of dishes that call for cooked chicken. Consider cooking an entire package of chicken breasts at once, slicing some into strips or nuggets and leaving some whole. (Be sure to pound the plumper breasts for faster cooking and increased portions.) Pre-portion into resealable bags and freeze. When a recipe calls for cooked chicken, just take what you need out of the freezer, thaw, and reheat. Simple as that.

1. In a wok or a large skillet, heat 1 teaspoon of the sesame oil over medium-high heat. Add the garlic and red pepper flakes and stir constantly using a wooden spoon or spatula for 1 minute, or until fragrant.

2. Increase the heat to high and add the chicken. Cook for 4 to 6 minutes, turning and moving the chicken constantly while cooking. Scrape the chicken and garlic onto a plate and set aside.

3. Microwave the rice according to the package directions. Set aside.

4. Add the remaining 1 teaspoon sesame oil to the pan. Once hot, add the onion, peas and carrots, and half of the green onions and stir-fry, constantly moving the mixture until the onion and carrots soften, 3 to 5 minutes.

5. Push the vegetables to the outer edges of the wok or skillet to open up the center. Crack the eggs into the pan and scramble. When the eggs are cooked through, combine with the vegetables. Reduce the heat to medium.

6. Add the reserved chicken, cooked brown rice, soy sauce, and oyster sauce to the vegetable mixture and stir to combine.

7. Serve garnished with the remaining green onions.

Calories 290 • Fat 7g • Carbohydrate 37g • Fiber 5g • Sugar 5g • Protein 23g

Sour Cream Enchiladas

In less than 1 hour from prep to the table, these rich and creamy enchiladas will be curing your family's craving for Mexican food. Even if you didn't have time to go to the grocery this week, chances are you've got all the ingredients to whip up this ultimate south-of-the-border favorite!

Prep Time: 10 minutes | **Cook Time:** 35 minutes
Serves: 8 | **Serving Size:** 1 enchilada

1 (10-ounce) can green enchilada sauce

1 pound boneless, skinless chicken breasts

½ cup light sour cream

1 (10.5-ounce) can Campbell's Healthy Request condensed cream of chicken soup

⅓ cup fat-free milk

1 teaspoon extra virgin olive oil

1 small onion, diced

1 (10-ounce) can Ro*Tel "Original" diced tomatoes and green chilies

1 (4.5-ounce) can chopped green chilies

1 teaspoon ground cumin

½ teaspoon salt

½ teaspoon black pepper

8 large low-carb, high-fiber tortillas, warmed (I like La Tortilla Factory; see Quick and Easy)

¾ cup shredded reduced-fat four-cheese Mexican blend (I like Sargento)

¼ cup chopped fresh cilantro

1. Preheat the oven to 350°F. Coat a 13 x 9-inch baking dish with cooking spray.

2. In a medium skillet, heat the enchilada sauce over medium-high heat. Add the chicken breasts and cook until cooked through, 7 to 8 minutes per side.

3. Transfer the chicken breasts to a plate to cool. After the chicken has slightly cooled, use two forks to shred the chicken and set aside.

4. Meanwhile, return the skillet of enchilada sauce to low heat. Add the sour cream, chicken soup, and fat-free milk. Stir frequently for 2 to 3 minutes, then remove from the heat.

5. In a separate large skillet, heat the olive oil over medium-high heat. Add the onion and cook until translucent, 2 to 3 minutes. Stir in the diced tomatoes, green chilies, cumin, salt, pepper, and the shredded chicken. Continue to stir frequently until the mixture is heated through, 2 to 3 minutes, then remove from the heat.

6. To assemble, fill each tortilla with a heaping ⅓ cup of the chicken mixture. Tightly roll each tortilla and place seam side down in the prepared baking dish.

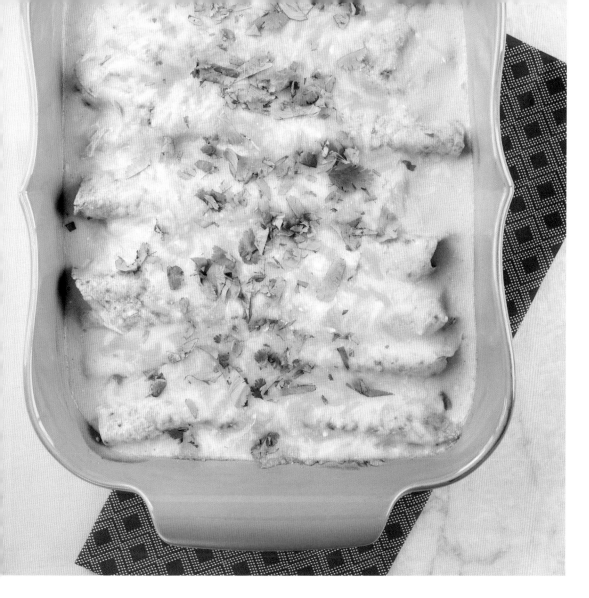

7. Pour and evenly spread the sour cream sauce over the enchiladas and sprinkle with the cheese. Bake until the cheese is melted and bubbly, 18 to 20 minutes.

8. Serve garnished with the cilantro.

Suggested Side Dish: Quinoa Mexi-Lime Salad (page 289)

quick and easy: Microwave tortillas on high for 30 seconds prior to filling and rolling them to soften them and make them more pliable.

Calories 250 • **Fat** 10g • **Carbohydrate** 28g • **Fiber** 13g • **Sugar** 5g • **Protein** 36g

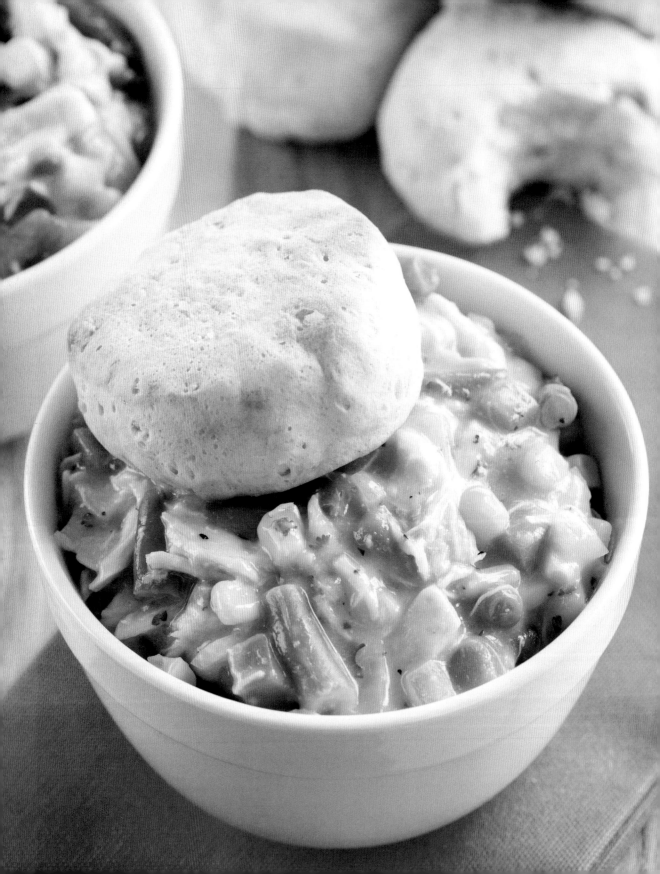

Slow-Cooker Chicken Pot Pie

The ingredients for this Southern supper are most likely staples in your home already. I love slow-cooker recipes because they're a great way to welcome my family home after a busy day. The aroma of a chicken pot pie in the air ushers in excitement and relaxation all at once. That's what I call a feel-good supper!

Prep Time: 10 minutes | **Cook Time:** 4 hours on high or 8 hours on low
Serves: 6 | **Serving Size:** Heaping 1 cup chicken mixture, 1 biscuit

1 pound boneless, skinless chicken breasts

1 small onion, diced

3½ stalks celery, diced

2 (10.5-ounce) cans Campbell's Healthy Request condensed cream of chicken soup

1 cup fat-free milk

1 teaspoon garlic powder

1 teaspoon dried thyme

½ teaspoon salt

½ teaspoon black pepper

1 (16-ounce) bag frozen mixed vegetables, thawed

2 tablespoons chopped fresh parsley

1 (12-ounce) can Pillsbury Grands! Jr. Golden Layers Flaky Biscuits

no slow cooker, no problem: Combine all the ingredients in a large pot or Dutch oven and cook over low heat until the chicken reaches an internal temperature of 145°F, 2 to 2½ hours. Continue with the recipe as directed.

1. Place the chicken breasts in a slow cooker. Top the chicken with the onion and celery.

2. In a small bowl, combine the chicken soup, milk, garlic powder, thyme, salt, and pepper and whisk until mixed well. Pour the mixture into the slow cooker.

3. Cover and cook on high heat for 4 hours or low heat for 8 hours.

4. About 30 minutes before serving, remove the chicken from the slow cooker with a slotted spoon and shred with two forks. Return the shredded chicken to the slow cooker and stir in the vegetables and parsley. Cook for an additional 30 minutes.

5. Preheat the oven to 400°F.

6. Bake the biscuits according to the package directions.

7. To serve, place a heaping 1 cup of the chicken mixture in each bowl and top with a biscuit.

Calories 380 • Fat 8g • Carbohydrate 47g • Fiber 4g • Sugar 12g • Protein 26g

Un-Sloppy Janes

Sloppy Joes have been around since at least the 1950s. Well, I decided it was time for a makeover. So, I've tweaked this American tradition and lightened it up by substituting lean ground turkey for fatty ground beef. I've also eliminated the mess by creating fun little pockets utilizing a biscuit. Now even the messiest eaters in your home can enjoy these lightened-up and mess-free Un-Sloppy Janes.

Prep Time: 25 minutes | **Cook Time:** 15 minutes
Serves: 10 | **Serving Size:** 1 filled biscuit

1 pound lean ground turkey breast

1 small onion, diced

½ red bell pepper, diced

1 (8-ounce) container baby bella (cremini) mushrooms, chopped

1 tablespoon minced garlic

½ tablespoon McCormick Grill Mates hamburger seasoning

¼ teaspoon salt

1 tablespoon red wine vinegar

1 tablespoon Worcestershire sauce

2 tablespoons Heinz reduced-sugar ketchup

2 cups tomato sauce

2 tablespoons tomato paste

1 (12-ounce) can Pillsbury Grands! Jr. Golden Homestyle Buttermilk Biscuits

½ cup shredded reduced-fat sharp cheddar cheese (I like Sargento)

1 egg white, beaten

1. Preheat the oven to 375°F. Coat a baking sheet with cooking spray.

2. In a large skillet over medium-high heat, cook the turkey, onion, bell pepper, mushrooms, and garlic until the turkey is browned and the vegetables have softened, 7 to 8 minutes. Use a wooden spoon to break the turkey up as it cooks.

3. Reduce the heat to low and add the hamburger seasoning, salt, vinegar, Worcestershire sauce, ketchup, tomato sauce, and tomato paste. Stir to evenly coat the ground turkey and vegetables. Cover and simmer over low heat for 3 to 4 minutes.

4. While the meat mixture is simmering, place the biscuits on the baking sheet and use a rolling pin to flatten and spread out each biscuit to increase the size to about 6 inches round and ¼ inch thick.

5. Spoon ¼ cup of the meat mixture onto the center of each biscuit round. Top with a heaping tablespoon of cheddar. Fold the dough in half over the filling and use your fingertips or the tines of a fork to press together and seal the dough.

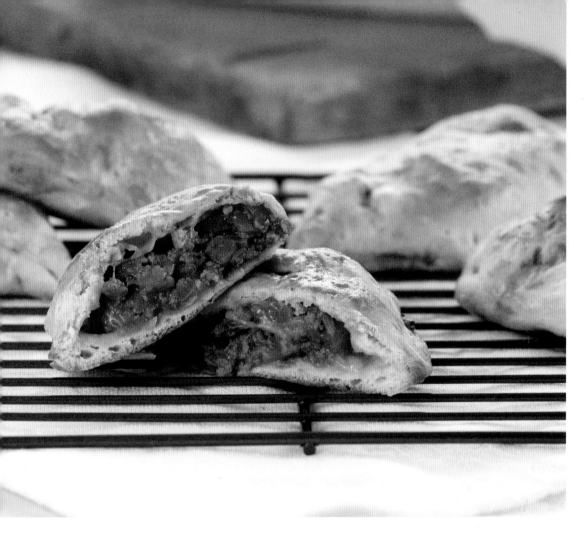

6. Use a knife to slice 3 slits through the top of the dough on each of the biscuits.

7. In a small bowl, whisk the egg white with 2 tablespoons of water to make an egg wash.

8. Lightly brush the tops of the biscuits with the egg white wash. Bake until the biscuits are golden brown, 10 to 15 minutes.

Suggested Side Dish: Skillet Corn (page 291)

quick and easy: Creating little "sandwich pockets" with biscuits is a fun way to jazz up any sandwich. Try this kid-friendly substitution any place you use bread, like grilled cheese or tuna! It makes an otherwise boring meal new and exciting.

Calories 219 • Fat 8g • Carbohydrate 22g • Fiber 2g • Sugar 5g • Protein 15g

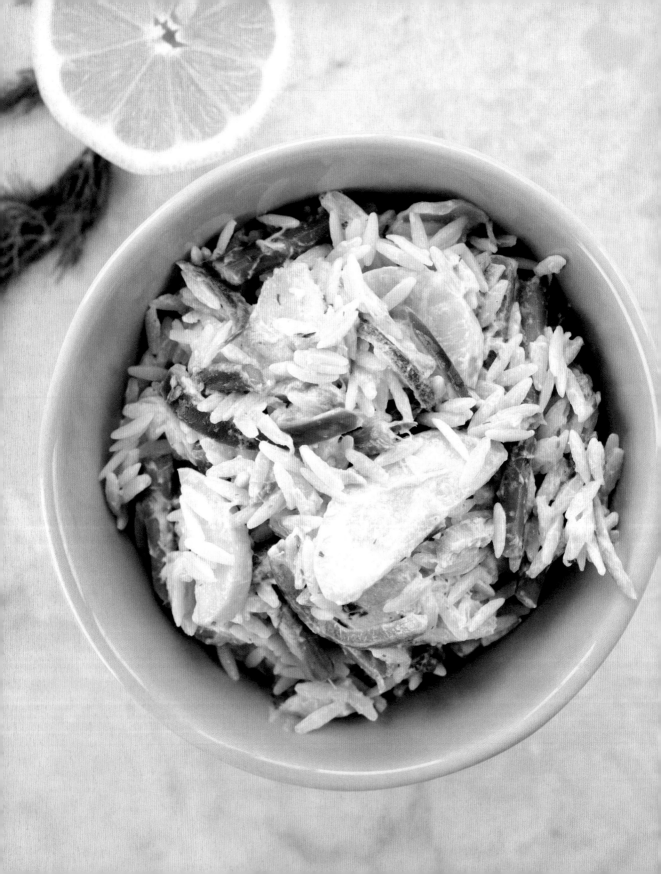

8 GOOD TO THE LAST SLURP
PASTA SUPPERS

Three-Cheese Penne

Do you get excited when you hear a recipe has three cheeses? I do! Couple ricotta, mozzarella, and cottage cheese with whole wheat pasta and my favorite no-sugar-added pasta sauce, and get this fill-you-up supper that will satisfy even the biggest appetites, without the big calorie count.

Prep Time: 5 minutes | **Cook Time:** 30 minutes
Serves: 8 | **Serving Size:** 1¼ cups

1 (13.25-ounce) box whole wheat penne pasta (I like Barilla)

1 teaspoon extra virgin olive oil

½ small onion, diced

1 tablespoon minced garlic

1 (23.25-ounce) jar Prego Light Smart Traditional pasta sauce

½ teaspoon dried basil

½ teaspoon dried oregano

¼ teaspoon salt

¼ teaspoon black pepper

½ cup low-fat cottage cheese

½ cup part-skim ricotta cheese

1½ cups shredded reduced-fat mozzarella cheese (I like Sargento)

2 tablespoons chopped fresh parsley

quick and easy: Why salt pasta water? Salted water flavors the pasta. As the pasta absorbs the liquid while it is cooking, the salt helps to season the pasta internally.

1. Bring a large pot of salted water to a boil over high heat. Cook the pasta to al dente according to the package directions. Drain and set aside.

2. In a large skillet, heat the olive oil over medium-high heat. Add the onion and garlic and cook until the onion has softened, 3 to 5 minutes.

3. Reduce the heat to low and pour in the pasta sauce. Stir in the basil, oregano, salt, and pepper. Cover and cook for 5 to 7 minutes, stirring occasionally, until heated through.

4. Preheat the oven to 350°F. Coat an 8 x 8-inch baking dish with cooking spray.

5. Meanwhile, in a medium bowl, combine the cottage cheese, ricotta, and 1 cup of the mozzarella.

6. Remove the sauce from the heat and stir in the cooked pasta.

7. Transfer half of the pasta to the baking dish. Evenly spread half of the cheese mixture on top. Then add the remaining pasta followed by the remaining cheese mixture. Sprinkle the remaining ½ cup mozzarella on top.

8. Bake uncovered until the cheese is melted, 18 to 20 minutes.

9. Serve garnished with the parsley.

Calories 284 · Fat 7g · Carbohydrate 44g · Fiber 7g · Sugar 8g · Protein 16g

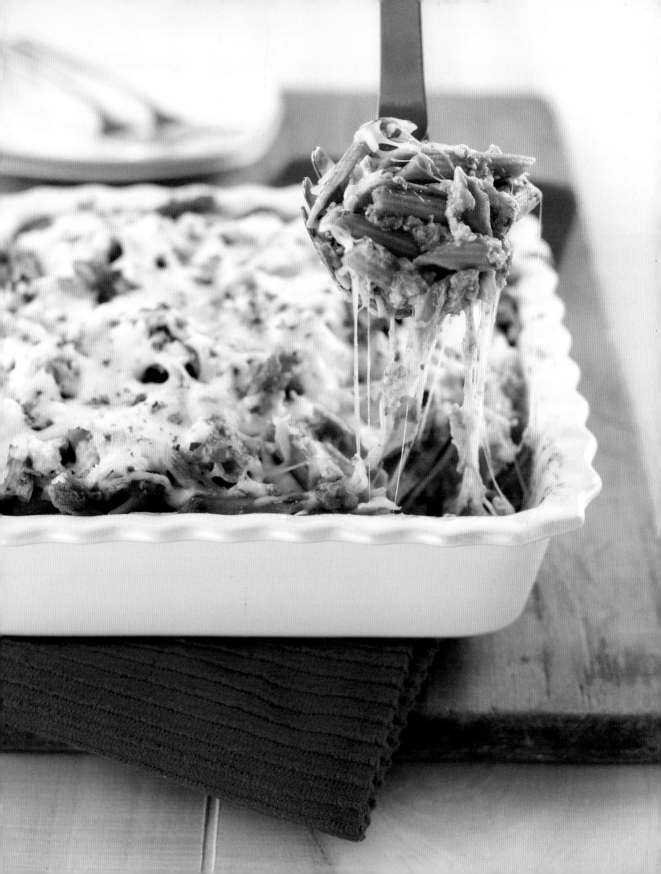

Chicken Pasta Primavera

Pasta dishes are notoriously calorie-dense. Well, not anymore! It's recipes like this one that continue to remind me that less is more. Simply swapping out lighter versions of cheese and milk here and using whole wheat flour allows me to create a creamy and satisfying pasta dish that can be whipped up in a flash, even on the craziest of nights.

Prep Time: 10 minutes | **Cook Time:** 20 minutes
Serves: 6 | **Serving Size:** 1½ cups

1 pound boneless, skinless chicken breasts

1 teaspoon salt

½ teaspoon black pepper

2 teaspoons extra virgin olive oil

8 ounces high-protein angel hair pasta (I like Barilla ProteinPLUS)

2 cups broccoli florets, cooked

1 red bell pepper, thinly sliced

1 (8-ounce) container baby bella (cremini) mushrooms, sliced

Alfredo Sauce:

2 tablespoons unsalted butter

2 tablespoons white whole wheat flour

1½ cups fat-free milk

4 ounces ⅓-less-fat cream cheese

¼ cup shredded Parmesan cheese (I like Sargento Artisan Blends)

1. Season the chicken with ½ teaspoon of the salt and ¼ teaspoon of the black pepper.

2. In a large skillet, heat 1 teaspoon of the olive oil over medium-high heat. Add the chicken breasts and cook until the chicken is no longer pink in the center but still juicy, 4 to 6 minutes per side. Set aside on a plate to rest.

3. Meanwhile, bring a large pot of salted water to a boil over high heat. Cook the pasta to al dente according to the package directions. Reserving ½ cup of the pasta water, drain and set aside.

4. Add the remaining 1 teaspoon of oil to the same skillet used for the chicken, and sauté the broccoli, bell pepper, and mushrooms for 5 to 7 minutes, until the vegetables soften. Season with the remaining ½ teaspoon salt and ¼ teaspoon black pepper. Remove the vegetables from the skillet and set aside.

5. To make the Alfredo sauce: In a medium saucepan, melt the butter over low heat. Whisk the flour into the butter for about 30 seconds, until smooth and the mixture smells nutty, making a roux. Whisk in the milk and bring to a boil over medium heat, stirring constantly.

6. Reduce the heat to low and stir in the cream cheese and Parmesan. Stir the Alfredo sauce frequently, until it is slightly thickened, 3 to 4 minutes.

7. Slice the chicken diagonally into thin strips. Return the chicken and vegetables to the skillet and toss to combine.

8. Transfer the pasta to the chicken and vegetables in the skillet. Coat the chicken and vegetables evenly with the Alfredo sauce and add the reserved pasta water as needed until the sauce reaches the desired consistency before serving. Serve warm.

Calories 375 • **Fat** 14g • **Carbohydrate** 37g • **Fiber** 6g • **Sugar** 6g • **Protein** 30g

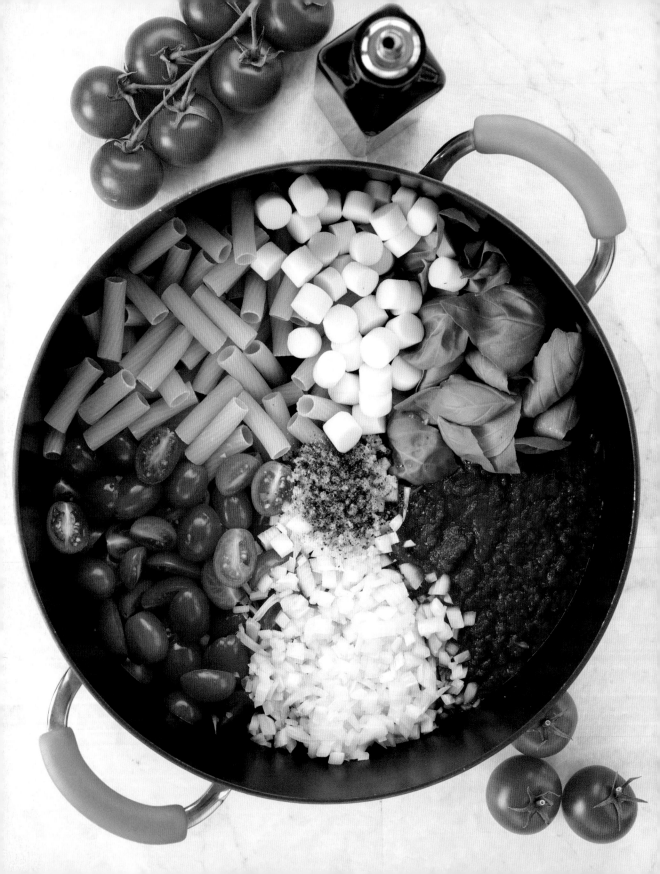

Easy One-Pot Caprese Pasta

I try not to use the word "easy" too loosely in my recipes. I can't tell you how many times I have perused cookbooks looking for the word "easy," only to become frustrated by overcomplicated recipes that make me want to give up. It truly doesn't get any easier than this one-pot sensation. Even on the busiest of nights, I have been able to prepare this palate-pleasing pasta supper with ease. Try this one out for "Meatless Mondays."

Prep Time: 5 minutes │ **Cook Time:** 25 to 30 minutes
Serves: 6 │ **Serving Size:** Heaping 1¾ cups

12 ounces whole wheat rigatoni pasta (I like Barilla)

1 (28-ounce) can crushed tomatoes with basil (I like Hunt's)

4 light string cheese sticks (I like Sargento), cut into ½-inch pieces

1 (10-ounce) container grape tomatoes, halved

½ small onion, diced

About 12 fresh basil leaves

1 tablespoon minced garlic

1 teaspoon salt

¼ teaspoon black pepper

¼ cup balsamic vinegar

About 6 fresh basil leaves, chopped (optional)

6 tablespoons shredded Parmesan cheese (optional; I like Sargento Artisan Blends)

1. In a large pot, combine 3 cups of water, the pasta, crushed tomatoes, cheese pieces, grape tomatoes, onion, basil, garlic, salt, and pepper and stir to combine.

2. Bring to a boil over medium-high heat, then reduce to a simmer and cook uncovered until the pasta has softened, 25 to 30 minutes. Much of the water will boil out.

3. Serve drizzled with balsamic vinegar. If desired, garnish with chopped basil and Parmesan.

quick and easy: Looking for big Italian flavor? Double the amount of garlic, onion, and basil in the recipe.

Calories 324 · **Fat** 3g · **Carbohydrate** 62g · **Fiber** 6g · **Sugar** 8g · **Protein** 15g
Nutrition does not include optional ingredients.

Cheesy Spinach and Mushroom Lasagna Rolls

A fun and effortless twist on the classic lasagna recipe that naturally controls portions (and mess): One roll is one serving. This is one of my favorites for getting my son cooking in the kitchen. Who doesn't love to play with lasagna?

Prep Time: 10 minutes | **Cook Time:** 40 minutes
Serves: 8 | **Serving Size:** 1 lasagna roll, ½ cup sauce, 1 tablespoon mozzarella cheese

8 whole wheat lasagna noodles

1 teaspoon extra virgin olive oil

1 (8-ounce) container baby bella (cremini) mushrooms, sliced

½ small onion, diced

1 tablespoon minced garlic

1 (23.25-ounce) jar Prego Light Smart Traditional pasta sauce

1 (14.5-ounce) can no-salt-added diced tomatoes (I like Hunt's)

½ teaspoon dried basil

¼ teaspoon dried oregano

1 (15-ounce) container part-skim ricotta cheese

½ cup grated Parmesan cheese (I like Sargento)

1 egg, beaten

¼ teaspoon salt

⅛ teaspoon black pepper

10 ounces frozen chopped spinach, thawed and drained

½ cup shredded reduced-fat mozzarella cheese (I like Sargento)

1. Preheat the oven to 350°F. Coat an 11 x 7-inch baking dish with cooking spray.

2. Bring a large pot of salted water to a boil over high heat. Cook the lasagna noodles to al dente according to the package directions. Drain the noodles and lay them out on a sheet of wax paper. Cover them with slightly damp paper towels until it is time to assemble the rolls.

3. In a large skillet, heat the olive oil over medium-high heat. Add the mushrooms, onion, and garlic and cook until the onion and mushrooms have softened, stirring occasionally, 3 to 4 minutes. Set the mushroom mixture aside.

4. In a large bowl, stir together the pasta sauce, diced tomatoes, basil, and oregano. Set aside.

5. In a medium bowl, mix together the ricotta, Parmesan, egg, salt, and pepper. Add the spinach and stir to evenly coat the spinach.

6. Spoon half of the pasta sauce into the bottom of the prepared baking dish.

7. Spread ⅓ cup of the cheese mixture and 1 tablespoon of the mushroom mixture onto each lasagna noodle. Carefully roll the covered lasagna noodles up and place them seam side down in the baking dish.

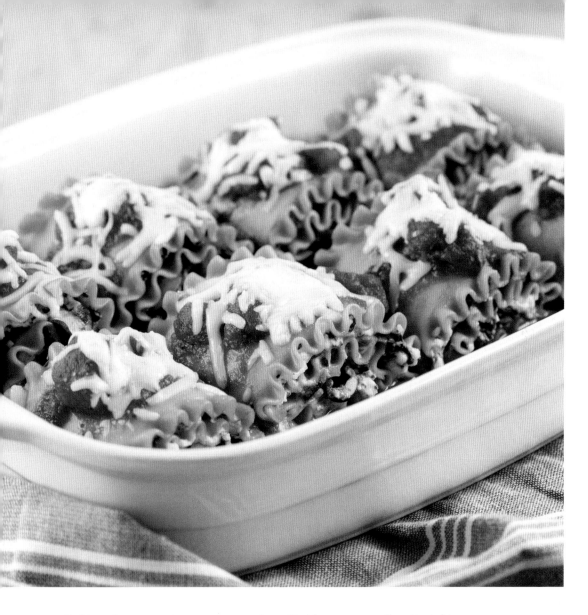

8. Pour the remaining sauce over the rolled lasagna noodles. Sprinkle 1 tablespoon mozzarella over each roll.

9. Lightly cover the baking dish with foil (to keep the lasagna moist and the cheese from browning) and bake until the cheese is melted, about 30 minutes.

skinny sense: Adding fresh mushrooms to the pasta sauce makes this vegetarian dish more filling and adds an extra serving of vegetables.

Calories 280 • **Fat** 9g • **Carbohydrate** 35g • **Fiber** 6g • **Sugar** 11g • **Protein** 17g

Veggie and Cheese "Manicotti"

This vegetarian-friendly meal is super simple and freezer-friendly, too. I like to make extra "manicotti" and freeze it in airtight containers or gallon-size freezer bags for quick access. Here I resolve a longtime dilemma of mine—manicotti noodles that rip and tear when I'm piping in stuffing. I've found lasagna noodles to be the perfect solution!

Prep Time: 15 minutes | **Cook Time:** 40 minutes
Serves: 8 | **Serving Size:** 2 rolls, ¼ cup sauce

16 Barilla oven-ready lasagna noodles

1 (23.25-ounce) jar Prego Light Smart Traditional pasta sauce

½ tablespoon extra virgin olive oil

1 tablespoon minced garlic

1 small onion, diced

½ cup shredded carrots

½ zucchini, julienned

1 yellow squash, julienned

1 (8-ounce) container baby bella (cremini) mushrooms, diced

1 red bell pepper, diced

1 (15-ounce) container part-skim ricotta cheese

1 egg white, beaten

1 teaspoon Italian seasoning

½ teaspoon salt

¼ teaspoon black pepper

¼ cup grated Parmesan cheese (I like Sargento)

¾ cup shredded reduced-fat mozzarella cheese (I like Sargento)

1. Preheat the oven to 375°F.

2. Fill a 13 x 9-inch baking dish with hot water. Line a baking sheet with parchment paper. Add the lasagna noodles one at a time to the hot water, making certain that the noodles are completely covered with water. Let soak until pliable, about 10 minutes. Remove the noodles from the water and arrange in a single layer on the parchment paper (pull apart gently if the noodles stick together, or use the tip of a knife to gently separate). Cover them with damp paper towels. (Discard the water.)

3. Coat the 13 x 9-inch baking dish with cooking spray. Evenly spread 1 cup of the pasta sauce in the bottom of the baking dish. Set aside.

4. In a large skillet, heat the olive oil over medium heat. Add the garlic, onion, carrots, zucchini, yellow squash, mushrooms, and bell pepper. Cook, stirring, until the veggies are tender, 3 to 5 minutes. Set aside and allow to cool for 1 to 2 minutes.

5. In a medium bowl, combine the ricotta, egg white, Italian seasoning, salt, black pepper, and Parmesan and mix well. Add the sautéed vegetables to the cheese mixture and gently stir to combine.

6. Using a spoon, spread 2 tablespoons of the vegetable mixture onto each noodle, keeping the mixture at one end. Roll the noodles and place seam side down in a single layer in the prepared baking dish.

7. Top the noodles evenly with the remaining pasta sauce, making certain that all of the noodles are completely covered.

8. Cover the baking dish with foil and bake for 30 minutes.

9. Remove the foil and sprinkle the noodles with the mozzarella. Bake, uncovered, until the cheese is melted, 5 to 7 minutes. Let the noodles rest for 5 minutes before serving.

Calories 380 · **Fat** 10g · **Carbohydrate** 56g · **Fiber** 9g · **Sugar** 13g · **Protein** 21g

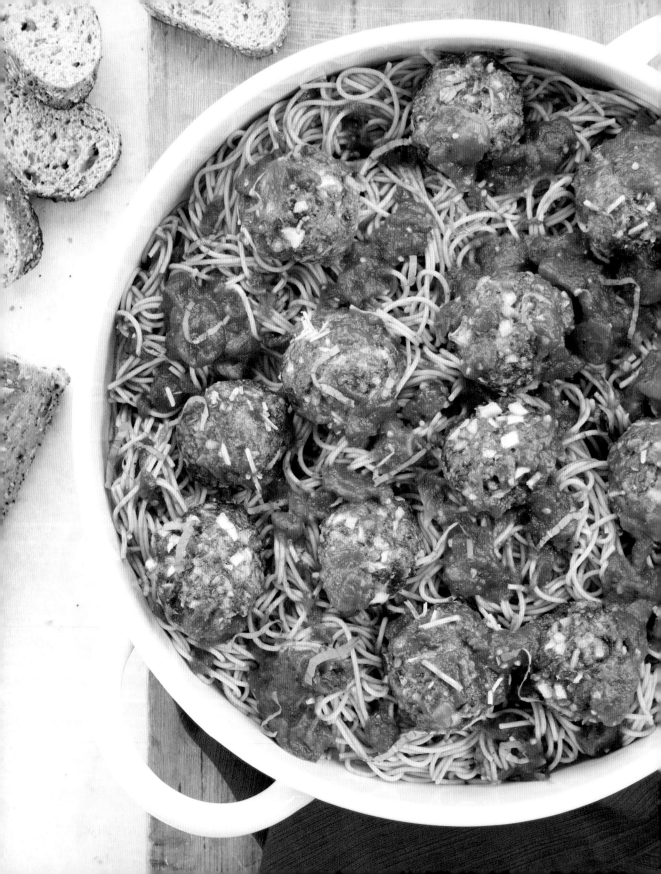

Old-Fashioned Spaghetti and Meatballs

2x

Sharing recipes with friends is a favorite pastime, and here is one of my all-time favorites: my aunt Tammy's meatball recipe. I grew up eating these tender and juicy meatballs every month at family dinners. But I've learned how to save a lot of time by starting with lighter versions of jarred pasta sauce and then adding my own unique Italian flavors. It's my version of "homemade." This is pure comfort food. I love serving it up with a big, colorful salad and a loaf of whole grain bread.

Prep Time: 10 minutes | **Cook Time:** 25 minutes
Serves: 6 | **Serving Size:** 1¼ cups cooked pasta, ⅔ cup sauce, 2 meatballs, 1 tablespoon Parmesan

Meatballs:

1 pound lean ground beef

2 links Italian turkey sausage, casings removed

¾ cup diced onion

¼ cup shredded Parmesan cheese (I like Sargento Artisan Blends)

¼ cup Italian-style bread crumbs

1 egg, beaten

2 tablespoons chopped fresh parsley

1 teaspoon garlic powder

¼ teaspoon salt

¼ teaspoon black pepper

Sauce:

1 teaspoon extra virgin olive oil

¼ cup diced onion

1 tablespoon minced garlic

1 (23.25-ounce) jar Prego Light Smart Traditional pasta sauce

1 (14.5-ounce) can no-salt-added diced tomatoes (I like Hunt's)

2 teaspoons stevia

1 teaspoon basil

½ teaspoon oregano

¼ teaspoon salt

½ teaspoon black pepper

For Serving:

12 ounces high-protein spaghetti (I like Barilla ProteinPLUS)

6 tablespoons shredded Parmesan cheese (I like Sargento Artisan Blends)

(recipe continues)

(continued from page 141)

suppertime chat: If you could have a conversation with any celebrity (past or present) and ask him or her anything you want, who would it be and what would you ask? Find out what musicians, actors, and athletes your kids are interested in learning more about.

1. To make the meatballs: Preheat the oven to 350°F. Line a large baking sheet with foil and generously coat the foil with cooking spray.

2. In a large bowl, using clean hands, combine the ground beef, sausage, onion, Parmesan, bread crumbs, egg, parsley, garlic powder, salt, and pepper. Combine all the ingredients and form into 12 meatballs (using about ¼ cup of meat mixture for each). Place the meatballs 1 inch apart on the baking sheet.

3. Bake the meatballs until browned and cooked through, about 25 minutes.

4. Meanwhile, to make the sauce: In a large pot, heat the olive oil over medium heat. Add the onion and garlic and cook until softened, 3 to 4 minutes. Add the pasta sauce, diced tomatoes, stevia, basil, oregano, salt, and pepper. Stir to combine, cover, reduce the heat to low, and simmer for 20 minutes.

5. While the sauce is simmering, bring a large pot of salted water to a boil over high heat. Cook the pasta to al dente according to the package directions. Drain.

6. Serve the spaghetti with the sauce and meatballs. Sprinkle each serving with 1 tablespoon of the Parmesan.

Calories 471 • Fat 14g • Carbohydrate 59g • Fiber 9g • Sugar 12g • Protein 34g

Salmon Orzo with Creamy Lemon Dill Sauce

Often, the old standby side dish for salmon is rice. I like to use orzo in place of rice to mix it up a little. And as a bonus, it cooks up in about half the time. Another added benefit of using orzo in this satiating supper is that although it is meant to be served warm, orzo tastes great cold. So this supper is fantastic as a chilled leftover, too! I often find myself preparing this dish almost nonstop in spring and summer. It's ideal for a picnic, and my favorite for a lazy afternoon by the pool.

Prep Time: 15 minutes | **Cook Time:** 20 minutes
Serves: 6 | **Serving Size:** 1¼ cups

1 pound skin-on salmon fillet

2 teaspoons extra virgin olive oil

¼ teaspoon salt

⅛ teaspoon black pepper

2 cups (1-inch) pieces asparagus

1 cup orzo pasta

1 medium yellow squash, halved lengthwise and sliced crosswise

½ small red onion, thinly sliced

Lemon-Dill Sauce:

⅔ cup plain 0% Greek yogurt

⅓ cup light mayonnaise

1 teaspoon grated lemon zest

1½ tablespoons lemon juice

1½ tablespoons minced fresh dill

½ tablespoon capers, rinsed and minced

½ teaspoon minced garlic

1. Preheat the oven to 425°F. Line a baking dish with aluminum foil.

2. Pat the salmon dry with a paper towel. Drizzle 1 teaspoon of the olive oil over the salmon and season with ⅛ teaspoon of the salt and the pepper.

3. Place the salmon in the baking dish skin side down. Bake until the salmon flakes easily when tested with a fork, 8 to 10 minutes. Keep in mind that the baking time will depend on the thickness of your salmon (as determined by the thickest part of the fillet). Set aside.

4. Meanwhile, set up a bowl of ice and water. In a large saucepan, bring 6 cups of water to a boil. Add the asparagus and cook for 3 minutes, just until it starts to get tender. Reserving the water in the pan, remove the asparagus with tongs or a slotted spoon and plunge into the ice water. Drain and set aside.

(recipe continues)

(continued from page 143)

skinny sense: Orzo is a versatile pasta shape and it absorbs flavors very well. Although its most traditional use is in soups, it performs great in casseroles and can be used in recipes like stuffed peppers, too.

5. Return the reserved water to a boil. Add the orzo and cook to al dente according to the package directions. Drain and set aside.

6. In a medium skillet, heat the remaining 1 teaspoon oil over medium-high heat. Add the squash, onion, and remaining ⅛ teaspoon salt. Sauté until soft and the onion is translucent, 4 to 6 minutes.

7. To make the lemon-dill sauce: In a small bowl, whisk together the yogurt, mayonnaise, lemon zest, lemon juice, dill, capers, and garlic.

8. Use 2 forks to break the salmon into large chunks (discard the skin). Transfer the salmon to a large bowl and add the orzo, asparagus, squash-onion mixture, and lemon-dill sauce and toss gently to coat.

9. Serve at room temperature or chilled.

Calories 379 • **Fat** 9g • **Carbohydrate** 49g • **Fiber** 4g • **Sugar** 5g • **Protein** 26g

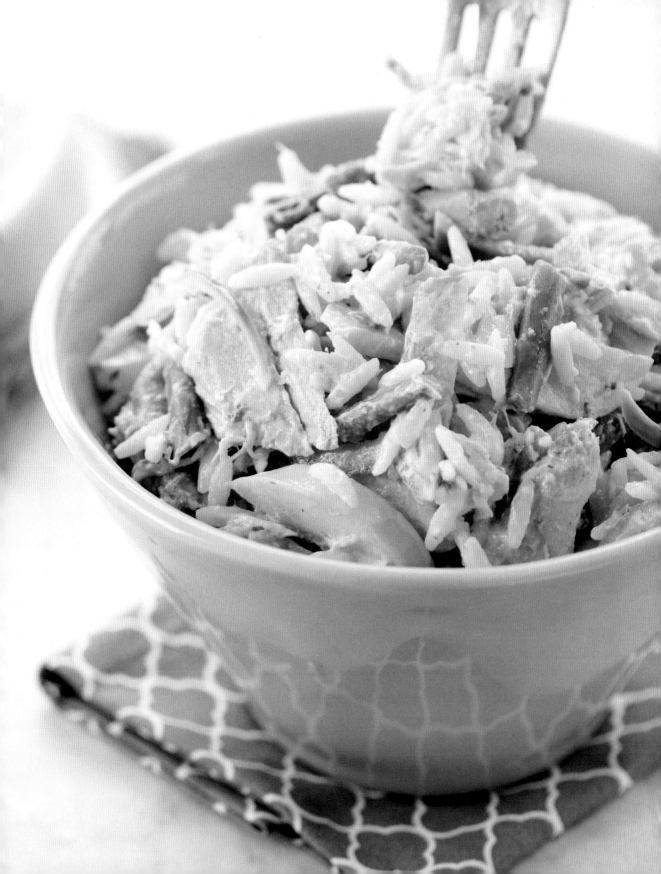

Creamy Seafood Stuffed Shells

This is a deliciously rich and cheesy supper the seafood lovers in my family often request. The use of light Alfredo sauce and low-fat mozzarella allows you to smother the shells in creamy goodness while still keeping the dish light and balanced. A word to the wise: Crabmeat should be light and flaky. Consider purchasing jumbo lump crab (usually found in tubs in the seafood section) instead of imitation for this and other recipes that call for crabmeat.

Prep Time: 25 minutes | **Cook Time:** 10 minutes
Serves: 6 | **Serving Size:** About 3 stuffed shells and ¼ cup sauce

20 jumbo pasta shells (I like Barilla)

1 tablespoon extra virgin olive oil

½ pound medium shrimp (about 20), peeled, deveined, and chopped into ½-inch pieces

1 teaspoon Old Bay seasoning

½ bunch asparagus, cut into ½-inch pieces

1 red bell pepper, diced

½ small onion, diced

¾ cup plain 0% Greek yogurt

¼ cup light mayonnaise

1 teaspoon grated lemon zest

¼ teaspoon salt

¼ teaspoon black pepper

⅛ teaspoon cayenne pepper

8 ounces lump crabmeat, picked over for shells

1 (14.5-ounce) jar Prego Light Homestyle Alfredo sauce or Make It Homemade (page 132)

½ cup shredded reduced-fat mozzarella cheese (I like Sargento)

2 tablespoons chopped fresh parsley

1. Preheat the oven to 350°F. Coat a 13 x 9-inch baking dish with cooking spray.

2. Bring a large pot of salted water to a boil over high heat. Cook the pasta to al dente according to the package directions. Drain and rinse the shells under warm water and transfer the shells to parchment paper to dry.

3. While the shells are cooking, in a medium skillet, heat ½ tablespoon of the olive oil over medium-high heat. Add the shrimp and sprinkle with the Old Bay seasoning. Cook until the shrimp is cooked through, 3 to 5 minutes, flipping the shrimp to cook both sides. Transfer the shrimp to a plate to cool.

4. Add the remaining ½ tablespoon olive oil to the skillet and set over medium-high heat. Add the asparagus, bell pepper, and onion. Cook until softened, 2 to 3 minutes. Remove from the heat to cool.

5. In a large bowl, combine the yogurt, mayonnaise, lemon zest, salt, black pepper, and cayenne. Stir until well mixed.

suppertime chat: Sometimes, a great conversation starter is the simple "On a scale of one to ten how was your day?" It's a way for me to get a glimpse of how my little man's day was before I probe any further.

6. Add the shrimp, crabmeat, and cooked vegetables to the mayonnaise mixture and stir to evenly coat.

7. Spread 1/3 cup of the Alfredo sauce into the bottom of the baking dish.

8. Choose the best 18 shells and fill each shell with a heaping 1 1/2 tablespoons of the seafood mixture and place in the casserole dish, seam side up. Cover the stuffed shells with the remaining Alfredo sauce.

9. Sprinkle the mozzarella on top of the shells and bake until the cheese is melted and the sauce is heated through, 10 to 15 minutes.

10. Serve garnished with the parsley.

Calories 332 • **Fat** 12g • **Carbohydrate** 33g • **Fiber** 2g • **Sugar** 5g • **Protein** 23g

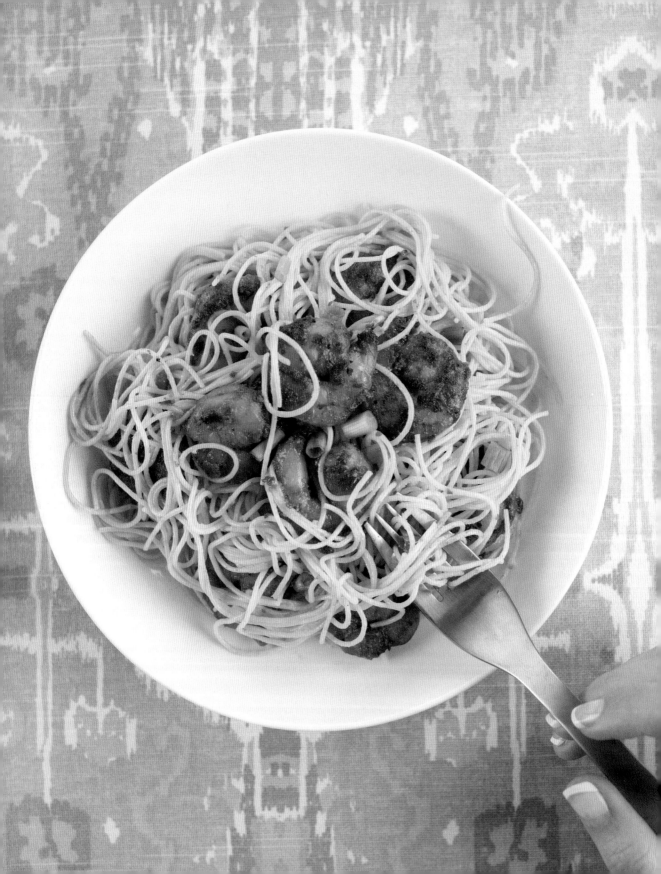

Bang Bang Shrimp Pasta

Bang! Bang! Dinner is on the table in less than 30 minutes from prep to your palate. You can do this! This pasta dish is light and creamy, with the right amount of zesty spice. Everyone's taste buds get a treat with this suppertime favorite.

Prep Time: 10 minutes | **Cook Time:** 10 minutes
Serves: 4 | **Serving Size:** Heaping ¾ cup pasta with sauce, 10 shrimp

8 ounces high-protein angel hair pasta (I like Barilla ProteinPLUS)

2 teaspoons cornstarch

½ tablespoon paprika

½ tablespoon chili powder

½ teaspoon salt

½ teaspoon black pepper

1 pound medium shrimp (about 40), peeled and deveined

3 tablespoons plain 0% Greek yogurt

3 tablespoons Thai Kitchen sweet red chili sauce

2½ tablespoons sesame oil

2 tablespoons lime juice

1½ teaspoons sriracha sauce

⅛ teaspoon red pepper flakes

3 green onions, thinly sliced

1. Bring a large pot of salted water to a boil over high heat. Cook the pasta to al dente according to the package directions. Drain and set aside.

2. In a large resealable bag, combine the cornstarch, paprika, chili powder, salt, and pepper. Add the shrimp, seal, and shake a few times to evenly coat the shrimp.

3. In a small bowl, whisk together the yogurt, sweet chili sauce, 1½ tablespoons of the sesame oil, the lime juice, sriracha, and pepper flakes. Pour the sauce over the pasta and toss to evenly coat the pasta. Set aside.

4. In a large skillet, heat the remaining 1 tablespoon sesame oil over medium-high heat. Add the shrimp and cook for 3 to 5 minutes, until the shrimp are pink, turning occasionally (see Quick and Easy).

5. Serve the shrimp over the pasta and garnish with the green onions.

quick and easy: Shrimp cook quickly—be sure not to overcook. Normally shrimp are cooked when they're pearly pink and opaque, but it's hard to tell in this recipe with the seasoning coating them. Use an instant-read thermometer to check the internal temperature: When the inside of a shrimp reaches 145°F, the shrimp are ready.

Calories 392 · Fat 12g · Carbohydrate 50g · Fiber 5g · Sugar 8g · Protein 27g

Cajun Chicken Pasta

Cajun seasoning is one of my favorite spices. I even like to sprinkle it on salads and veggies. This pasta dish is an old family recipe that has been passed down for generations and is decadent and creamy. This dish is just spicy enough to satisfy all the taste buds in our house.

Prep Time: 10 minutes | **Cook Time:** 15 minutes
Serves: 6 | **Serving Size:** 1½ cups

¼ cup fat-free milk

1½ tablespoons white whole wheat flour

2 tablespoons ⅓-less-fat cream cheese

¼ cup light sour cream

1½ pounds boneless, skinless chicken breasts, sliced into thin strips

4 teaspoons Cajun seasoning or Make It Homemade (page 299)

8 ounces whole wheat linguine (I like Barilla)

1 tablespoon extra virgin olive oil

2 tablespoons minced garlic

1 red bell pepper, thinly sliced

1 yellow bell pepper, thinly sliced

1 green bell pepper, thinly sliced

1 small onion, sliced

1 (14.5-ounce) can no-salt-added diced tomatoes (I like Hunt's)

2 links Al Fresco andouille-style chicken sausage, sliced into 1-inch pieces

1 cup low-sodium chicken broth (I like Pacific Organic)

¼ teaspoon salt

¼ teaspoon black pepper

1 teaspoon cayenne pepper

2 tablespoons chopped fresh parsley

1. In a blender, combine the milk, flour, cream cheese, and sour cream and blend until smooth. Set the sour cream sauce aside.

2. Toss the chicken strips with 2 teaspoons of the Cajun seasoning.

3. Bring a large pot of salted water to a boil over high heat. Cook the pasta to al dente according to the package directions. Drain and set aside.

4. Meanwhile, in a large nonstick skillet, heat ½ tablespoon of the olive oil over medium-high heat. Add the seasoned chicken strips in a single layer and cook until golden, 3 to 5 minutes on each side. Transfer the chicken to a plate.

5. Return the skillet to medium heat and add the remaining ½ tablespoon olive oil. When hot, add the garlic, bell

(recipe continues)

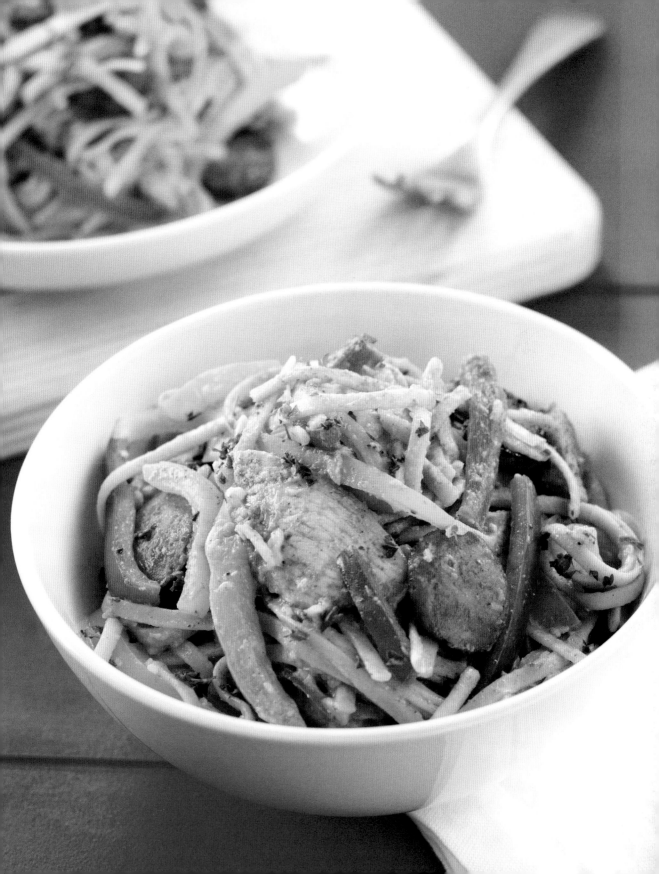

(continued from page 150)

suppertime chat: Begin by thinking of a character trait you would like to instill and see firmly rooted in your children. Talk with them about that character trait and ask them to name someone who possesses that trait. For instance, "Who is the most 'patient' person you know? What makes him or her patient? How does patience help him or her?" The goal is to help your children recognize the importance of a character trait, such as patience, and how it could benefit, or even reward, them in life.

peppers, and onion and sauté for 2 to 3 minutes. Add the diced tomatoes (with juice) and chicken sausage and cook 2 to 3 minutes. Stir in the remaining 2 teaspoons Cajun seasoning.

6. Pour the sour cream sauce and the chicken broth into the skillet and stir for 2 to 3 minutes, making sure the vegetables and chicken sausage are evenly coated. Add the salt and black pepper.

7. Return the cooked chicken to the skillet and stir to evenly coat. Add the pasta and toss lightly to coat with the sauce.

8. Serve sprinkled with the cayenne and garnished with the parsley.

Calories 403 • **Fat** 11g • **Carbohydrate** 41g • **Fiber** 8g • **Sugar** 8g • **Protein** 36g

Creamy Mac and Alfredo

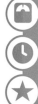

Face it, Popeye ate spinach for a reason! For those who don't have the taste for this ultrahealthy vegetable, the creamy combination of cottage cheese and mozzarella will disguise the spinach so well, no one will ever know how healthy they're eating.

Prep Time: 10 minutes │ **Cook Time:** 20 minutes
Serves: 6 │ **Serving Size:** Heaping 1½ cups

12 ounces whole wheat penne pasta (I like Barilla)

1 (14.5-ounce) jar Prego Light Homestyle Alfredo sauce or Make It Homemade (page 132)

½ cup low-fat cottage cheese

½ cup fat-free milk

2 egg whites

1 teaspoon garlic powder

½ teaspoon salt

¼ teaspoon black pepper

10 ounces frozen chopped spinach, thawed and drained

½ cup shredded reduced-fat mozzarella cheese (I like Sargento)

1. Preheat the oven to 350°F. Coat a 13 x 9-inch baking dish with cooking spray.

2. Bring a large pot of salted water to a boil over high heat. Cook the pasta to al dente according to the package directions. Drain and set aside.

3. In a large bowl, whisk together the Alfredo sauce, cottage cheese, milk, egg whites, garlic powder, salt, and pepper. Stir in the spinach to combine.

4. Gently fold the cooked pasta into the Alfredo mixture until evenly covered.

5. Transfer the mixture to the prepared baking dish. Sprinkle the mozzarella on top.

6. Bake uncovered until the cheese is melted, about 20 minutes.

suppertime chat: What's your favorite vegetable and why? What's your least favorite vegetable and why? Get ready to giggle yourself silly when the kiddos talk about how much they hate spinach, but love your Mac and Alfredo!

Calories 310 • Fat 8g • Carbohydrate 47g • Fiber 7g • Sugar 5g • Protein 17g

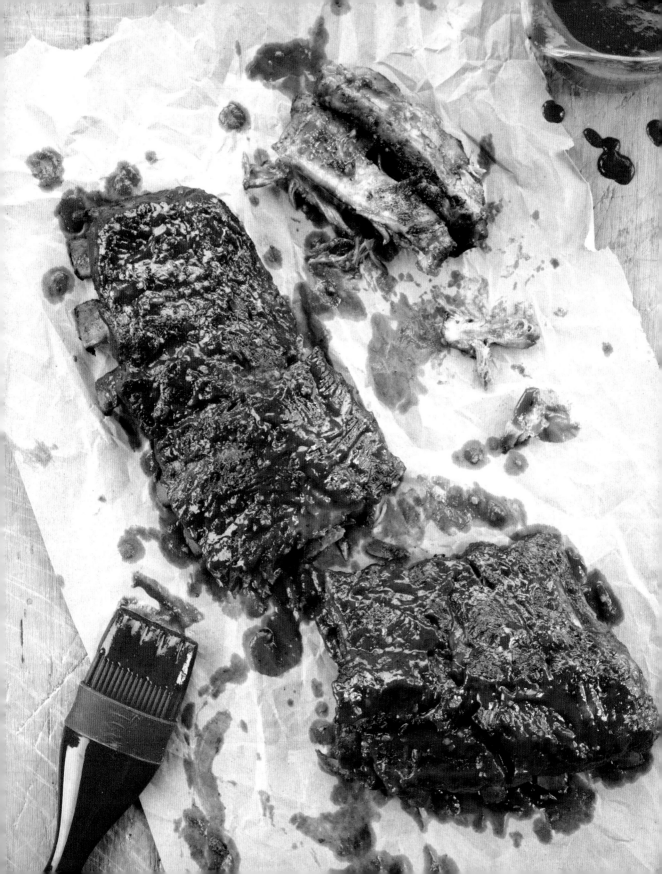

Apple-Stuffed Pork Tenderloin with Dijon Mustard Sauce

I grew up eating baked apples. I remember vividly the sweet smells of cinnamon and sugar filling the whole house as I'd come running through my granny's back door after school. In some ways, those warm aromas provided comfort and security for me growing up. It's one of the reasons I long to fill my kitchen with comforting smells as my little guy comes home after a long day at school. In this recipe, those heavenly scents are paired with a succulent pork tenderloin topped with a sweet Dijon sauce your family won't soon forget!

Prep Time: 10 minutes | **Cook Time:** 35 minutes
Serves: 6 | **Serving Size:** 4 ounces stuffed pork, 1½ tablespoons sauce

1½ teaspoons extra virgin olive oil

1 large Golden Delicious apple (or other sweet baking apple), peeled and diced

½ cup golden raisins

½ teaspoon cinnamon

2 tablespoons apple cider vinegar

1½ pounds pork tenderloin, trimmed of fat

1 teaspoon kosher salt

½ teaspoon black pepper

3 wedges Laughing Cow Creamy Swiss Light cheese

Dijon Mustard Sauce:

2 tablespoons unsalted butter

2 tablespoons white whole wheat flour

2 tablespoons apple cider vinegar

1 cup reduced-sugar apple juice

(ingredients continue)

1. In a large skillet, heat 1 teaspoon of the olive oil over medium-low heat. Add the apple, raisins, cinnamon, and 2 tablespoons of the vinegar. Stir and cook until the apples have softened, 8 to 10 minutes. Remove from the heat and set aside.

2. Preheat the oven to 400°F. Coat a roasting pan with cooking spray.

3. Butterfly the tenderloin by slicing it lengthwise, but not cutting it all the way through. The tenderloin will open up like a book. Place it between two pieces of plastic wrap and flatten it out with a meat mallet to a ¼- to ½-inch thickness.

4. Season both sides of the pork with the salt and pepper.

5. Spread the cheese wedges evenly over the surface of the pork. Layer the cooked apple mixture lengthwise on top of the cheese, leaving 1 inch without filling on one side.

6. Begin rolling the tenderloin up lengthwise with the grain.

2 teaspoons Dijon mustard

2 teaspoons sugar-free maple-flavor syrup (I like Maple Grove Farms)

⅛ teaspoon salt

⅛ teaspoon black pepper

Special Equipment:

Butcher's twine

skinny sense: Ever wonder how to choose the leanest cut of meat? Remember this little "skinny phrase": loin means lean. The word "loin" will always guide you to the leanest cut in a meat family. If you're looking for a lean steak, choose a sirloin; for a lean cut of pork, go for the tenderloin, as I did here.

7. With the seam side down, tie the tenderloin in several places with the butcher's twine so it keeps its shape.

8. In the same skillet used to prepare the apple mixture, add the remaining ½ teaspoon olive oil over medium-high heat. Once heated, add the tenderloin and sear for 2 to 3 minutes on all sides. Transfer the tenderloin to the prepared roasting pan.

9. Bake until the internal temperature in the thickest part of the tenderloin reaches 145°F, 25 to 30 minutes. Let the tenderloin rest for 3 to 5 minutes.

10. Meanwhile, prepare the Dijon mustard sauce: In a small saucepan, melt the butter over low heat. Whisk the flour into the butter for about 30 seconds, until smooth and the mixture smells nutty, making a roux.

11. Gradually whisk in the vinegar and apple juice. Increase the heat to medium-high and bring the mixture to a boil, then immediately reduce the heat to low, making sure to constantly whisk the sauce. Stir in the mustard, syrup, salt, and pepper and cook until thickened. Remove from the heat.

12. To serve, cut the butcher's twine off the tenderloin and slice the meat. Serve with the sauce.

Suggested Side Dish: Caramelized Brussels Sprouts with Pecans (page 298)

Calories 267 • Fat 8g • Carbohydrate 20g • Fiber 2g • Sugar 16g • Protein 25g

Carnitas Veggie Bowl

Although the word "carnitas" literally means "little meats," it most often references pork. This dish was inspired by a favorite of mine from Chipotle. I've learned that the best way to get the fork-tender meat like they serve up is to use a slow cooker. And the use of the slow cooker makes it a simple recipe to get started in the morning, especially on days when I know ahead of time I'll be rushed when I come back through the door.

Prep Time: 10 minutes │ **Cook Time:** 4 hours on high or 8 hours on low
Serves: 6 │ **Serving Size:** 1 carnitas veggie bowl

---

1 teaspoon ground cumin

1 tablespoon minced garlic

1 teaspoon kosher salt

1 teaspoon black pepper

3 pounds pork shoulder, fat trimmed and cut into 2-inch cubes

2 chipotle peppers in adobo sauce

1 (4.5-ounce) can chopped green chilies

3 tablespoons lime juice

¼ cup apple cider vinegar

1 cup low-sodium chicken broth (I like Pacific Organic)

2 tablespoons sugar-free maple-flavor syrup (I like Maple Grove Farms)

2 teaspoons extra virgin olive oil

1 medium red onion, sliced

2 red bell peppers, sliced

2 green bell peppers, sliced

Pico de Gallo:

4 Roma (plum) tomatoes, diced

½ cup red onion, diced

1 jalapeño pepper, seeded and diced

2 teaspoons lime juice

2 teaspoons chopped fresh cilantro

¼ teaspoon kosher salt

Optional Garnishes:

3 tablespoons shredded reduced-fat four-cheese Mexican blend (I like Sargento)

3 tablespoons light sour cream

---

1. Lightly coat the liner of a slow cooker with cooking spray.

2. In a large bowl, combine the cumin, garlic, salt, and black pepper. Add the pork and generously cover the pork with the spices on all sides. Place the pork in the slow cooker.

3. Finely mince the chipotle peppers in adobo sauce and transfer to a small bowl. Add the green chilies, lime juice, vinegar, chicken broth, and maple syrup. Pour over the pork.

4. Cover the slow cooker and cook on low heat for 8 hours or on high heat for 4 hours.

(recipe continues)

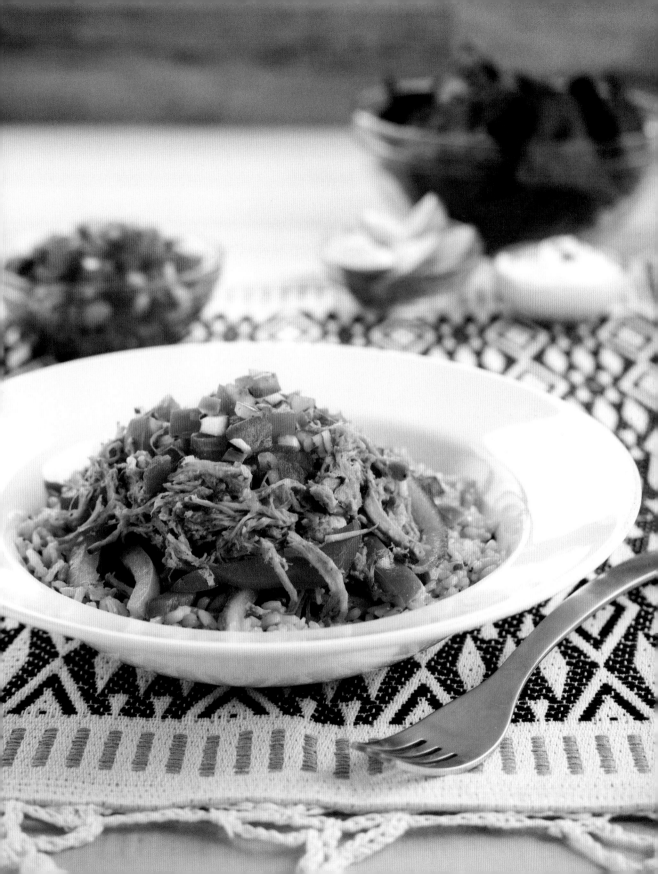

(recipe continued from page 158)

suppertime chat: **Describe your idea of a perfect day. What would you do? Who would be there? What would you eat? It's a great way to persuade everyone at the table that daydreaming is a good thing!**

5. Just before the pork is done, in a medium skillet, heat the olive oil over medium-high heat. Add the red onion and bell peppers and cook for 3 to 5 minutes to soften.

6. Once the pork is fork-tender, remove from the slow cooker and shred (discard the cooking liquid).

7. For the pico de gallo: In a medium bowl, combine the tomatoes, red onion, jalapeño, lime juice, cilantro, and salt. Refrigerate until ready to serve.

8. To assemble the bowls, fill each bowl with a heaping ¹/2 cup onion and peppers, then cover with a ¹/2 cup pork and 2 tablespoons pico de gallo. If desired, garnish with ¹/2 tablespoon each Mexican blend cheese and sour cream.

Suggested Side Dish: Cilantro-Lime Rice (page 271)

no slow cooker, no problem: **Season the pork as directed and place it in the bottom of a large pot or Dutch oven. Prepare the liquid as directed and pour over the pork. Cover and cook over low heat until the pork is fork-tender, 2 to 3 hours. Follow the rest of the recipe as directed.**

Calories 340 • **Fat** 13g • **Carbohydrate** 15g • **Fiber** 3g • **Sugar** 7g • **Protein** 38g
Nutrition does not include optional garnishes (or the Cilantro-Lime Rice shown in the photo).

Kentucky Bourbon Fall-off-the-Bone Ribs

Ninety-five percent of the country's bourbon is distilled, aged, and bottled right here in Kentucky. A few years ago, I learned how to cook with the state native. To this day, I've not found a better base for my fall-off-the-bone ribs, and I have grown to truly appreciate the luscious, caramel sweetness you get when you cook with it. This dish takes only 10 minutes to prep, but will need 8 hours to reach its flawless state.

Prep Time: 10 minutes | **Cook Time:** 8 hours on low plus 3 minutes broil time
Serves: 6 | **Serving Size:** 2 ribs

2½ pounds baby back ribs
   (see Quick and Easy, page 163)

Dry Rub:

1 tablespoon brown sugar

1 tablespoon chili powder

1½ teaspoons paprika

1 teaspoon kosher salt

1 teaspoon black pepper

Sauce:

¾ cup Heinz reduced-sugar ketchup

¼ cup bourbon or substitute
   ¼ cup sparkling apple cider
   and 2 teaspoons vanilla extract

3 tablespoons apple cider vinegar

3 tablespoons sugar-free maple-
   flavor syrup (I like Maple Grove
   Farms)

2 tablespoons Worcestershire sauce

1 tablespoon minced garlic

½ teaspoon chili powder

½ teaspoon onion powder

¼ teaspoon salt

¼ teaspoon black pepper

1. Cut the ribs so they'll fit in your slow cooker (I use kitchen shears to cut the rack in half). Pat the ribs dry with a paper towel to remove excess moisture.

2. To make the rub: Using a shallow baking dish as a work surface, combine the brown sugar, chili powder, paprika, salt, and pepper and mix well.

3. Generously cover both sides of the ribs with the dry rub.

4. Coat a slow cooker with cooking spray. Place the ribs standing up around the sides of the slow cooker.

5. To make the sauce: In a medium bowl, whisk together the ketchup, bourbon, vinegar, syrup, Worcestershire sauce, garlic, chili powder, onion powder, salt, and pepper. Pour the sauce into the slow cooker.

6. Cover and cook the ribs on low heat for 8 hours.

7. A few minutes before the ribs have finished cooking, turn on the broiler. Coat a baking sheet with cooking spray.

(recipe continues)

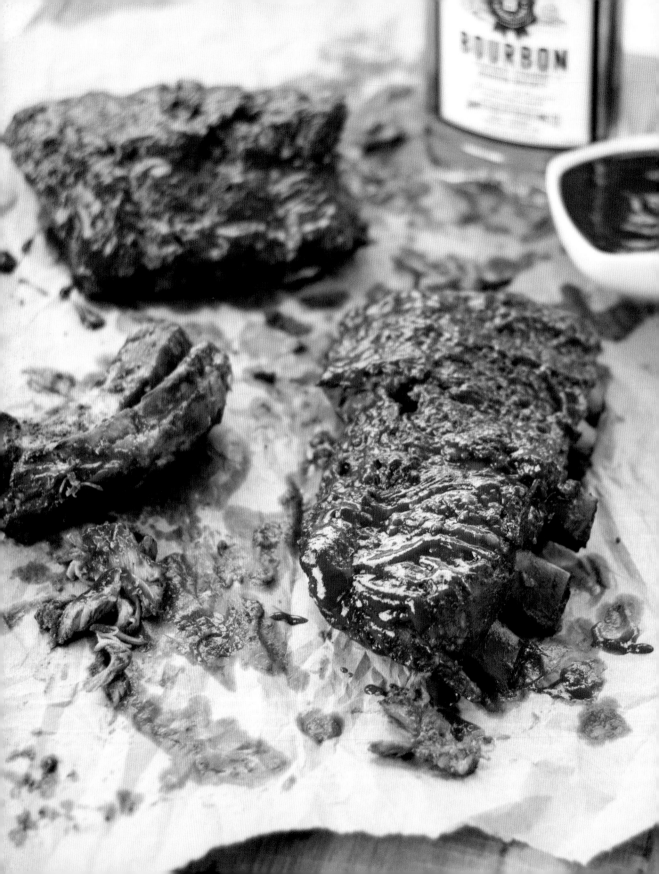

(recipe continued from page 161)

quick and easy: When purchasing ribs, ask the butcher to remove the outer membrane, or you can do this at home before cooking. Here's how: Flip the ribs over so they're bone side up and pat dry with paper towels. Starting at one end of the rack, slide the tip of a paring knife between the membrane and the bone, then lift and cut through the membrane. Grasping the membrane with a paper towel, pull it toward the other end of the rack and completely remove it.

8. Carefully remove the ribs from the slow cooker and arrange on the baking sheet, meat side up.

9. Transfer the sauce from the slow cooker to a small saucepan. Cook over medium-low heat for 5 to 8 minutes, stirring constantly, until the sauce thickens. Brush a thick coat of the sauce onto the ribs.

10. Broil the ribs for 2 to 4 minutes, being careful not to burn the ribs.

11. Serve with the remaining sauce.

Suggested Side Dish: Skillet Corn (page 291)

no slow cooker, no problem: Preheat the oven to 300°F. Coat two 13 x 9-inch baking dishes with cooking spray. Arrange the seasoned ribs, meat side down, in the baking dishes. Evenly cover the ribs with the prepared sauce. Cover the baking dishes with foil and bake until the rib meat is fork-tender, 3½ to 4 hours. Continue with the recipe as directed.

Calories 380 • **Fat** 21g • **Carbohydrate** 6g • **Fiber** 0g • **Sugar** 4g • **Protein** 39g

Deep-Dish BBQ Hawaiian Skillet Pizza

Do you ever get a hankering for a deep-dish pizza? Me, too! In this recipe, I use low-sodium, reduced-fat, whole grain, and overall quality ingredients that allow you (and me) to savor this deep-dish sensation! The foundation of the red sauce is the perfect bed for my favorite toppings and tangy BBQ sauce. One bite of this and it's "Bye-bye, delivery!"

Prep Time: 5 minutes | **Cook Time:** 20 minutes
Serves: 6 | **Serving Size:** 1 slice

1 (13.8-ounce) can Pillsbury Artisan whole grain pizza dough

3 slices lower-sodium turkey bacon

½ cup Prego Veggie Smart pizza sauce

1 cup shredded reduced-fat mozzarella cheese (I like Sargento)

2 thick-cut slices lower-sodium ham (I like Boar's Head Branded Deluxe), cut into quarters

¼ cup thinly sliced red onion

½ cup juice-packed pineapple tidbits (I like Del Monte), drained

2 tablespoons Stubb's Original All-Natural Bar-B-Q Sauce

¼ cup chopped fresh cilantro

1. Preheat the oven to 400°F. Generously coat a 12-inch cast iron skillet or other ovenproof skillet with cooking spray.

2. On a large cutting board, roll out the pizza dough and stretch to make it larger all around. Lift the dough and transfer it to the skillet, covering the bottom. Trim off any excess dough and use the trimmings to cover the skillet walls and any holes by pinching together the dough.

3. Prebake the crust for 8 minutes.

4. Meanwhile, place the turkey bacon slices in a single layer on a microwave-safe plate lined with paper towels. Microwave on high for 1½ to 2½ minutes until crisp. When cool enough to handle, crumble the bacon and set aside.

5. Remove the crust from the oven. Spread the pizza sauce over the crust. Cover with the mozzarella, followed by the ham, red onion, pineapple, and bacon. Drizzle the barbecue sauce evenly over the top of the pizza.

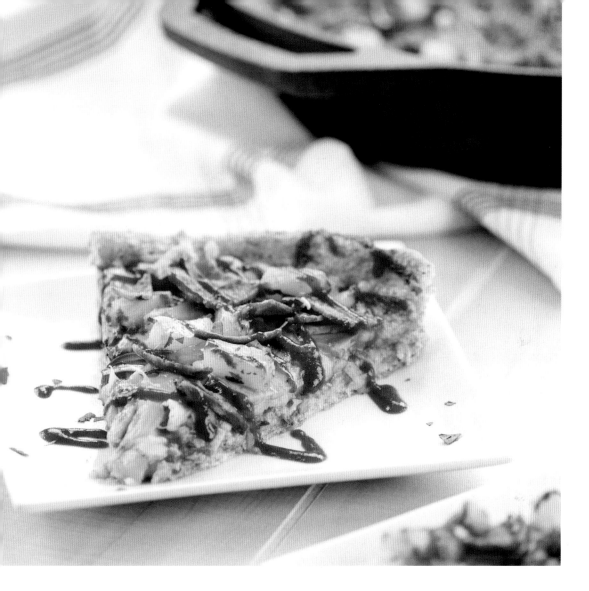

6. Return the pan to the oven and bake until the cheese is melted and bubbling, 10 to 12 minutes.

7. Remove from the oven and garnish with the cilantro. Cut into 6 slices.

suppertime inspiration: "What's your 'why'?" Why do you want to prepare lighter and balanced meals for your family? Why is suppertime important to you? Remembering each and every day "why" you want to prepare lighter and healthier meals for your family will keep you motivated and moving forward. Never forget your "why"!

Calories 297 · **Fat** 11g · **Carbohydrate** 39g · **Fiber** 3g · **Sugar** 9g · **Protein** 12g

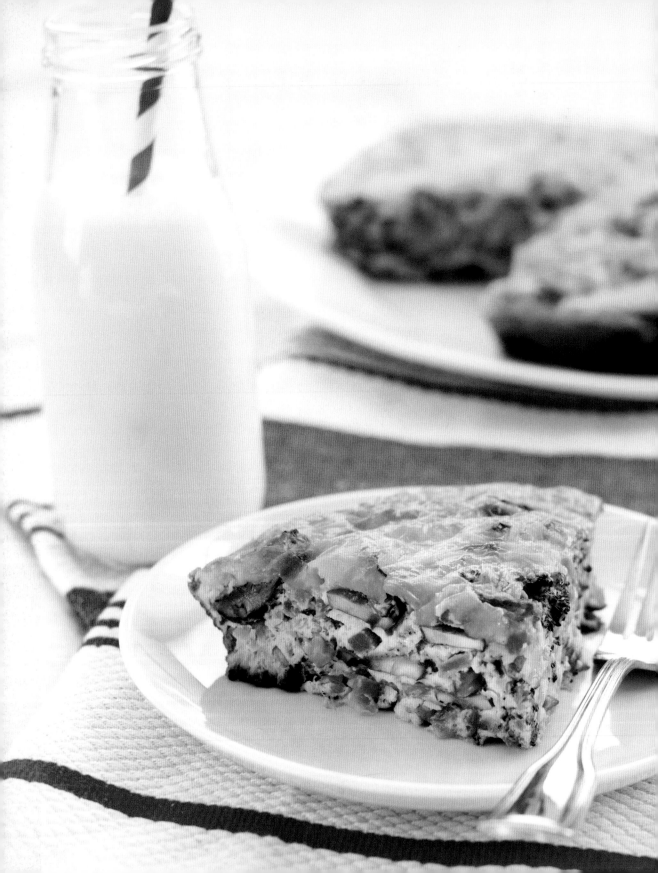

Crustless Broccoli, Ham, and Cheese Quiche

One of the best ways to avoid the extra calories is to shave off the excess portions. By eliminating the bottom and side crusts in this quiche, you'll save hundreds of unwanted calories and fat without sacrificing the savory goodness of the broccoli, ham, and cheese that are on the inside. After all, everyone knows it's what's on the inside that counts!

Prep Time: 10 minutes | **Cook Time:** 50 minutes
Serves: 6 | **Serving Size:** 1/6 of the quiche

½ tablespoon extra virgin olive oil

2 teaspoons minced garlic

2 cups chopped broccoli

1 small onion, diced

1 (8-ounce) container baby bella (cremini) mushrooms, sliced

1 cup diced ham

5 eggs

4 egg whites

⅓ cup fat-free milk

2 tablespoons white whole wheat flour

½ teaspoon salt

½ teaspoon black pepper

½ cup shredded reduced-fat sharp cheddar cheese (I like Sargento)

1. Preheat the oven to 350°F. Coat a 9-inch pie pan with cooking spray.

2. In a large skillet, heat the olive oil over medium heat. Add the garlic, broccoli, onion, and mushrooms. Sauté until the vegetables are tender and the liquid has cooked out of the mushrooms, 8 to 10 minutes.

3. Arrange the sautéed vegetables and diced ham in the bottom of the prepared pie pan. In a small bowl, whisk together the whole eggs, egg whites, milk, flour, salt, and pepper. Pour over the vegetables and ham.

4. Cover with the cheddar and bake until the middle has set, 30 to 35 minutes. Let cool before cutting into 6 wedges.

Suggested Side Dish: Carrot and Raisin Salad (page 268)

quick and easy: Is that crisper drawer of yours full of veggies on the verge of being tossed into the trash? Make a quiche! Combine eggs with virtually any combination of veggies, mixed with a little meat and cheese.

Calories 180 • Fat 8g • Carbohydrate 11g • Fiber 3g • Sugar 4g • Protein 19g

Grilled Pineapple Teriyaki Pork Chops

The pineapple topping on these succulent pork chops provides a bold, sweet twist that will have you feeling like you're on a tropical vacation. Just fire up the indoor grill and imagine yourself under the palm trees.

Prep Time: 10 minutes, plus 2 hours marinating time | **Cook Time:** 10 minutes
Serves: 4 | **Serving Size:** 1 pork chop, 1 pineapple slice

⅓ cup Tropicana Trop50 orange juice

2 tablespoons less-sodium soy sauce

1 tablespoon rice vinegar

1 tablespoon brown sugar

½ teaspoon ground ginger

½ teaspoon onion powder

½ teaspoon garlic powder

4 (4-ounce) boneless pork chops, trimmed of fat

2 teaspoons cornstarch

4 thickly sliced fresh pineapple rings

1. In a small bowl, whisk together the orange juice, soy sauce, rice vinegar, brown sugar, ground ginger, onion powder, and garlic powder to make a marinade.

2. Place the pork chops in a large resealable bag and add the marinade to coat. Seal the bag and place in the refrigerator for at least 2 hours or up to overnight. If possible, turn the bag every hour or so to evenly coat the pork chops with the marinade.

3. Transfer the pork chops to a shallow dish. Pour the marinade into a small saucepan.

4. In a small bowl, dissolve the cornstarch in 2 teaspoons of cold water to make a slurry. Place the saucepan of marinade over medium heat and bring to a boil. Reduce the heat to low and whisk in the slurry. Cook, whisking, until the sauce thickens, about 2 minutes. Remove from the heat and set aside to use as a basting for the grilled pork chops and pineapple.

5. Preheat an indoor grill, grill pan, or outdoor grill to medium-high heat. Lightly coat the grill rack of the indoor grill or grill pan with cooking spray.

suppertime chat: If you could go anywhere in the world, where would you go and why? Don't be surprised if you get some "out of this world" answers from your three-year-old (or your teen for that matter). Roll with it, it's all about the conversation!

6. Place the pork chops on the grill and cook until the internal temperature reaches 145°F, 4 to 5 minutes per side, brushing often with the basting as you grill.

7. Add the pineapple slices to the grill and cook for 1 to 2 minutes on both sides.

8. Let the pork chops rest for 2 to 4 minutes before serving.

9. To serve, place one grilled pineapple slice on top of each pork chop and serve with any remaining basting.

Suggested Side Dish: Sweet and Spicy Coleslaw (page 287)

Calories 210 • **Fat** 9g • **Carbohydrate** 13g • **Fiber** 0g • **Sugar** 9g • **Protein** 24g

Country Pork Chops and Gravy

The older I get, the more I realize how much my cooking is influenced by my granny. She fried everything she could get her hands on and then put heaping spoonfuls of her special gravy on it. Well, I don't fry (at least in lard) or smother too many of my dishes anymore, but I have preserved my granny's down-home goodness and special seasonings in this country creation.

Prep Time: 10 minutes │ **Cook Time:** 30 minutes
Serves: 4 │ **Serving Size:** 1 pork chop, 2 tablespoons gravy

1 tablespoon white whole wheat flour

2 egg whites

1 tablespoon fat-free milk

½ cup panko bread crumbs

⅓ cup shredded Parmesan cheese (I like Sargento Artisan Blends)

1½ tablespoons Old Bay seasoning

½ teaspoon salt

½ teaspoon black pepper

4 (4-ounce) boneless pork chops

Granny's Gravy:

1 tablespoon unsalted butter

1 tablespoon white whole wheat flour

¾ cup fat-free milk

⅛ teaspoon salt

⅛ teaspoon black pepper

1. Preheat the oven to 400°F. Line a baking sheet with foil and coat generously with cooking spray.

2. Place the flour in a shallow dish. In a separate shallow dish, beat the egg whites, then whisk in the milk. In a third shallow dish, combine the panko, Parmesan, Old Bay, salt, and pepper.

3. Pat the pork chops dry with a paper towel to remove excess moisture. Dredge each pork chop in the flour and shake off the excess. Dip each pork chop in the egg mixture, then generously coat both sides in the panko mixture, and transfer to the prepared baking sheet.

4. Bake for 25 to 30 minutes, or until the internal temperature reaches 145°F.

5. Meanwhile, to make Granny's gravy: In a small saucepan, melt the butter over low heat. Whisk the flour into the butter for about 30 seconds, until smooth and the mixture smells nutty, making a roux. Whisk in the milk and bring to a boil over medium heat, making sure to stir constantly. Season with the salt and pepper. Turn the heat to low and continue to stir until the gravy is thickened, 5 to 8 minutes.

6. Serve each pork chop with 2 tablespoons gravy.

Suggested Side Dish: Skinny Fried Apples (page 297)

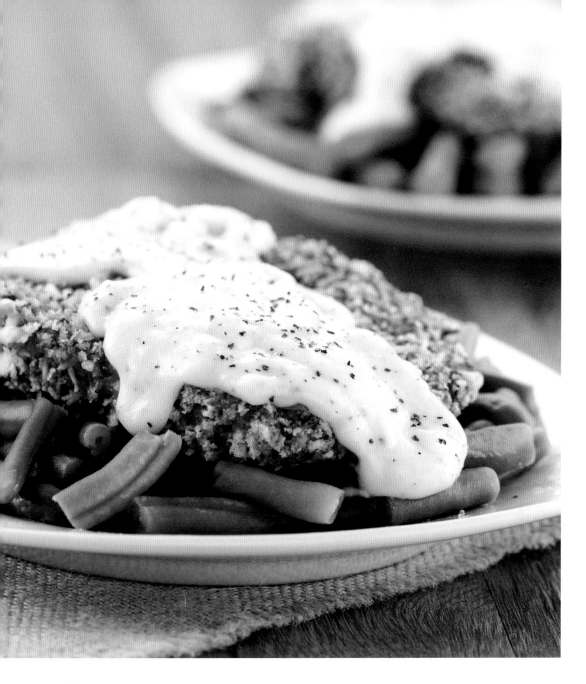

skinny sense: Don't be afraid to experiment with the seasonings in your pantry! Old Bay seasoning, usually reserved for seafood, pairs well with the pork in this dish. It has a zesty flavor that is a perfect topper for everything from salad to soups to pizza.

Calories 334 · **Fat** 18g · **Carbohydrate** 14g · **Fiber** 1g · **Sugar** 5g · **Protein** 33g

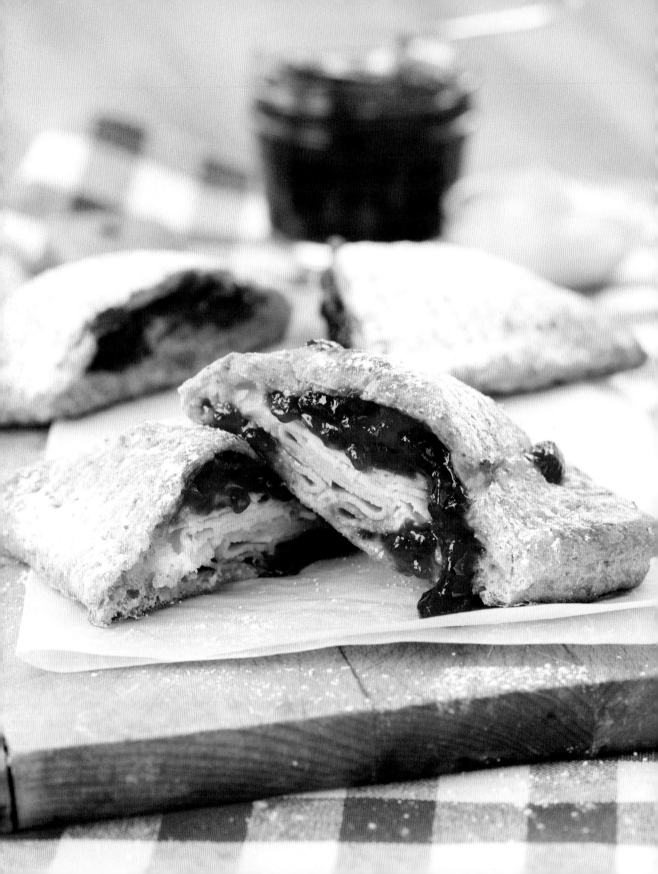

Lightened-Up Monte Cristo Calzone

(2x)

The traditional Monte Cristo sandwich gained wide fame and popularity in the 1960s when The Blue Bayou restaurant in Anaheim, California, began serving it up. For those of you who have never tasted a Monte Cristo, it's basically a ham and cheese sandwich that is battered, deep-fried, and sometimes sprinkled with powdered sugar, then drizzled with preserves for dipping. I decided to lighten it up, using a whole grain pizza crust, lean and flavorful deli meats, and part-skim cheeses. More of a calzone than a sandwich, these are so much fun to serve up to hungry kids after school or as a party food.

Prep Time: 10 minutes | **Cook Time:** 12 minutes
Serves: 8 | **Serving Size:** 1 calzone, 2 teaspoons raspberry preserves, ⅛ teaspoon powdered sugar

1 (13.8-ounce) can Pillsbury Artisan whole grain pizza dough

8 teaspoons Dijon mustard

16 teaspoons no-sugar-added raspberry preserves (I like Smucker's)

8 thin slices lower-sodium ham (I like Boar's Head Branded Deluxe)

8 thin slices lower-sodium turkey breast (I like Boar's Head)

8 slices Sargento Ultra Thin sliced provolone cheese

1 teaspoon powdered sugar

suppertime inspiration:
A diamond is a piece of coal that has undergone intense pressure. So, if you're feeling more pressure than you think you can handle, just remember you're about to shine!

1. Preheat the oven to 350°F. Coat a baking sheet with cooking spray.

2. Roll out the pizza crust on the prepared baking sheet and cut evenly into 8 squares. Roll each square into about a 5 x 7-inch rectangle.

3. Spread each rectangle with 1 teaspoon mustard. Spread 2 teaspoons preserves over the mustard. On one half of each rectangle, place 1 slice each of the ham, turkey, and provolone. Fold over the top half of the dough rectangle to cover the meat and cheese and pinch the edges closed with the tines of a fork.

4. Place the calzones on the prepared baking sheet. Bake until golden brown, 10 to 12 minutes. Let rest for 5 minutes.

5. To serve, sprinkle ⅛ teaspoon powdered sugar lightly over the top of each calzone.

Suggested Side Dish: Asparagus Fries with Garlic Lemon Aioli (page 262)

Calories 239 • Fat 7g • Carbohydrate 27g • Fiber 4g • Sugar 3g • Protein 15g

Savory Stromboli Muffin Cups

Calling all meat lovers! Finding a way to lighten up dishes like this one was a priority. I love meat, cheese, and bread, and that's a dangerous trio. The portion-control aspect of the cups is key in this recipe, but not to be outdone by the smart combination of turkey pepperoni, bacon, and salami, which I purposely slice into quarters for portion control.

Prep Time: 20 minutes | **Cook Time:** 15 minutes
Serves: 6 | **Serving Size:** 2 stromboli muffin cups, ¼ cup pizza sauce

1 (13.8-ounce) can Pillsbury Artisan whole grain pizza dough

2 egg whites, beaten

½ teaspoon Italian seasoning

2 tablespoons grated Parmesan cheese (I like Sargento)

6 slices Canadian bacon (I like Boar's Head), cut into quarters

24 slices turkey pepperoni

6 slices Sargento Ultra Thin sliced provolone cheese, cut into quarters

6 slices hard salami (I like Boar's Head), cut into quarters

1½ cups Prego Veggie Smart pizza sauce

3 tablespoons shredded reduced-fat mozzarella cheese (I like Sargento)

24 pepperoncini slices

1. Preheat the oven to 350°F. Get out a 12-cup muffin tin and set aside.

2. Roll the pizza crust out to a 12-inch square. Using a 3½-inch round cutter (or the rim of a juice glass), cut 12 rounds from the crust. Flip the muffin tin over (so the top of the muffin tin is facing down) and coat the outsides of the muffin cups with cooking spray. Firmly press each dough round down and around each muffin cup.

3. Place the upside-down muffin tin into the oven and bake for 5 minutes. Remove from the oven and allow to cool for 2 to 3 minutes. (Leave the oven on.)

4. Gently peel the dough cups off the bottom of the muffin tin. Flip the muffin tin over (hole side up) and lightly coat with cooking spray before placing the dough cups in each of the muffin cups.

5. In a small bowl, whisk together the egg whites, Italian seasoning, and Parmesan. Lightly brush the egg white mixture on the insides and the walls of the muffin cups.

(recipe continues)

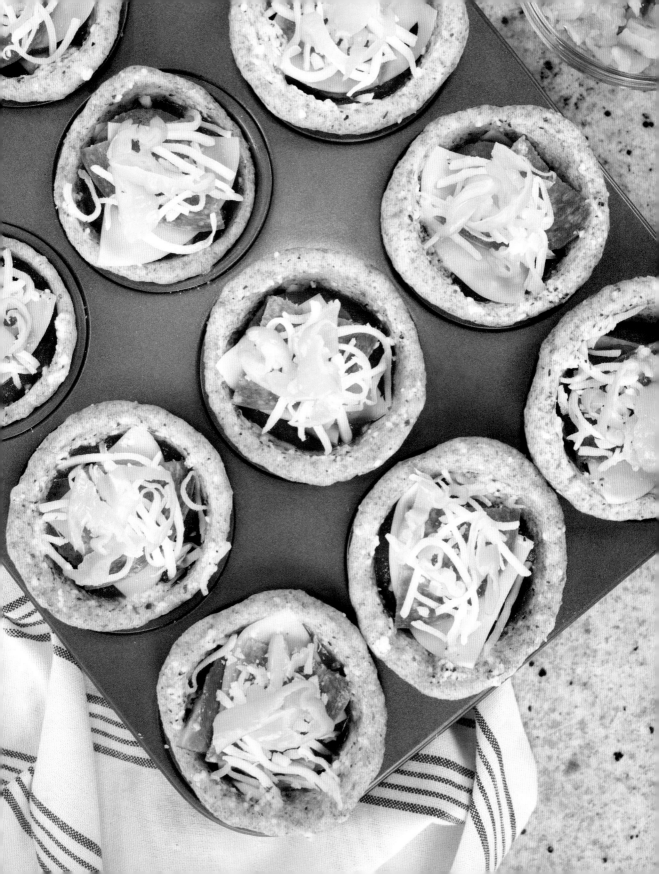

(recipe continued from page 174)

suppertime inspiration:

The K.I.S.S. Method is often used in reference to weight loss. It stands for Keep It Simple Sweetie and it can be a very powerful motivating force. Work to educate and inspire the family with small steps. Create family goals that are attainable for everyone: Drink more water today, eat an apple today instead of a cookie, or move your body 5 minutes more today than yesterday. Keeping it simple can go a long way to improving your health, shrinking your waistline, and building family bonds.

6. In the bottom of each cup, layer ¼ slice Canadian bacon, 1 slice pepperoni, ¼ slice provolone, ¼ slice salami, and 1 tablespoon pizza sauce. Repeat the layering.

7. Top each cup with a scant teaspoon of the mozzarella and 2 pepperoncini slices.

8. Bake for 15 minutes and serve warm.

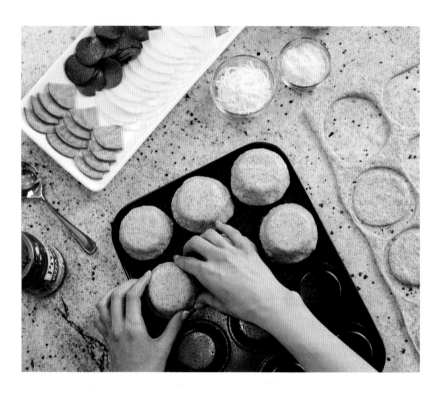

Calories 420 • Fat 19g • Carbohydrate 40g • Fiber 4g • Sugar 10g • Protein 22g

Slow-Cooker Chili Peach Glazed Pork Tenderloin

Growing up, I was taught to "waste not, want not." In other words, find ways to use everything you have for something; don't waste it. So creating sauces and gravies with the juices cooking off the meats I prepare is a skill I learned and have honed over the years. The sauce that cooks up from the pork in this dish is my favorite part of the supper. There is just something about the way the peach juice blends with the brown sugar and forms a glaze that coats this pork tenderloin to perfection.

Prep Time: 10 minutes | **Cook Time:** 2½ to 3 hours on high or 5 to 6 hours on low
Serves: 6 | **Serving Size:** 4 ounces pork, 2½ tablespoons sauce, and 3 peach slices

1½ pounds pork tenderloin, trimmed of fat

3 tablespoons brown sugar

2 teaspoons chili powder

½ teaspoon kosher salt

½ teaspoon black pepper

1 teaspoon extra virgin olive oil

1 (14.5-ounce) can no-sugar-added sliced peaches (I like Del Monte)

¼ cup no-sugar-added peach preserves (I like Smucker's)

1 cup low-sodium chicken broth (I like Pacific Organic)

1 tablespoon cornstarch

1. Coat the liner of a slow cooker with cooking spray.

2. Pat the tenderloin dry with a paper towel to remove excess moisture.

3. Using a shallow baking dish as a work surface, generously rub the meat with 2 tablespoons of the brown sugar, the chili powder, salt, and pepper.

4. In a large skillet, heat the olive oil over medium-high heat. Add the pork tenderloin and sear for 1 to 2 minutes on each side and repeat until all sides are seared.

5. Reserving the juice, drain the peach slices. Add the peaches to the slow cooker. Arrange the seared pork tenderloin on top of the peaches.

6. In a medium bowl, whisk together the reserved peach juice, peach preserves, and chicken broth. Pour the peach mixture into the slow cooker. Cover and cook on high heat for 2¹/2 to 3 hours or on low heat for 5 to 6 hours, or until the

(recipe continues)

(recipe continued from page 177)

quick and easy: **For best results when searing: Take the meat from the refrigerator and set it out at room temperature for just a few minutes before searing it. Using clean hands and paper towels, pat the roast dry to remove as much moisture as possible. Make sure the pan that will be used for searing is hot, then sear the meat as directed in the recipe for a delicious and flavorful roast!**

internal temperature in the thickest part of the pork reaches 145°F.

7. Remove the pork from the slow cooker and allow to rest for 5 minutes. Spoon the peaches from the slow cooker onto a plate and set aside.

8. In a small bowl, dissolve the cornstarch in 1 tablespoon of cold water to make a slurry. Pour the liquid from the slow cooker into a small saucepan and add the slurry and the remaining 1 tablespoon brown sugar. Whisk the sauce over medium-high heat until it thickens to a glaze, 2 to 3 minutes.

9. Slice the pork into medallions and serve with the peach glaze and cooked peaches.

Suggested Side Dish: Southern Sweet Beets (page 296)

no slow cooker, no problem: **Add the seasoned and seared pork tenderloin, peaches, and prepared peach mixture to a large pot or Dutch oven and cook over low heat for 3 to 4 hours, or until the internal temperature in the thickest part of the pork reaches 145°F. Remove the pork and continue as directed.**

Calories 186 • Fat 3g • Carbohydrate 15g • Fiber 2g • Sugar 10g • Protein 24g

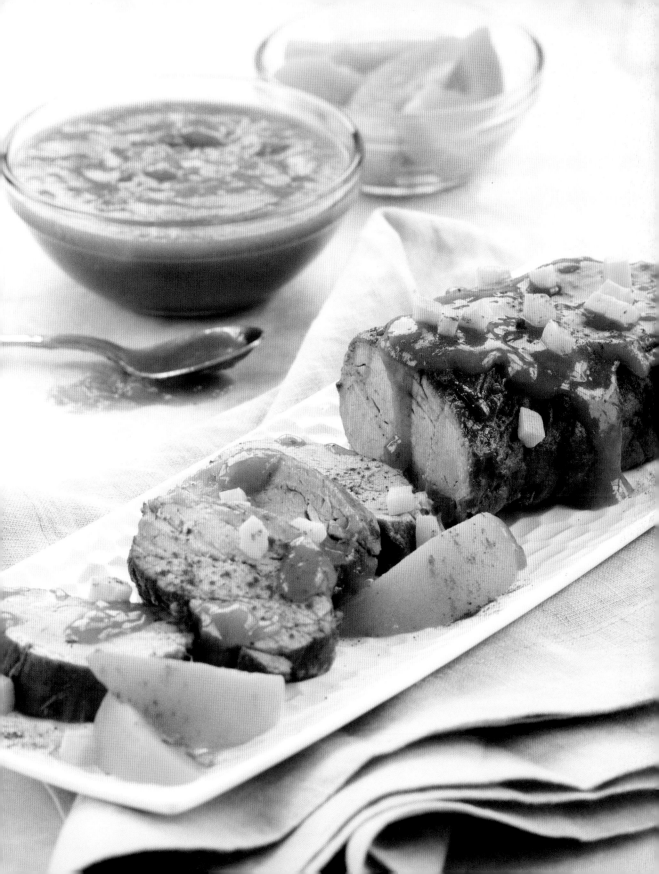

Slow-Cooker BBQ Pulled Pork Quesadillas

This recipe was inspired by my uncle, a celebrity in my hometown as the master of the best BBQ. At local festivals and family gatherings, he served up the best pulled pork I had ever tasted. Although he never released his secret recipe, I learned one thing from him growing up: It's all about the rub. Here, I combine my very own Tex-Mex rub with the tried-and-true method for the juiciest pulled pork—slow cooking.

Prep Time: 10 minutes | **Cook Time:** 4 hours on high or 8 hours on low, plus 10 minutes
Serves: 8 | **Serving Size:** 1 quesadilla, ½ tablespoon light sour cream

Rub:

1 tablespoon brown sugar

1 tablespoon chili powder

1 tablespoon minced garlic

2 teaspoons kosher salt

1 teaspoon ground cumin

1 teaspoon paprika

Pulled Pork:

1 medium onion, thinly sliced

1 cup low-sodium chicken broth
(I like Pacific Organic)

2¼ pounds boneless center-cut
pork loin roast, trimmed of fat

1 cup Stubb's Original All-Natural
Bar-B-Q Sauce

Quesadillas:

8 large low-carb, high-fiber
whole wheat tortillas
(I like La Tortilla Factory)

½ cup shredded reduced-fat
four-cheese Mexican blend
(I like Sargento)

¼ cup light sour cream

2 tablespoons chopped
fresh cilantro

1. To make the rub: In a bowl, whisk together the brown sugar, chili powder, garlic, salt, cumin, and paprika.

2. To make the pulled pork: Coat the liner of a slow cooker with cooking spray. Place the onion in the bottom of the slow cooker. Pour the chicken broth over the onion to cover.

3. Using paper towels, pat the pork loin roast to remove any moisture. With clean hands, rub the spice mixture generously over the pork loin roast to cover completely.

4. Place the pork loin roast on top of the sliced onion in the slow cooker. Cover and cook for 8 hours on low heat or 4 hours on high heat, until the pork easily shreds.

5. Remove the pork from the slow cooker and set on a cutting board. Strain the cooking liquid from the slow cooker through a fine-mesh strainer set over a large bowl (discard the solids).

6. Shred the cooked pork and return it to the slow cooker.

no slow cooker, no problem: Place the onion, chicken broth, and seasoned pork loin roast into the bottom of a large pot or Dutch oven and cook over low heat for 3 to 4 hours until the internal temperature reaches 145°F and the pork is fork-tender. Remove the pork and continue as directed.

7. Add the barbecue sauce to the slow cooker along with enough of the reserved strained cooking liquid to moisten the pork, 1/4 to 1/2 cup. Mix gently to evenly coat the pork.

8. To make the quesadillas: Preheat an indoor grill, grill pan, or panini maker to medium-high heat. Generously coat with cooking spray.

9. Spoon a heaping 1/2 cup pulled pork evenly onto 1 half of each tortilla. Top the pork with 1 tablespoon cheese. Fold the tortillas in half, pressing gently to seal.

10. Place the quesadillas on the indoor grill, grill pan, or panini maker and cook the quesadillas for 2 to 3 minutes on each side until golden brown.

11. To serve, cut each quesadilla in half and garnish with 1/2 tablespoon sour cream and some chopped cilantro.

Suggested Side Dish: Sweet and Spicy Coleslaw (page 287)

suppertime chat: Play a little game called "Guess what makes me happy?" Each person takes turns guessing what makes their family members happy. It's a playful way to learn about the "little things" that make your family members smile.

Calories 332 • **Fat** 11g • **Carbohydrate** 28g • **Fiber** 13g • **Sugar** 8g • **Protein** 51g

Spicy Cashew Pork Stir-Fry

This stir-fry emerged from needing to lighten up one of my favorite guilty pleasures from a restaurant in Cincinnati. This modified recipe is delicious, but much lighter in fat and calories. The standout element is definitely the all-original sauce. It's hard to find a stir-fry sauce that has just the right combination of sweet and tangy without all the added sodium, but this blend does the trick!

Prep Time: 10 minutes, plus 30 minutes marinating time │ **Cook Time:** 25 minutes
Serves: 6 │ **Serving Size:** Heaping 1 cup

Pork and Marinade:

1 tablespoon cornstarch

2 tablespoons rice vinegar

1½ tablespoons less-sodium soy sauce

1 pound pork tenderloin, cut into 1-inch pieces

Sauce:

1 tablespoon cornstarch

⅓ cup Tropicana Trop50 orange juice

3 tablespoons less-sodium soy sauce

2 tablespoons rice vinegar

1 tablespoon Stubb's Original All-Natural Bar-B-Q Sauce

½ teaspoon red pepper flakes

½ teaspoon ground ginger

1 tablespoon sugar-free maple-flavor syrup (I like Maple Grove Farms)

Stir-Fry:

1 tablespoon sesame oil

1 tablespoon minced garlic

(ingredients continue)

1. To marinate the pork: In a small bowl, whisk together the cornstarch, vinegar, and soy sauce. Place the pork pieces in a large resealable bag, cover with the marinade, and refrigerate for at least 30 minutes and up to 2 hours.

2. To make the sauce: In a small saucepan, dissolve the cornstarch in the orange juice. Cook over medium-high heat, whisking constantly, for 1 minute. Reduce the heat to low and stir in the soy sauce, vinegar, barbecue sauce, pepper flakes, ginger, and syrup. Cook, stirring, for 2 to 3 minutes. Remove from the heat and set aside.

3. To make the stir-fry: In a wok or large skillet, heat ½ tablespoon of the sesame oil over high heat. Add the garlic and cook until softened, 1 to 2 minutes. Add the frozen vegetables and cook until softened, 6 to 8 minutes. Remove the cooked vegetables from the wok and set aside.

4. Return the wok to high heat and add the remaining ½ tablespoon sesame oil. Remove the pork from the marinade and cook until cooked through, 8 to 10 minutes. (Discard any remaining marinade.) Reduce the heat to low, return the vegetables to the pan, and add the cashews, stirring well to combine.

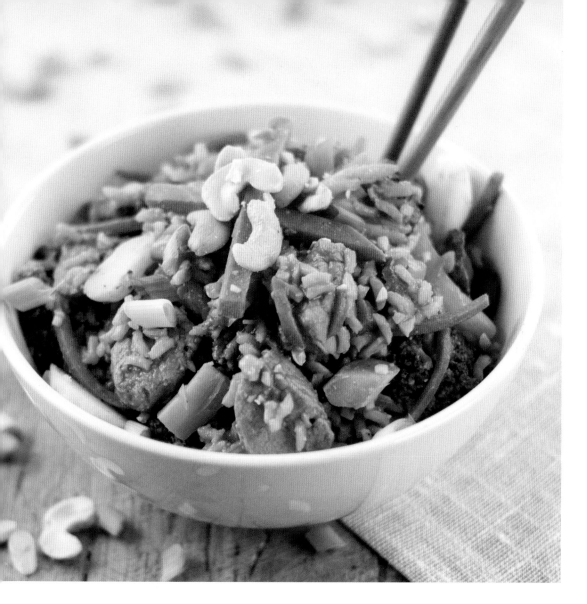

5. Microwave the rice according to the package directions. Add the cooked rice to the wok with the pork and vegetables.

6. Add the reserved sauce to the pan and gently stir to evenly coat the ingredients. Simmer over low heat for 2 to 3 minutes.

7. Serve garnished with the green onions.

2 (14-ounce) bags frozen broccoli stir-fry mix

½ cup raw cashews, coarsely chopped

1 (8.8-ounce) pouch Uncle Ben's Ready Rice brown rice

3 green onions, thinly sliced

Calories 293 · Fat 10g · Carbohydrate 29g · Fiber 5g · Sugar 5g · Protein 22g

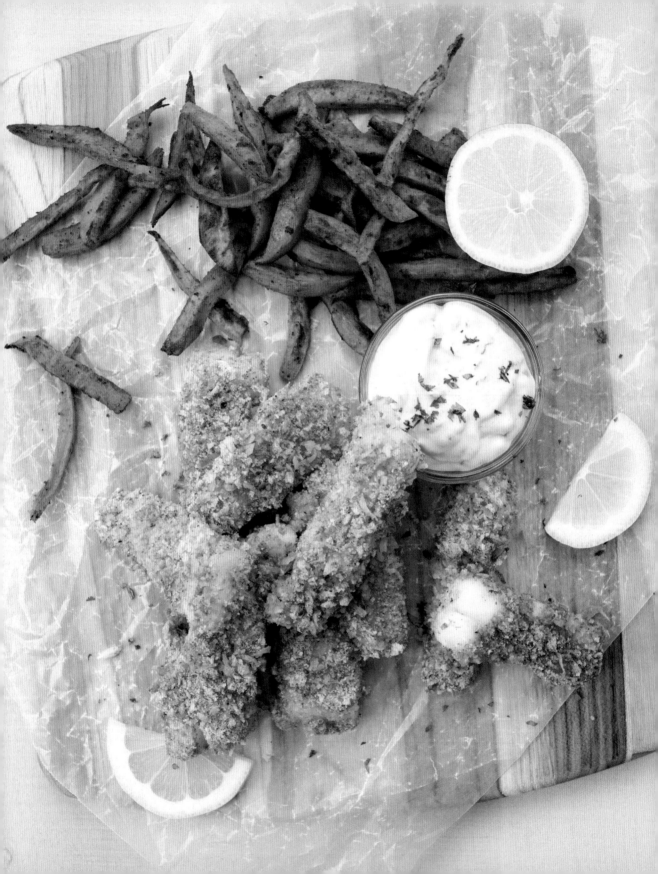

Shrimp and Sausage Jambalaya

This recipe is a tribute to my dad. Back in 2005, shortly after Hurricane Katrina, he felt the call to serve in Louisiana, helping out any way he could. During his short stay there, he fell in love with the authentic foods of the bayou, specifically the hallmark of Creole cuisine: jambalaya. Since true Creole foods are difficult to come by in Kentucky, I decided to create a jambalaya just for him. It packs a little heat (which my dad loves), and I call him up every time I make it.

Prep Time: 10 minutes | **Cook Time:** 20 minutes
Serves: 6 | **Serving Size:** Heaping 1¾ cups

2 teaspoons extra virgin olive oil

1 small onion, diced

1 green bell pepper, diced

3 stalks celery, chopped

1 tablespoon minced garlic

2 (14.5-ounce) cans no-salt-added diced tomatoes (I like Hunt's)

3 cups low-sodium chicken broth (I like Pacific Organic)

1 (6-ounce) can tomato paste

1 tablespoon Old Bay seasoning

1½ teaspoons salt

½ teaspoon Frank's RedHot Sauce

¼ teaspoon cayenne pepper

¼ teaspoon dried thyme

¼ teaspoon black pepper

3 links Al Fresco andouille-style chicken sausage, cut into 1-inch slices

1½ pounds medium shrimp (about 60), peeled and deveined

1 (8.8-ounce) pouch Uncle Ben's Ready Rice brown rice

3 green onions, thinly sliced

¼ cup chopped fresh parsley

1. In a large soup pot or Dutch oven, heat the olive oil over medium-high heat. Add the onion, bell pepper, celery, and garlic. Cook until the onion is translucent and the vegetables have softened, 8 to 10 minutes.

2. Add the diced tomatoes, chicken broth, and tomato paste. Stir to mix well. Season with the Old Bay, salt, hot sauce, cayenne, thyme, and black pepper. Bring the mixture to a boil, then reduce the heat to medium-low and simmer for 3 to 5 minutes.

3. Add the chicken sausage, shrimp, and rice to the pan and gently stir to combine. Simmer until the shrimp are cooked through and the rice has softened, 5 to 7 minutes longer.

4. To serve, ladle the jambalaya into bowls. Garnish with the green onions and parsley.

Suggested Side Dish: Cheesy Jalapeño Cornbread (page 270)

quick and easy: Feel free to modify the spices to your liking. Remember, you can add spice later, but you can't take it away.

Calories 317 • Fat 7g • Carbohydrate 34g • Fiber 7g • Sugar 10g • Protein 29g

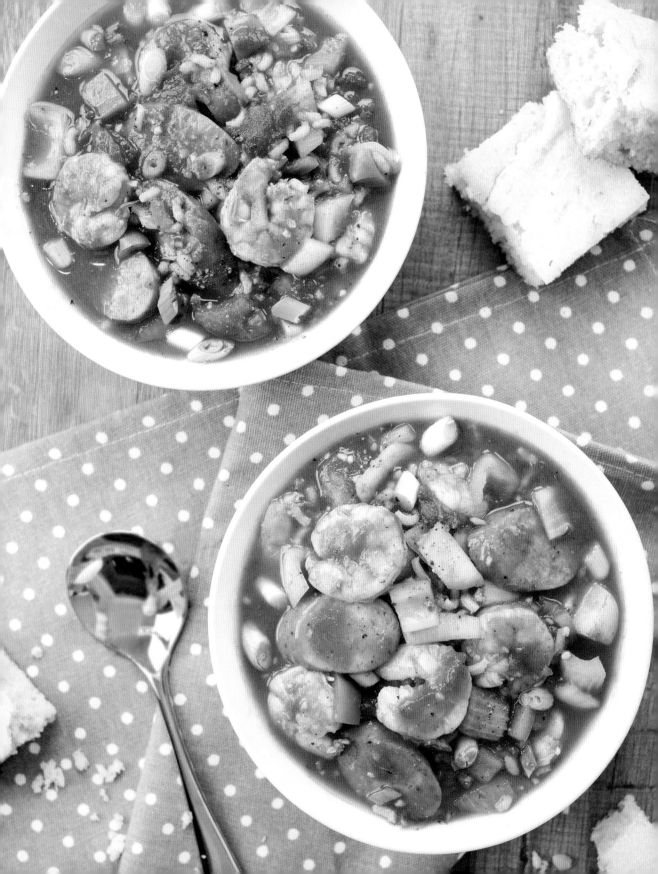

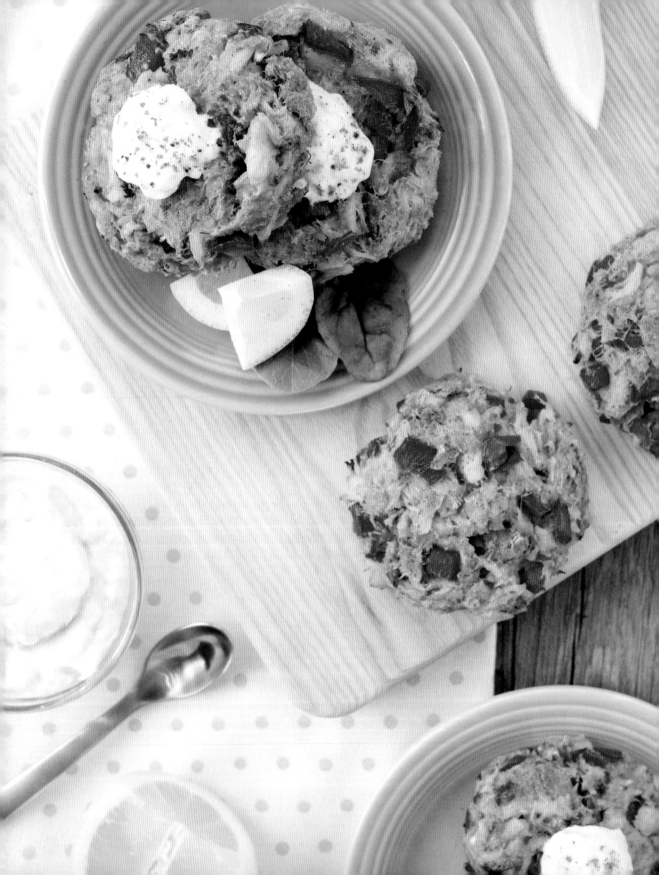

Baked Lump Crab Cakes

The last time I prepared this dish, my son overheard me say "crab cakes for dinner," and he thought I planned to cook his pet hermit crab, Hermie. I quickly assured him Hermie would never ever be dinner! While I don't want you to cook your kid's Hermie, I do want you to use real crabmeat to craft the perfect, restaurant-quality cake!

Prep Time: 10 minutes, plus 1 hour chilling time | **Cook Time:** 15 minutes
Serves: 4 | **Serving Size:** 2 crab cakes, 1 tablespoon tartar sauce

Crab Cakes:

3 green onions, thinly sliced

1 red bell pepper, diced

¼ cup plain bread crumbs

½ cup crushed whole wheat Ritz Crackers (about 13)

1 egg

2 egg whites

2 tablespoons light mayonnaise

1 teaspoon Worcestershire sauce

1 teaspoon garlic powder

1 tablespoon Old Bay seasoning

1 teaspoon grated lemon zest

½ teaspoon salt

½ teaspoon black pepper

1½ pounds jumbo lump crabmeat, picked over for shells

Quick Tartar Sauce:

2 tablespoons light mayonnaise

2 tablespoons plain 0% Greek yogurt

1 tablespoon no-sugar-added sweet relish

1 teaspoon Dijon mustard

¼ teaspoon onion powder

Pinch each of salt and black pepper

1. To make the crab cakes: At least 1 hour before baking, in a large bowl, combine the green onions, bell pepper, bread crumbs, crushed crackers, whole egg, egg whites, mayonnaise, Worcestershire sauce, garlic powder, Old Bay, lemon zest, salt, and black pepper. Mix well, then fold in the crabmeat. Gently shape into 8 cakes, about ¾ cup mixture each.

2. Line a plate with parchment paper. Transfer the crab cakes to the lined plate and refrigerate until chilled, at least 1 hour.

3. Meanwhile, to make the tartar sauce: In a small bowl, whisk together the mayonnaise, yogurt, relish, mustard, onion powder, salt, and pepper until well combined. Refrigerate until ready to serve.

4. Preheat the oven to 400°F. Coat a baking sheet with cooking spray.

5. Transfer the crab cakes to the baking sheet and bake until golden brown, 12 to 15 minutes per side.

6. Serve the crab cakes with the tartar sauce.

Suggested Side Dish: The Creamiest Mac 'n' Cheese Dish You Will Ever Make (page 264)

Calories 311 • Fat 10g • Carbohydrate 17g • Fiber 1g • Sugar 3g • Protein 36g

Blackened Fish Tacos with Cilantro-Lime Slaw

I first fell in love with fish tacos years ago on an annual family vacation to Destin, Florida. We would head down to one of those little unpretentious places right on the beach; you know the ones—wooden walls, wooden floors, metal tables and chairs, and a wall of windows that overlooks the ocean. I've re-created this summer memory, but added a little flair with my vibrant, tangy slaw.

Prep Time: 10 minutes | **Cook Time:** 10 minutes
Serves: 4 | **Serving Size:** 2 tacos

Cilantro-Lime Slaw:

1 (10-ounce) bag shredded red cabbage

½ red onion, thinly sliced

2 tablespoons chopped fresh cilantro

1 tablespoon rice vinegar

3 tablespoons light mayonnaise

1 teaspoon sugar-free maple-flavor syrup (I like Maple Grove Farms)

2 tablespoons lime juice

⅛ teaspoon salt

Avocado-Chile Sauce:

½ avocado

2 tablespoons plain 0% Greek yogurt

3 tablespoons chopped canned green chilies

1 tablespoon chopped fresh cilantro

1 teaspoon lime juice

¼ teaspoon salt

Pinch of black pepper

(ingredients continue)

1. To make the cilantro-lime slaw: In a medium bowl, combine the cabbage, onion, and cilantro. In a small bowl, whisk together the vinegar, mayonnaise, syrup, lime juice, and salt. Pour over the slaw and gently toss with tongs.

2. To make the avocado-chile sauce: In a food processor or blender, combine the avocado, Greek yogurt, green chilies, cilantro, lime juice, salt, and black pepper and pulse or blend.

3. To cook the fish tacos: In a small shallow dish, mix together the blackened seasoning and brown sugar. Sprinkle the seasoning onto both sides of the fish.

4. In a large skillet, heat the olive oil over medium-high heat. Add the fish and cook on both sides for 4 to 5 minutes, or until the outside is blackened and the fish flakes apart easily. Set aside.

5. Wipe the skillet clean and heat each tortilla in the skillet over high heat, about 30 seconds on each side.

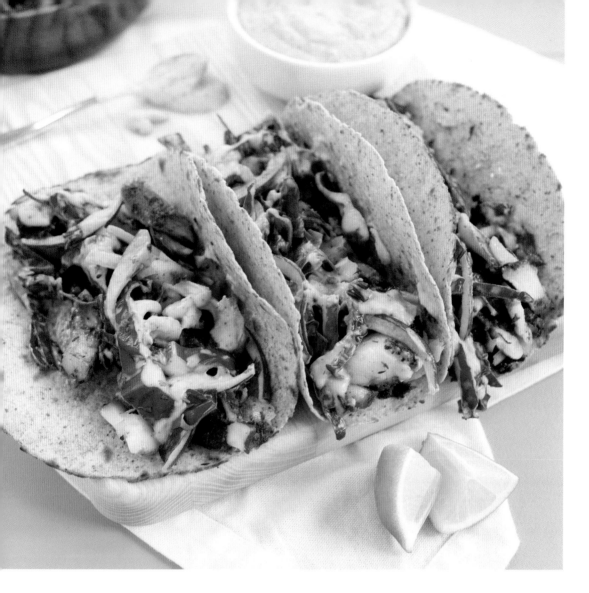

6. Assemble the tacos by filling each tortilla with 2 pieces of fish, ½ cup slaw, and 2 tablespoons avocado-chile sauce.

suppertime inspiration: Regularly planning and preparing healthy meals can be quite a stretch with my busy schedule, even though it's just the two of us. A great quote that I discovered a few years ago is "When you feel like quitting, think about why you started." It's a powerful way to get reenergized and refocused.

Fish Tacos:

3 tablespoons blackened seasoning

½ teaspoon light brown sugar

1 pound lean white fish fillets, such as cod, halibut, or flounder, cut into 1-inch strips

2 teaspoons extra virgin olive oil

8 mini whole wheat tortillas (I like La Tortilla Factory)

Calories 307 • Fat 12g • Carbohydrate 30g • Fiber 16g • Sugar 5g • Protein 28g

Pistachio-Crusted Salmon

The unique blend of ground pistachios, bread crumbs, butter, and brown sugar gives this flaky salmon a sweet and salty coating that is out-of-this-world delicious!

Prep Time: 10 minutes │ **Cook Time:** 20 minutes
Serves: 4 │ **Serving Size:** 1 fillet

3 tablespoons sugar-free maple-flavor syrup (I like Maple Grove Farms)

2 teaspoons sriracha sauce

¼ cup pistachios

1 teaspoon extra virgin olive oil

¼ cup panko bread crumbs

1 teaspoon light brown sugar

4 (4-ounce) salmon fillets

skinny sense: Pistachios contain fewer calories and more potassium and vitamin K per serving than other nuts. A 1-ounce serving of dry-roasted pistachios contains 160 calories, 6 grams of protein, 3 grams of fiber, and 15 grams of fat, including only 2 grams of saturated fat. Now that's a healthy nut!

1. Preheat the oven to 375°F. Line a baking sheet with foil and coat with cooking spray.

2. In a medium bowl, mix together the syrup and sriracha. Set aside.

3. In a food processor, pulse the pistachios 1 to 2 times, until crushed. Add the olive oil, panko, and brown sugar. Pulse 3 to 4 more times, until the mixture is crumbly.

4. Place the salmon fillets skin side down on the foil-lined baking sheet. Evenly spoon the syrup mixture over the top of the salmon fillets. Evenly distribute the pistachio crumble among the fillets and lightly press down to adhere.

5. Bake until the internal temperature reaches 145°F, 15 to 20 minutes (the bake time will depend on the thickness of the fillets).

Suggested Side Dish: Quick Cauliflower Couscous (page 286)

Calories 196 • **Fat** 8g • **Carbohydrate** 6g • **Fiber** 0g • **Sugar** 2g • **Protein** 24g

Dijon Baked Tilapia

I've had many tilapia fails over the years, so creating this little masterpiece has inspired me to never give up. Working with tilapia is interesting because it's such a mild fish; it takes just the right seasoning to give it the flair I'm looking for. Wedges of Laughing Cow cheese provide the perfect binder for the bread crumbs and add sharp contrast in flavor to the lemon-pepper foundation. It's a burst of lemon-pepper heaven right in your mouth!

Prep Time: 10 minutes │ **Cook Time:** 15 minutes
Serves: 6 │ **Serving Size:** 1 fillet

6 (4-ounce) tilapia fillets

1 tablespoon lemon-pepper seasoning

3 wedges Laughing Cow Creamy Swiss Light cheese

1 tablespoon Dijon mustard

1 tablespoon unsalted butter

¾ cup panko bread crumbs

3 tablespoons grated Parmesan cheese (I like Sargento)

suppertime chat: Have you ever persevered in school or in a sport when you wanted to give up? How did it make you feel to "stick with it"? What does that teach you about when times get tough?

1. Preheat the oven to 375°F. Line a baking sheet with foil and coat with cooking spray.

2. Use paper towels to blot the tilapia fillets to remove any excess moisture. Sprinkle the tops of the fillets with the lemon-pepper seasoning.

3. Gently spread the cheese wedges evenly over all of the fillets using the back of a spoon. Evenly spread the mustard over the cheese.

4. In a microwave-safe bowl, melt the butter in the microwave. Add the bread crumbs and Parmesan to the bowl and gently stir together to moisten the bread crumbs.

5. Gently press the bread crumb mixture onto the tops of the fillets.

6. Transfer the fillets to the prepared baking sheet. Bake until golden brown and the fish flakes easily with a fork, 10 to 15 minutes.

Suggested Side Dish: Italian Chickpea Salad (page 278)

Calories 174 • **Fat** 5g • **Carbohydrate** 6g • **Fiber** 0g • **Sugar** 1g • **Protein** 25g

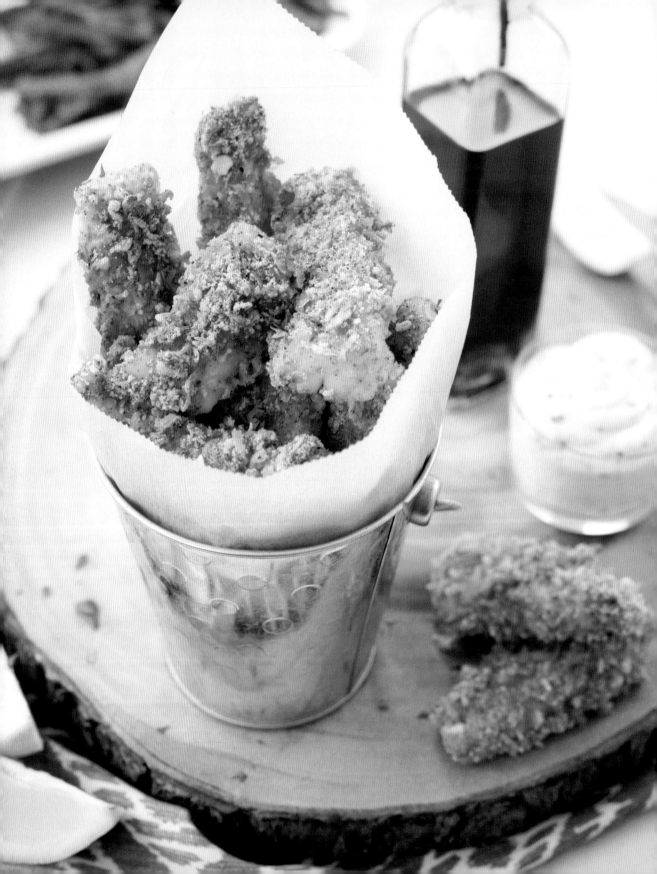

Crispy Coconut Fish Sticks

I hear from a lot of moms who say the only kind of fish they can get their kids to eat is frozen fish sticks (yours truly included). This recipe allows you to continue serving up fun finger food without stopping by the freezer aisle. The crunchy, flaky coating created by the panko bread crumbs and coconut flakes provides just the right texture. Pair these fish sticks with some fresh fruit and pat yourself on the back for a job well done!

Prep Time: 30 minutes | **Cook Time:** 20 minutes
Serves: 6 | **Serving Size:** 4 fish sticks

1 pound lean white fish fillets, such as cod, flounder, or halibut, cut into 3 x 1-inch strips (see Quick and Easy)

1 (13.5-ounce) can lite coconut milk (I like Thai Kitchen)

¾ cup plain bread crumbs

½ cup panko bread crumbs

½ cup sweetened coconut flakes

2 teaspoons chili powder

½ teaspoon salt

½ teaspoon black pepper

Optional Ingredients:

Malt vinegar

Quick Tartar Sauce (from Baked Lump Crab Cakes, page 189)

quick and easy: Be accurate and consistent when cutting fish for fish sticks. Uniform size is the key to fish cooking evenly.

1. Preheat the oven to 400°F. Coat a baking sheet with cooking spray.

2. Place the fish in a large bowl and cover with the coconut milk. Allow the fish to marinate in the coconut milk for 20 minutes in the refrigerator.

3. In a shallow bowl, combine the plain bread crumbs, panko, coconut flakes, chili powder, salt, and pepper.

4. After the fish has marinated, dip each piece of fish into the bread crumb mixture to cover evenly. Arrange the fish on the prepared baking sheet.

5. Bake on one side for 8 to 10 minutes and then flip over. Bake the fish until it starts to brown and is cooked through, 8 to 10 minutes longer.

6. If desired, serve with malt vinegar and tartar sauce.

Suggested Side Dish: Cajun-Style Sweet Potato Fries (page 267)

Calories 213 • **Fat** 8g • **Carbohydrate** 21g • **Fiber** 2g • **Sugar** 5g • **Protein** 16g
Nutrition does not include optional ingredients.

Easy Asian Salmon with Orange Sweet Glaze

This is by far the best salmon I have ever prepared! Utilizing the marinade and other juices that cook out from the salmon, you can create a sweet orange glaze that is phenomenal. To top that, the salmon gets marinated in the baking dish, so it literally goes from refrigerator to oven.

Prep Time: 10 minutes, plus 30 minutes to 1 hour marinating time | **Cook Time:** 22 minutes
Serves: 4 | **Serving Size:** 1 salmon fillet, 2 tablespoons orange glaze

¼ cup sugar-free maple-flavor syrup (I like Maple Grove Farms)

2 tablespoons less-sodium soy sauce

1 tablespoon brown sugar

1 tablespoon sesame oil

1 tablespoon rice vinegar

½ teaspoon garlic powder

2 teaspoons sriracha sauce

½ teaspoon ground ginger

4 (4-ounce) salmon fillets

1 teaspoon cornstarch

¼ cup Tropicana Trop50 orange juice

1 teaspoon sesame seeds

3 green onions, thinly sliced

1. Coat a 13 x 9-inch baking dish with cooking spray.

2. In a small bowl, whisk together the syrup, soy sauce, brown sugar, sesame oil, vinegar, garlic powder, sriracha, and ginger.

3. Place the salmon fillets skin side down in the baking dish. Using a knife, gently cut 3 shallow slits into the tops of the salmon fillets to seal in the marinade flavor. Pour the marinade evenly over the salmon. Cover the dish with foil and refrigerate for at least 30 minutes and up to 1 hour.

4. Preheat the oven to 375°F.

5. Remove the salmon from the refrigerator and bake covered for 8 minutes. Uncover and bake until it flakes easily with a fork, 5 to 7 minutes longer (the baking time will depend on the thickness of the salmon).

6. Transfer the salmon to a plate, reserving the cooking juices and marinade in the baking dish.

7. In a small saucepan, dissolve the cornstarch in the orange juice. Whisk constantly over medium-high heat for 1 minute. Add the reserved juices from the baking dish. Bring to a boil, then immediately reduce the heat to medium-low, and cook, continuing to whisk, until the sauce thickens to a glaze, 2 to 3 minutes.

8. Serve the salmon fillets with the orange glaze. Garnish with the sesame seeds and green onions.

Suggested Side Dish: Mango Slaw (page 281)

suppertime chat: If you could start your own restaurant, what type of food would you serve and why? Who knows, maybe there's an entrepreneur in the making in your house. Did you know that Subway was founded by a seventeen-year-old who thought he'd open a small "sub shop" for a few years to earn money for medical school?

Calories 210 • **Fat** 9g • **Carbohydrate** 8g • **Fiber** 0g • **Sugar** 5g • **Protein** 24g

Greek-Style Crab-Stuffed Portobello Mushrooms

This recipe is full of yummy Greek flavors and it is oh so colorful. When purchasing portobellos, look for a firm, plump mushroom with a pleasant smell. That will ensure the perfect nest for the crab stuffing!

Prep Time: 10 minutes | **Cook Time:** 25 minutes
Serves: 6 | **Serving Size:** 1 stuffed mushroom

1 cup quinoa, rinsed

2 cups low-sodium chicken broth (I like Pacific Organic)

1 tablespoon extra virgin olive oil

½ cup frozen chopped spinach, thawed and drained

½ red bell pepper, diced

1 teaspoon minced garlic

½ cup diced red onion

½ cup canned chickpeas, drained and rinsed

½ teaspoon salt

¼ teaspoon black pepper

1 pound lump crabmeat, picked over for shells

¼ cup reduced-fat feta cheese crumbles

½ cup Kalamata olives, finely chopped

2 teaspoons fresh dill

1 tablespoon lemon juice

6 large (5-inch diameter) portobello mushrooms, stems and gills removed (see Quick and Easy)

3 tablespoons grated Parmesan cheese (I like Sargento)

3 tablespoons plain 0% Greek yogurt (optional)

1. Preheat the oven to 350°F. Coat a baking sheet with cooking spray.

2. In a medium saucepan, combine the quinoa and chicken broth and bring to a boil. When it comes to a boil, cover, reduce the heat to medium-low, and simmer until the seeds are translucent and have "spiraled out," 10 to 15 minutes. Uncover and set aside.

3. In a medium skillet, heat ½ tablespoon of the olive oil over medium-high heat. Add the spinach, bell pepper, garlic, and onion. Cook until soft, 5 to 7 minutes. Add the chickpeas and season with ¼ teaspoon of the salt and the pepper. Sauté for an additional minute.

4. In a large bowl, combine the cooked quinoa, crabmeat, sautéed vegetables, feta, olives, dill, lemon juice, and remaining ½ tablespoon olive oil and ¼ teaspoon salt. Gently fold the ingredients together until well combined.

5. Place the mushrooms stem side up on the baking sheet. Fill each mushroom with ¾ cup of the crab mixture. Sprinkle the top of each mushroom with ½ tablespoon Parmesan cheese. Bake for 12 to 15 minutes to heat through.

6. If desired, serve with ½ tablespoon Greek yogurt.

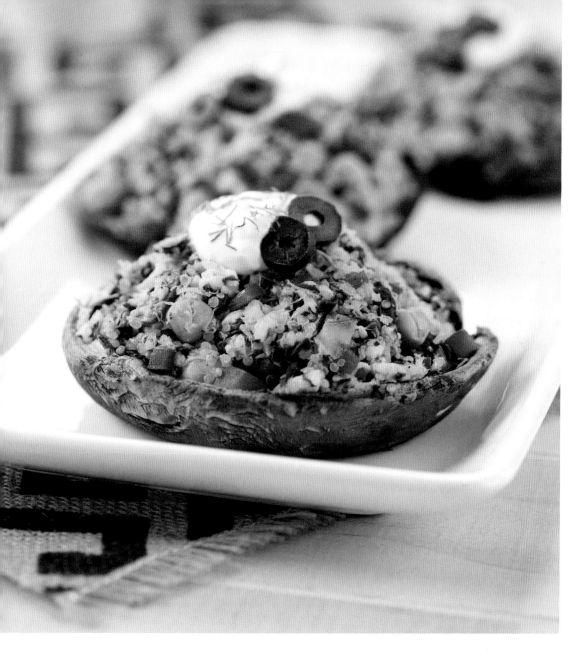

quick and easy: To remove the stems, lay the mushrooms stem side up and gently bend and pull up the stems. Discard the stems. To remove the gills, cradle the mushroom in one hand, use a spoon to gently scrape and scoop out the gills, moving all around the mushroom. Do not apply a lot of pressure, as the mushrooms are very fragile and can easily be broken. Discard the gills.

Calories 289 • **Fat** 10g • **Carbohydrate** 29g • **Fiber** 5g • **Sugar** 3g • **Protein** 16g
Nutrition does not include optional ingredient.

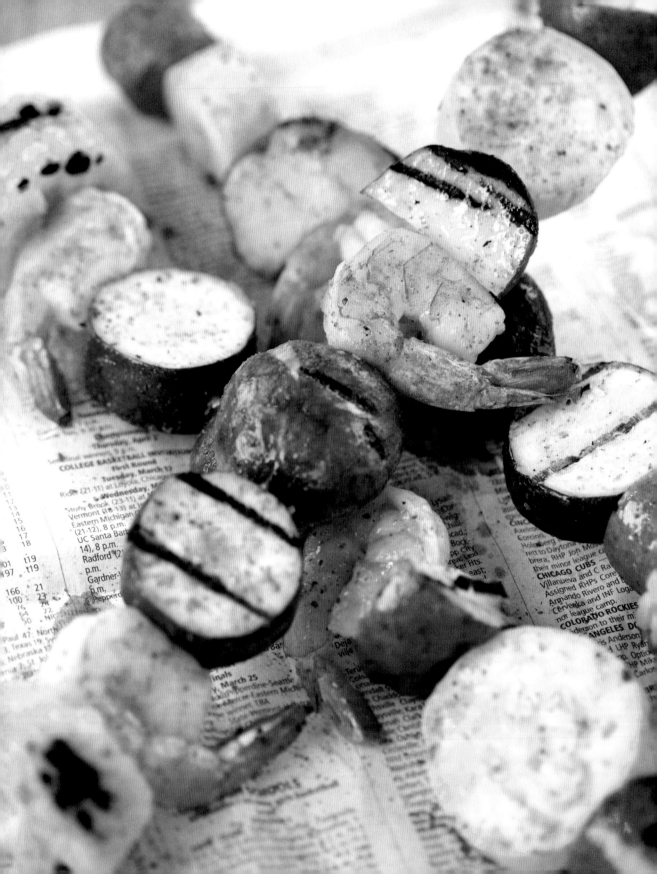

Low Country Boil Kabobs

If you're from the South, you know what "Low country boil" means. This style of cooking was made famous in the Low country, which stretches from South Carolina to the coasts of Georgia. But it definitely made its way up to Kentucky and was by far my family's favorite way to cook for summer holidays, like Memorial Day and the Fourth of July.

Prep Time: 10 minutes │ **Cook Time:** 10 minutes
Serves: 5 │ **Serving Size:** 2 kabobs

½ pound red new potatoes

2 ears of corn, cut into 2-inch sections

½ pound large shrimp (about 10), peeled and deveined

2 teaspoons Old Bay seasoning

3 links Al Fresco andouille-style chicken sausage, cut into 1-inch slices

2 medium zucchini, cut into 2-inch slices

1 (8-ounce) container baby bella (cremini) mushrooms

3 tablespoons lemon juice

1 tablespoon unsalted butter, melted

2 teaspoons Frank's RedHot Sauce

½ teaspoon garlic powder

Optional Ingredients:

5 lemon wedges

½ cup cocktail sauce

Special Equipment:

10 skewers

1. In a large pot, combine the potatoes with water to cover and bring to a boil. Boil for 6 minutes. Add the corn and continue to boil for 3 to 4 minutes longer. Drain and set aside to cool.

2. Season the shrimp with 1 teaspoon of the Old Bay.

3. Thread 10 skewers with the potatoes, shrimp, corn, sausage, zucchini, and mushrooms.

4. In a small bowl, whisk together the lemon juice, melted butter, hot sauce, garlic powder, and remaining 1 teaspoon Old Bay. Brush the mixture onto the skewers.

5. Preheat an indoor grill, grill pan, or outdoor grill to medium-high heat. Coat the grill pan or indoor grill with cooking spray. Add the skewers and cook until the shrimp are cooked through and the vegetables have grill marks, 6 to 8 minutes, turning occasionally and brushing with the remaining Old Bay mixture.

6. If desired, serve with lemon wedges and cocktail sauce.

Suggested Side Dish: Sweet and Spicy Coleslaw (page 287)

Calories 244 • Fat 8g • Carbohydrate 26g • Fiber 4g • Sugar 6g • Protein 20g
Nutrition does not include optional ingredients.

Quick Shrimp and Vegetable Stir-Fry

Stir-fries make for a fast and flexible supper. Plus, even the pickiest of eaters can be satisfied with this quick and easy dish by swapping out the shrimp for chicken, pork, steak, or more vegetables.

Prep Time: 5 minutes | **Cook Time:** 10 minutes
Servings: 4 | **Serving Size:** 1/3 cup cooked rice, 1 heaping cup stir-fry

2 teaspoons sesame oil

2 (14-ounce) bags frozen broccoli stir-fry mix

1 (8-ounce) container baby bella (cremini) mushrooms, sliced

1/2 cup low-sodium chicken broth (I like Pacific Organic)

2 tablespoons less-sodium soy sauce

1 tablespoon minced garlic

2 1/2 tablespoons rice vinegar

1 teaspoon oyster sauce

1 tablespoon light brown sugar

1/2 teaspoon ground ginger

1 tablespoon cornstarch

1 pound medium shrimp (about 40), peeled and deveined

1 (8.8-ounce) pouch Uncle Ben's Ready Rice brown rice

1/2 teaspoon sesame seeds

3 green onions, thinly sliced

1. In a wok or large skillet, heat the sesame oil over medium-high heat. Add the broccoli stir-fry mix and mushrooms. Sauté the vegetables for 5 minutes, until the vegetables have started to soften.

2. In a small bowl, whisk together the chicken broth, soy sauce, garlic, vinegar, oyster sauce, brown sugar, ginger, and cornstarch.

3. Add the shrimp to the vegetables and mix. Pour the sauce over the shrimp mixture to evenly cover, and stir frequently until the sauce has thickened and the shrimp are pink and cooked through, 3 to 5 minutes.

4. Microwave the rice according to the package directions.

5. To serve, place 1/3 cup cooked rice in the bottom of a bowl, top with a heaping 1 cup of the stir-fry mixture, and garnish with sesame seeds and green onions.

suppertime chat: Stir-fry dishes can be a fun mix of different veggies and meats. What's the craziest food combination you've eaten or made? What flavor combos do you think would be really tasty together?

Calories 196 · Fat 3g · Carbohydrate 25g · Fiber 5g · Sugar 3g · Protein 16g

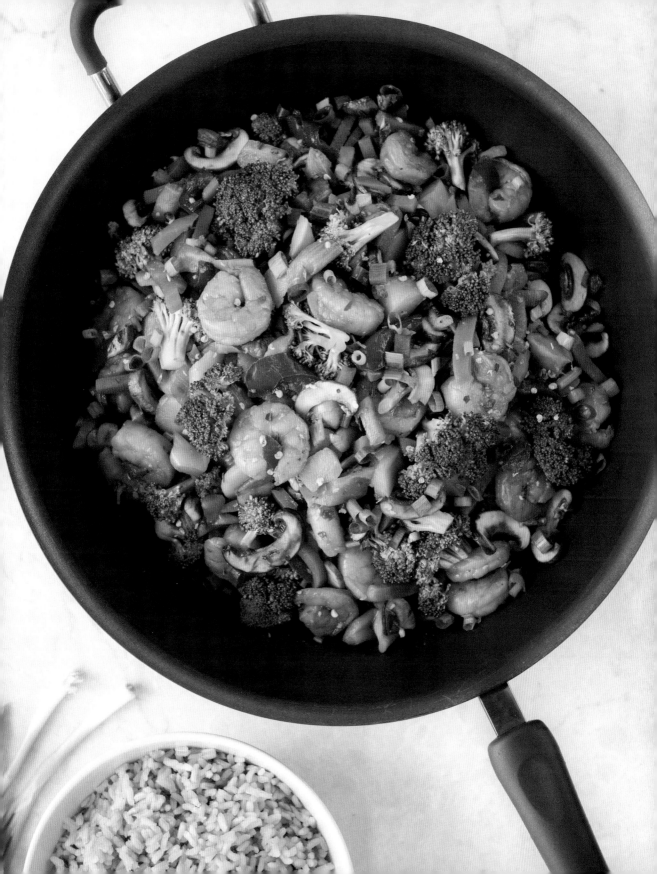

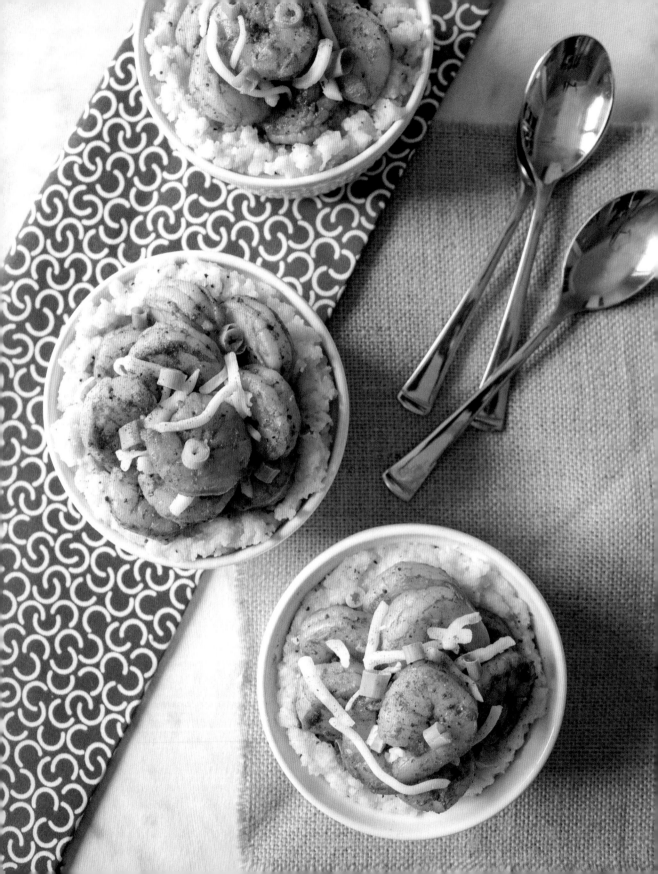

Southern Shrimp and Grits

In the South, grits are more of a dinner staple than a breakfast side dish. It wasn't until I moved up North that I noticed how often they're served for breakfast. These grits are so creamy and cheesy, you'll want to serve them up for breakfast, lunch, and dinner!

Prep Time: 5 minutes | **Cook Time:** 10 minutes
Serves: 4 | **Serving Size:** 1 cup of grits, 10 shrimp

2¼ cups low-sodium chicken broth (I like Pacific Organic)

1½ cups fat-free milk

1¼ cups Quaker Quick 5-Minute Grits

½ teaspoon salt

1 cup shredded Wisconsin sharp white cheddar cheese (I like Sargento Artisan Blends)

½ teaspoon black pepper

1 pound medium shrimp (about 40), peeled and deveined

1 tablespoon Old Bay seasoning

1 tablespoon extra virgin olive oil

2 teaspoons minced garlic

4 green onions, thinly sliced

1. In a medium saucepan, bring the chicken broth and milk to a boil. Gradually whisk in the grits and salt. Reduce the heat to medium-low, cover, and cook the grits, stirring occasionally, until they start to thicken, about 5 minutes. Remove from the heat and stir in the cheddar and pepper.

2. Put the shrimp and Old Bay in a large resealable bag. Seal the bag and give it a few shakes to evenly coat the shrimp with the seasoning.

3. In a large skillet, heat the olive oil over medium heat. Add the garlic and green onions and cook until the green onions begin to soften, 1 to 2 minutes.

4. Add the shrimp to the skillet and cook on both sides until cooked through, 3 to 5 minutes.

5. To serve, spoon 1 cup grits into a bowl and top with about 10 shrimp.

skinny sense: Do you know how shrimp get their pink color? A crazy little thing called astaxanthin! It's a carotenoid that can also act as a potent antioxidant, which protects the skin from premature aging. Do you need another reason to prepare this dish?

Calories 425 • Fat 14g • Carbohydrate 46g • Fiber 3g • Sugar 5g • Protein 31g

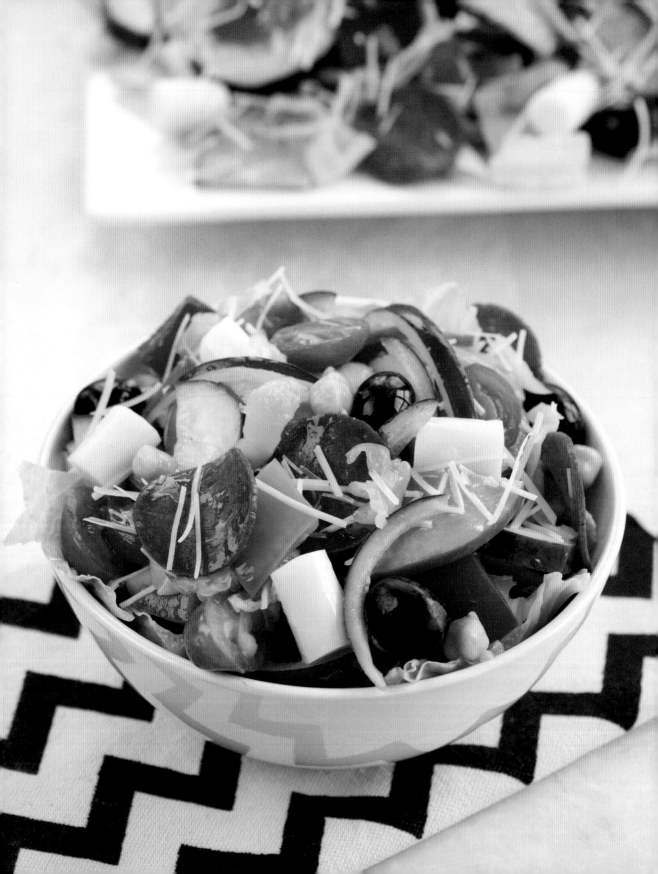

11 HEARTY ONE-BOWL MEALS
SKINNY SOUPS AND SALADS

Grilled Chicken and Fruit Salad Wraps

When you're trying to eat light, salads can become mundane and "ho-hum" quickly. Not to mention that most of us don't normally get excited about salad for dinner. Well, hold that thought! I've found a way to make salad fun *and* portable! These wraps aren't just simple, they're also the perfect solution to eating on the go without the drive-thru calories. And the unique combination of grilled chicken, avocado, and fruit is a great balance of nutrition, too: lean protein, healthy fats, and carbs.

Prep Time: 10 minutes, plus 20 minutes marinating time | **Cook Time:** 10 minutes
Serves: 6 | **Serving Size:** 1 cup salad, 1/3 cup chicken, 1 flatbread

1 pound boneless, skinless chicken breasts

1/4 cup lemon juice

1/2 teaspoon salt

1/2 teaspoon black pepper

2 cups spinach leaves

2 cups chopped romaine lettuce

12 strawberries, sliced

3/4 cup canned no-sugar-added mandarin oranges (I like Del Monte), drained

3/4 cup blueberries

1 avocado, chopped

1/3 cup sliced almonds

1/2 cup Bolthouse Farms Classic balsamic vinaigrette

6 Flatout Light Original flatbreads

1. Place the chicken breasts in a large resealable bag. Use a rolling pin to pound the chicken to about a 1/2-inch thickness. Add the lemon juice to the chicken, seal the bag, and refrigerate for 20 minutes to marinate.

2. Heat the grill pan, indoor grill, or outdoor grill to medium-high heat. Generously coat the pan or grill with cooking spray. Remove the chicken breasts from the bag and season with the salt and pepper. Cook until the internal temperature reaches 165°F, 4 to 6 minutes on each side.

3. Remove the chicken and allow to rest for 2 to 3 minutes. Cut the cooked chicken into 1-inch pieces.

4. In a large bowl, combine the spinach, romaine, strawberries, mandarin oranges, blueberries, avocado, and almonds. Pour in the balsamic dressing and toss gently to combine all of the ingredients and coat with the dressing.

(recipe continues)

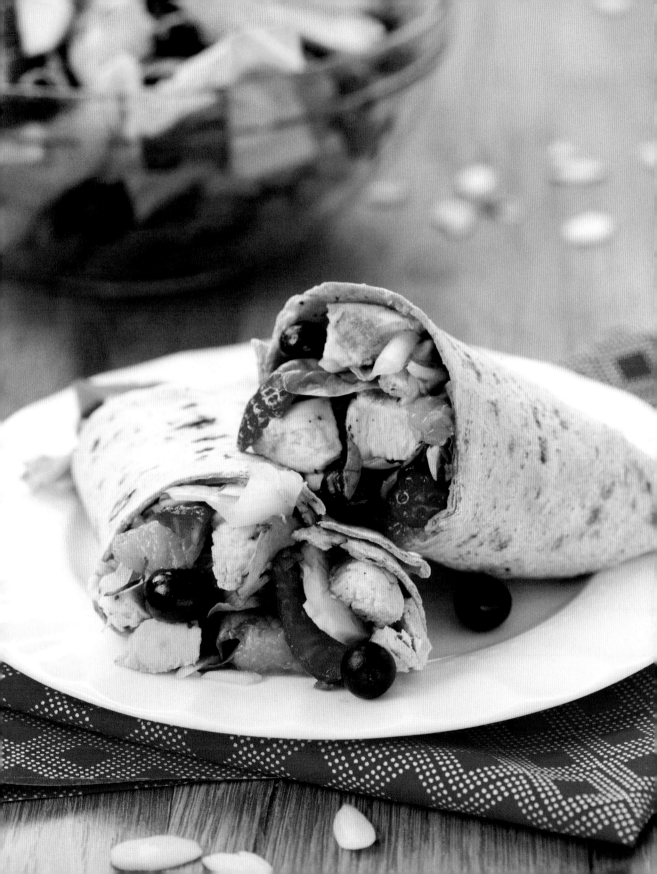

(recipe continued from page 208)

suppertime inspiration:
Feeling exhausted at the end of the day? Even though it's the last thing on your mind, a brisk walk has been proven to fight fatigue more effectively than caffeine or even a power nap. It's also a great way to model healthy behaviors for your kids.

5. To assemble, top each flatbread with a generous amount of salad (about 1 cup) across the middle, add 1/3 cup of the grilled chicken, and tightly roll the wrap. To serve, slice the wraps in half.

Suggested Side Dish: Old Bay Deviled Eggs (page 282)

suppertime chat: What makes you feel safe and secure? A personal or private space at home? In your room? Why do you think you feel safe and secure there? This is an opportunity to remind your children and yourself how important home is.

Calories 319 • Fat 13g • Carbohydrate 34g • Fiber 10g • Sugar 9g • Protein 27g

Superfood Salad

I've become a fan of the prepackaged chopped salads at my local grocery. The simplicity of the flavors and dressing all in one bag is very attractive to my busy lifestyle. That's where the inspiration for this powerhouse salad originated. But I struggled to find just the right blend of flavors and nutrients, and a dressing that I really loved. Shaving the Brussels sprouts for this salad lessens their bitterness but keeps a crunch that I love without adding a carb-dense crouton. My homemade poppy seed dressing adds a perfect punch of sweetness.

Prep Time: 10 minutes
Serves: 4 | **Serving Size:** About 2½ cups

Light Poppy Seed Dressing

¼ cup light mayonnaise

3 tablespoons apple cider vinegar

2 tablespoons sugar-free maple-flavor syrup (I like Maple Grove Farms)

1 teaspoon stevia

½ teaspoon poppy seeds

⅛ teaspoon salt

Salad:

6 cups kale, finely chopped

3 cups Brussels sprouts (about 6 large), shaved

½ cup Reduced Sugar Craisins Dried Cranberries

¼ cup raw unsalted sunflower seeds

1 large Fuji apple, thinly sliced (see Quick and Easy)

1. To make the dressing: In a small bowl, whisk together the mayonnaise, vinegar, syrup, and stevia until smooth. Whisk in the poppy seeds and salt until combined. Refrigerate until ready to serve.

2. To assemble the salad: In a large bowl, toss together the kale, shaved Brussels sprouts, Craisins, sunflower seeds, apple, and dressing.

3. Serve chilled.

quick and easy: Instead of sliced fresh apples, try this salad with apple chips that you can make at home. Start by removing the core of the apple with an apple corer and thinly slicing rings by hand or with a mandoline. Lay the rings out on a baking sheet lined with parchment paper and bake at 200˚F until dried and crispy, about 45 minutes. They're great to snack on, too!

Calories 214 • Fat 8g • Carbohydrate 36g • Fiber 10g • Sugar 14g • Protein 5g

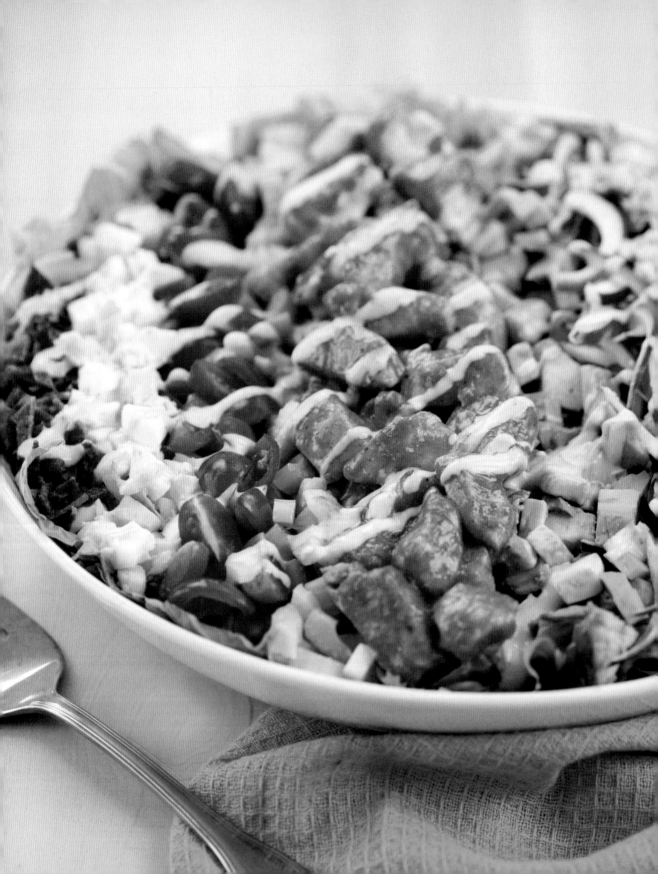

Buffalo Chicken Cobb Salad

I put hot sauce on just about everything. This recipe marries my love of salads and spicy flavor. Adding hot sauce to the ranch dressing and chicken gives this salad a little fire, but you can modify it to suit the taste buds you're feeding.

Prep Time: 10 minutes | **Cook Time:** 10 minutes
Serves: 6 | **Serving Size:** 2½ cups salad

Chicken:

½ pound boneless, skinless chicken breasts

¼ teaspoon salt

¼ teaspoon black pepper

½ tablespoon extra virgin olive oil

¼ cup Frank's RedHot Sauce

Buffalo Ranch Dressing:

½ cup Bolthouse Farms Classic Ranch Yogurt Dressing

1 tablespoon Frank's RedHot Sauce

Salad:

4 cups chopped romaine lettuce

3 cups chopped iceberg lettuce

2 hard-boiled eggs, chopped

¾ cup shredded carrots

3 stalks celery, diced

½ red onion, julienned

3 tablespoons reduced-fat blue cheese crumbles

1 avocado, chopped

4 slices turkey bacon, cooked and crumbled

1 cup halved grape tomatoes

1. To make the chicken: Cut the chicken breasts into 1-inch cubes. Season with the salt and pepper.

2. In a large skillet, heat the olive oil over medium-high heat. Add the chicken and cook, turning occasionally, until cooked through, 7 to 8 minutes. Add the hot sauce and use a spatula to stir, making sure the chicken is evenly coated. Set aside.

3. Meanwhile, to make the Buffalo ranch dressing: In a small bowl, whisk together the ranch dressing and hot sauce. Refrigerate until ready to serve.

4. To assemble the salad: In a large shallow bowl or on a large platter, combine the romaine lettuce and the iceberg lettuce. Layer the chicken pieces, chopped eggs, carrots, celery, red onion, blue cheese crumbles, avocado, turkey bacon, and grape tomatoes in neat rows over the lettuce.

5. To serve, drizzle with the dressing.

skinny sense: Hot sauce has been noted for its ability to boost metabolism and keep it revved for hours after eating. In addition, the February 2013 issue of the *European Journal of Nutrition* reported that eating a meal with hot sauce reduces levels of ghrelin, which is the hormone that stimulates hunger. Adding a little fire is a win-win!

Calories 205 • Fat 13g • Carbohydrate 11g • Fiber 5g • Sugar 5g • Protein 14g

"Anti-Pasta" Salad

Every small town has a little mom-and-pop pizza shop on its edge, and ours was famous for their antipasto salad. I learned early on that the secret behind its bold taste was marinating the veggies in Italian dressing for hours to soak up the rich, vibrant flavors of garlic and oregano. I've retained the great taste but slashed the carbs by serving the salad over a bed of romaine instead of pasta, making this the perfect "anti-pasta" salad.

Prep Time: 10 minutes, plus 30 minutes marinating time
Serves: 6 | **Serving Size:** 3 cups salad

2 cups grape tomatoes, halved

1 cup canned chickpeas, drained and rinsed

1 green bell pepper, cut into ½-inch pieces

1 red bell pepper, cut into ½-inch pieces

1 cup canned artichoke hearts, drained, rinsed, and quartered

1 small red onion, thinly sliced

1 large cucumber, halved lengthwise and sliced crosswise

1 cup fat-free Italian salad dressing

6 cups chopped romaine lettuce

½ cup pepperoncini slices

1 (4-ounce) can sliced black olives, drained and rinsed

3 light string cheese sticks (I like Sargento), quartered

½ cup quarterd Canadian bacon slices (I like Boar's Head)

18 slices turkey pepperoni, quartered

3 tablespoons shredded Parmesan cheese (I like Sargento Artisan Blends)

1. In a large bowl, combine the tomatoes, chickpeas, bell peppers, artichoke hearts, onion, and cucumber. Cover with the Italian dressing and toss to evenly combine. Refrigerate for at least 30 minutes but up to 4 hours to marinate the vegetables.

2. In a large bowl, toss together the lettuce, pepperoncinis, olives, cheese, Canadian bacon, and turkey pepperoni. Add the marinated vegetables and toss gently to evenly combine all of the ingredients. Top with the Parmesan.

suppertime chat: Name someone you'd like to start a tradition with. Who is it and what would the tradition be? Why? (I'll share mine: I'd like to start a tradition of cuddling up with my five-year-old at least once a week after school on the couch and taking a nap. Doesn't that sound heavenly?)

Calories 229 • Fat 9g • Carbohydrate 24g • Fiber 6g • Sugar 9g • Protein 14g

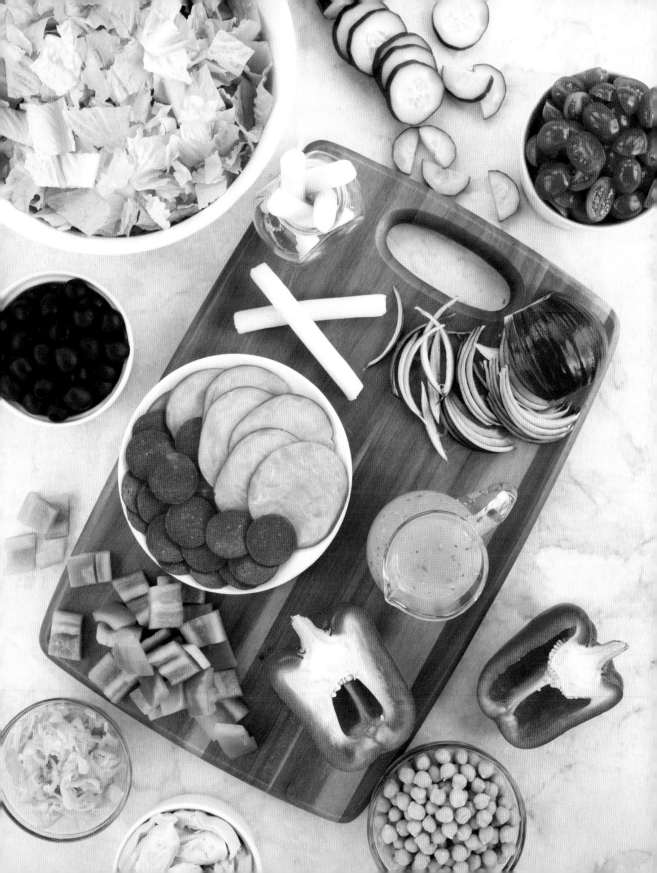

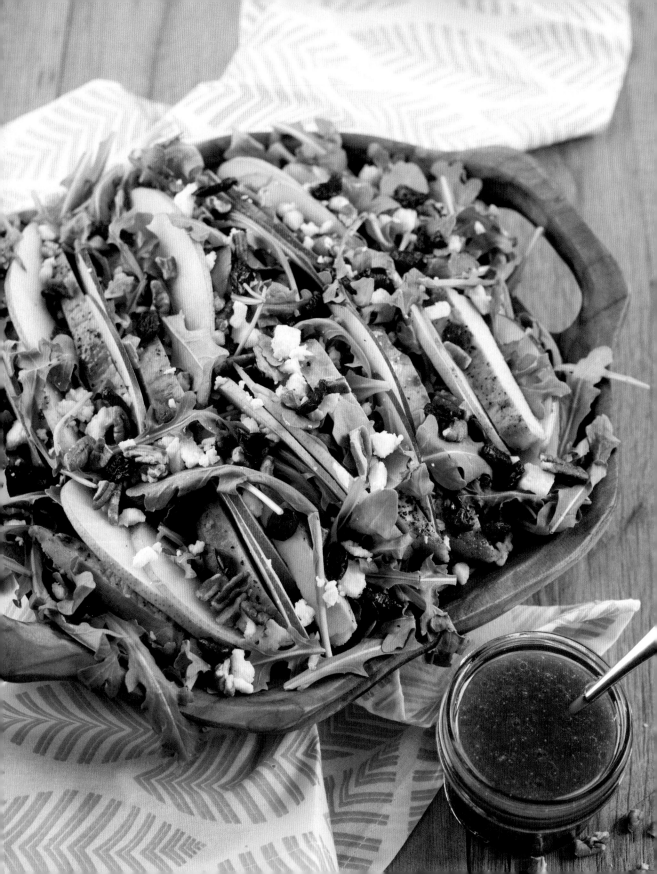

Autumn Chopped Salad

Freshly harvested apples and warm cider capture the essence of fall flavors in this pork-chop topped salad. It's satisfying, light, and full of tangy sweetness.

Prep Time: 10 minutes | **Cook Time:** 10 minutes
Serves: 4 | **Serving Size:** 2½ cups salad

Pork:

1 teaspoon extra virgin olive oil

1 pound boneless pork chops

¼ teaspoon salt

¼ teaspoon black pepper

1 tablespoon sugar-free maple-flavor syrup (I like Maple Grove Farms)

1 tablespoon apple cider vinegar

½ teaspoon light brown sugar

Harvest Vinaigrette:

½ tablespoon apple cider vinegar

1 tablespoon sugar-free maple-flavor syrup (I like Maple Grove Farms)

1 tablespoon sugar-free blackberry jam (I like Smucker's)

1 teaspoon lemon juice

⅛ teaspoon salt

⅛ teaspoon black pepper

1½ tablespoons extra virgin olive oil

Salad:

6 cups baby arugula

1 Anjou or Bartlett pear, sliced

1 Fuji or Honeycrisp apple, sliced

¼ cup reduced-fat feta cheese crumbles

¼ cup Reduced Sugar Craisins Dried Cranberries

2 tablespoons coarsely chopped pecans

1. To make the pork: In a large skillet, heat the olive oil over medium-high heat. Season the pork chops with the salt and pepper. Add the pork chops to the skillet, brushing both sides with the syrup and vinegar. Sprinkle the brown sugar evenly over the pork chops and cook for 4 to 6 minutes, until golden brown on each side or until the internal temperature in the thickest part of the pork reaches 145°F. Set the pork chops aside to rest, then slice against the grain into strips.

2. Meanwhile, to make the vinaigrette: In a small bowl, whisk together the vinegar, syrup, blackberry jam, lemon juice, salt, and pepper. Gradually whisk in the olive oil. Refrigerate the vinaigrette until ready to serve.

3. To assemble the salad: In a large bowl, combine the arugula, pear, apple, feta, Craisins, and pecans. Drizzle with the vinaigrette and then toss to mix all of the ingredients together. Serve with the sliced pork on top.

Suggested Side Dish: Southern Sweet Beets (page 296)

Calories 355 · Fat 19g · Carbohydrate 26g · Fiber 6g · Sugar 15g · Protein 26g

Pink Detox Salad

I'm a girly girl, so I definitely love pink. This salad takes all my favorite pink fruits and swirls them together to form a beautiful detox salad that will cleanse the crankiest of colons. The sweet pomegranate dressing is the perfect topping to the tart grapefruit and tender baby kale. This is one of my faves and a must-try for any girly event on your calendar.

Prep Time: 10 minutes | **Serves:** 4
Serving Size: About 2½ cups salad, 1½ tablespoons dressing

Creamy Pomegranate Dressing:

½ cup plain 0% Greek yogurt

¼ cup pomegranate juice

2 tablespoons apple cider vinegar

½ teaspoon grated lemon zest

1 teaspoon stevia

⅛ teaspoon salt

Salad:

1 pink grapefruit, peeled, segmented (see Quick and Easy), and seeded

½ teaspoon stevia

6 cups baby kale, chopped

1 (16-ounce) container strawberries, sliced

2 cups (1-inch-cubed) watermelon

½ cup pomegranate seeds

¼ cup walnuts, coarsely chopped

½ cup reduced-fat feta cheese crumbles

1. To make the dressing: In a small bowl, whisk together the yogurt, pomegranate juice, vinegar, lemon zest, stevia, and salt until well combined. Refrigerate until ready to serve.

2. To make the salad: In a small bowl, sprinkle the grapefruit segments with the stevia. Set aside.

3. When ready to serve, divide the baby kale among 4 plates. Top each serving with the strawberries, watermelon, grapefruit slices, pomegranate seeds, walnuts, and feta cheese.

4. Drizzle each salad with 1½ tablespoons of the pomegranate dressing.

quick and easy: To segment a grapefruit, slice the top and bottom off the grapefruit, so it sits flat on the cutting board. Then, carefully slice off the peel and membrane from all sides of the grapefruit, exposing the fruit. Holding the grapefruit in one hand, use a paring knife to cut along the membranes on either side of a segment, meeting in the middle. This will loosen the fruit segment and it will lift out easily. Be sure to do this over a bowl or the sink. Grapefruits are extremely juicy; it can get a little messy!

Calories 254 • Fat 8g • Carbohydrate 35g • Fiber 6g • Sugar 19g • Protein 11g

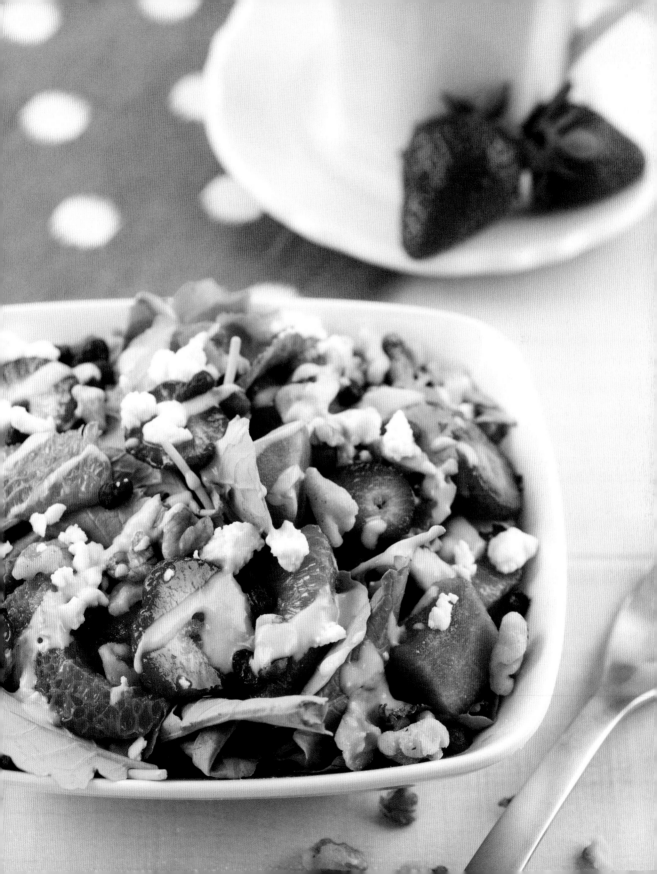

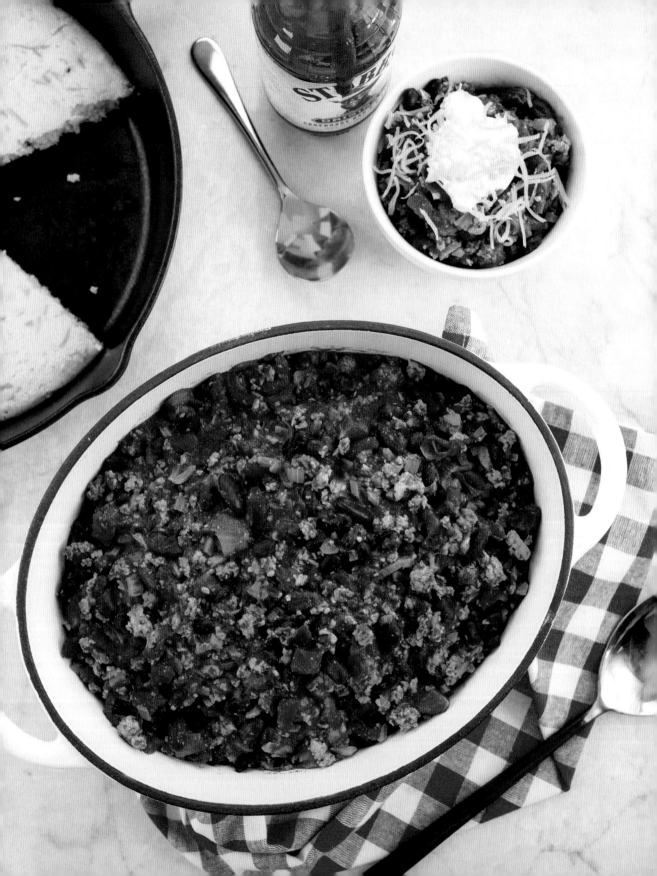

BBQ Turkey Chili

2x

I live right outside of Cincinnati, Ohio, and this town is crazy famous for chili. Many restaurants—and residents—boast their tried-and-true recipes. I decided to put my own little twist on the famous tailgating staple, and what resulted is a bold taste with a sweet, smoky flavor.

Prep Time: 10 minutes | **Cook Time:** 30 minutes
Serves: 6 | **Serving Size:** 1⅓ cups

½ tablespoon extra virgin olive oil

1 pound lean ground turkey

1 small onion, diced

1 tablespoon minced garlic

3 stalks celery, diced

½ cup carrots, diced

1 (15-ounce) can reduced-sodium black beans, drained and rinsed

1 (15-ounce) can reduced-sodium dark red kidney beans, drained and rinsed

2 (14.5-ounce) cans no-salt-added diced tomatoes (I like Hunt's)

1 cup Stubb's Original All-Natural Bar-B-Q Sauce

½ tablespoon chili powder

1 teaspoon ground cumin

¼ teaspoon salt

¼ teaspoon black pepper

Optional Ingredients:

3 tablespoons shredded reduced-fat cheddar cheese (I like Sargento)

3 tablespoons light sour cream

1. In a large soup pot or Dutch oven, heat the olive oil over medium-high heat. Add the turkey, onion, garlic, celery, and carrots. Cook until the ground turkey is browned, 7 to 8 minutes. Use a wooden spoon to break up the turkey as it cooks.

2. Add the black beans, kidney beans, diced tomatoes, barbecue sauce, chili powder, cumin, salt, and pepper and stir to combine.

3. Cover, reduce the heat to low, and simmer for 20 minutes. Uncover and taste, adjusting the seasoning if needed.

4. Ladle the chili into bowls. If desired, top each serving with ½ tablespoon cheddar and ½ tablespoon sour cream.

Suggested Side Dish: Cheesy Jalapeño Cornbread (page 270)

skinny sense: Did you know that draining and rinsing your canned vegetables and beans can reduce sodium by up to 40 percent?

quick and easy: Chili is almost always just as good (if not better) the second time around. If you find yourself with leftovers, do what we do in Cincinnati, make a three-way: Cook spaghetti to al dente and serve topped with chili and shredded cheddar cheese.

Calories 320 · **Fat** 7g · **Carbohydrate** 44g · **Fiber** 10g · **Sugar** 11g · **Protein** 23g
Nutrition does not include optional ingredients.

Slow-Cooker Creamy Chicken and Wild Rice Soup

My goal with this recipe was to maintain the creamy texture of this classic soup, while keeping it low in fat and calories. It's a challenge to create the creaminess without the cream, but after much trial and error, this soup turned out just right. It is one of my favorite go-to soup recipes on busy weeknights.

Prep Time: 10 minutes | **Cook Time:** 7½ hours on low or 3½ hours on high
Serves: 6 | **Serving Size:** 1⅓ cups

1 small onion, diced

2 large carrots, diced

3 stalks celery, diced

1 (8-ounce) container baby bella (cremini) mushrooms, stemmed and sliced

1 pound boneless, skinless chicken breasts

2½ cups low-sodium chicken broth (I like Pacific Organic)

2 (10.5-ounce) cans Campbell's Healthy Request condensed cream of mushroom soup

¼ teaspoon poultry seasoning

½ teaspoon salt

¼ teaspoon black pepper

½ cup fat-free milk

2 teaspoons cornstarch

1 (8.5-ounce) pouch Uncle Ben's Brown and Wild Rice Medley

3 tablespoons chopped fresh parsley

1. Coat the liner of a slow cooker with cooking spray.

2. Place the onion, carrots, celery, and mushrooms evenly into the slow cooker. Place the chicken breasts on top of the vegetables. Add the chicken broth, mushroom soup, poultry seasoning, salt, and pepper and stir gently. Cover and cook on high heat for 3 hours or on low heat for 7 hours.

3. Uncover and use 2 forks to shred the chicken.

4. In a small bowl, add the milk to the cornstarch and stir to dissolve the slurry. Add the slurry and rice to the slow cooker and stir to combine. Cook uncovered for an additional 30 minutes on high heat until the soup has thickened.

5. Ladle the soup into bowls and garnish with the parsley.

Suggested Side Dish: Rustic Rosemary Root Vegetables (page 290)

no slow cooker, no problem: Combine all of the ingredients except the fat-free milk, cornstarch, rice, and parsley in a large soup pot or Dutch oven and cook over low heat for 1 to 2 hours, stirring regularly, until the chicken is cooked through. Shred the chicken and continue as directed.

Calories 230 • Fat 4g • Carbohydrate 29g • Fiber 4g • Sugar 6g • Protein 21g

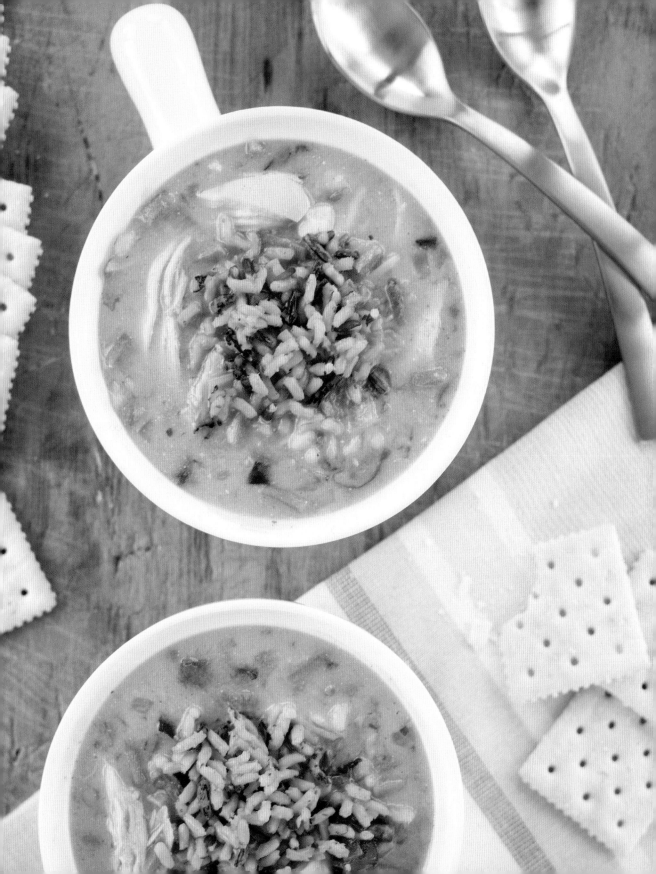

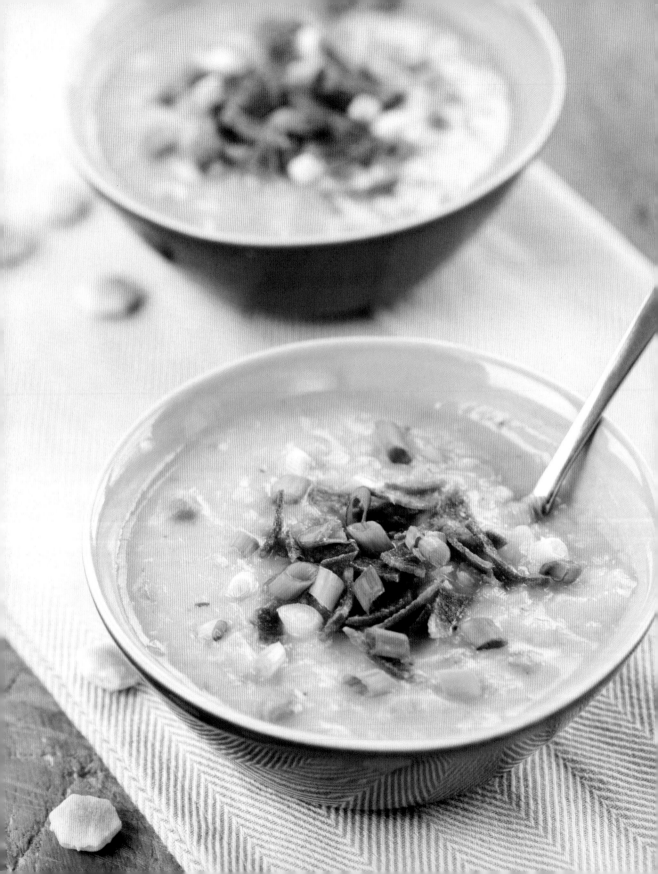

New England Clam Chowder

I usually reserve clams for when I'm eating out. But since clam chowder is such a comfort food for me, I decided it was time for a homemade version. Even though I reserve the juice from the clams for later use in the recipe, rinsing the clams before using helps to reduce overall sodium content.

Prep Time: 10 minutes │ **Cook Time:** 30 minutes
Serves: 4 │ **Serving Size:** 1¼ cups

½ tablespoon extra virgin olive oil

1 small onion, diced

3 stalks celery, diced

½ cup diced carrots

1 teaspoon minced garlic

1 (12-ounce) bag frozen cauliflower florets

1½ cups low-sodium chicken broth (I like Pacific Organic)

¼ teaspoon black pepper

¼ teaspoon red pepper flakes

1 bay leaf

3 (6-ounce) cans chopped clams, drained, juice reserved

1 (12-ounce) can fat-free evaporated milk

½ tablespoon Worcestershire sauce

1 tablespoon cornstarch

3 slices turkey bacon, cooked and crumbled

2 green onions, thinly sliced

1. In a large soup pot or Dutch oven, heat the olive oil over medium-high heat. Add the onion, celery, carrots, and garlic and cook until softened, 5 to 6 minutes.

2. Steam the cauliflower in the microwave, according to the package directions. Then chop into bite-size pieces.

3. Add the chopped cauliflower, chicken broth, black pepper, pepper flakes, bay leaf, and 1 cup of the juice reserved from the canned clams to the pot. Reduce the heat to medium-low and simmer for 20 minutes, stirring occasionally.

4. Meanwhile, in a small bowl, whisk together the evaporated milk, Worcestershire sauce, and cornstarch.

5. After the soup has simmered for 20 minutes, add the Worcestershire mixture along with the drained clams. Stir to combine and simmer for 10 minutes longer.

6. Ladle the soup into bowls and garnish with the crumbled bacon and green onions.

skinny sense: Iron deficiency is common among women, so it's vital that women eat iron-rich foods. Clams are one of the most iron-rich foods, even beating out beef liver and steak.

Calories 231 • Fat 3g • Carbohydrate 32g • Fiber 2g • Sugar 17g • Protein 17g

Loaded Nacho Soup

Is it a soup? Is it a dip? It's both! Everyone in the family will be ready to dive into this hearty "loaded" soup. No utensils necessary!

Prep Time: 5 minutes | **Cook Time:** 20 minutes
Serves: 6 | **Serving Size:** 1⅓ cups soup, 1 tablespoon light sour cream, 1 tablespoon green onions, and 5 tortilla chips

1 pound lean ground beef

1 small onion, diced

1 tablespoon minced garlic

2 cups low-sodium beef broth
(I like Pacific Organic)

1 (15-ounce) can fat-free refried beans

1 (15-ounce) can reduced-sodium black beans, drained and rinsed

1 (10.5-ounce) can Campbell's Healthy Request condensed cheddar cheese soup

1 (10-ounce) can Ro*Tel Original Diced Tomatoes and Green Chilies

1 cup frozen corn kernels

1 (4.5-ounce) can chopped green chilies

1 (1-ounce) packet less-sodium taco seasoning or Make It Homemade (page 299)

3 tablespoons light sour cream

3 green onions, thinly sliced

30 whole grain tortilla chips

Optional Ingredients:

3 tablespoons reduced-fat shredded sharp cheddar cheese (I like Sargento)

½ tomato, diced

¼ cup sliced black olives

1. In a large soup pot or Dutch oven over medium-high heat, cook the beef, onion, and garlic until the beef is no longer pink, 7 to 8 minutes. Use a wooden spoon to break up the beef as it cooks. Drain any excess fat and return the skillet to the stovetop, turning the heat down to low.

2. Add the beef broth, refried beans, black beans, cheddar cheese soup, diced tomatoes, corn, green chilies, and taco seasoning. Stir and bring to a boil. Reduce the heat to low and simmer for 10 minutes before serving.

3. To serve, ladle the soup into bowls. Top each serving with ½ tablespoon sour cream and some green onions. Serve with tortilla chips and, if desired, garnish with additional optional ingredients.

skinny sense: Be careful to portion out tortilla chips, though; calories can add up quickly!

quick and easy: Have a "no-fork night" and serve this soup up with other finger foods like fruits and veggies and have fun. Less mess to clean up, too!

Calories 412 · **Fat** 13g · **Carbohydrate** 58g · **Fiber** 12g · **Sugar** 10g · **Protein** 30g
Nutrition does not include optional ingredients.

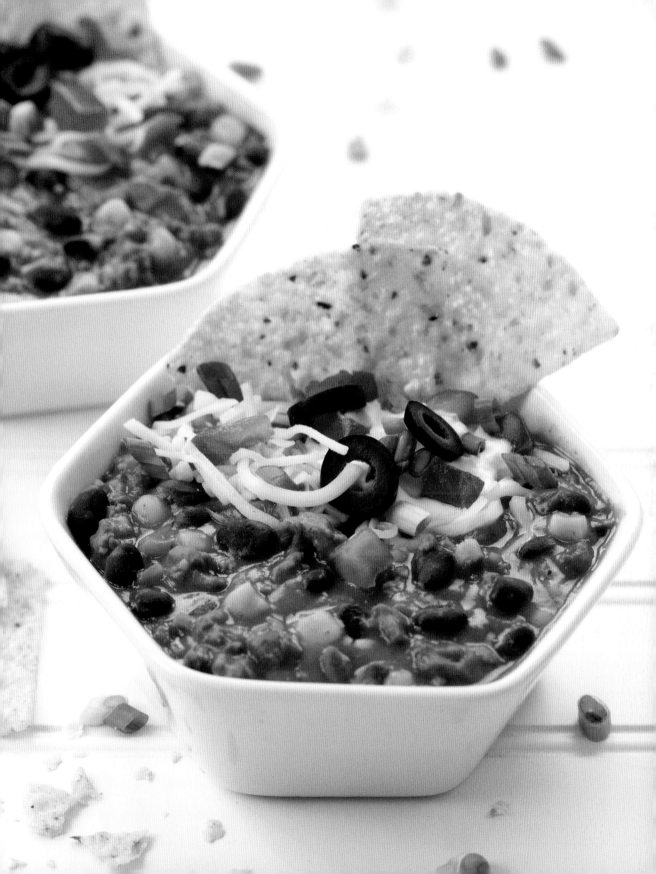

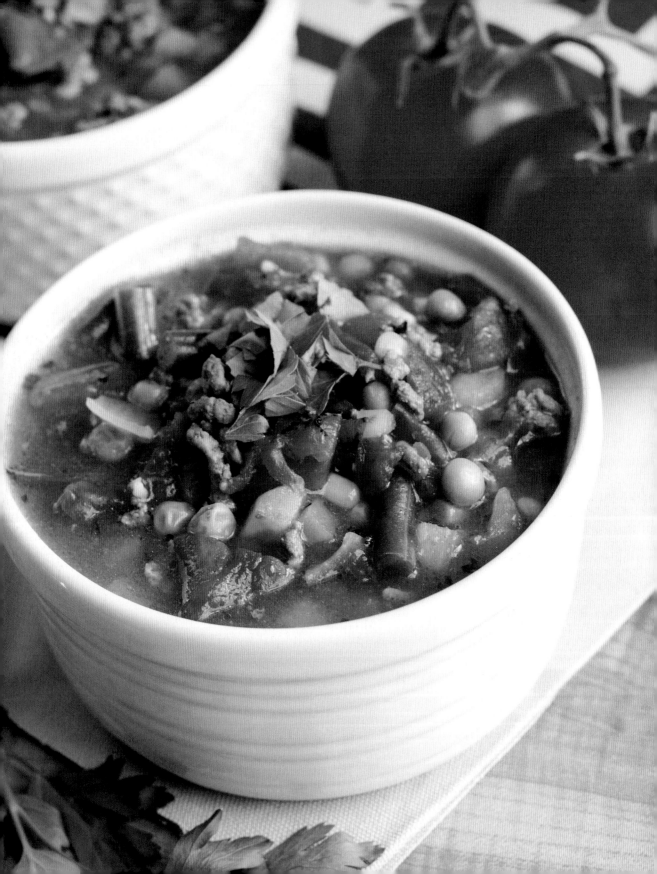

Rustic Beef and Vegetable Soup

This one is straight out of my momma's kitchen. It's her classic hearty, beefy, vegetable soup, a comfort food that exudes warm sentiments of home and family. Outside of purchasing leaner ground beef, I changed nothing. As they say in the South, "If it ain't broke, don't fix it."

Prep Time: 5 minutes | **Cook Time:** 25 minutes
Serves: 6 | **Serving Size:** 1½ cups

1 pound lean ground beef

1 small onion, diced

2 tablespoons minced garlic

2 stalks celery, chopped

1 (32-ounce) container low-sodium beef broth (I like Pacific Organic)

1 (16-ounce) bag frozen Birds Eye Classic mixed vegetables

2 (14.5-ounce) cans no-salt-added diced tomatoes (I like Hunt's)

2 bay leaves

1 teaspoon Italian seasoning

1½ teaspoons salt

1 teaspoon black pepper

2 teaspoons Frank's RedHot Sauce

3 tablespoons chopped fresh parsley

1. In a large soup pot or Dutch oven over medium-high heat, cook the beef, onion, garlic, and celery until the beef is no longer pink, 7 to 8 minutes. Use a wooden spoon to break up the beef as it cooks. Drain any excess fat and return the pot to the stovetop, turning the heat down to low.

2. Add the beef broth, mixed vegetables, and diced tomatoes and stir to combine. Add the bay leaves. Season with the Italian seasoning, salt, pepper, and hot sauce. Stir to combine and simmer over medium heat for 15 minutes, until heated through.

3. Discard the bay leaves and serve garnished with the parsley.

Suggested Side Dish: Skinny Sweet Potato Biscuits (page 272)

suppertime inspiration: As parents, we often agonize over the decisions we have to make. The following verse gives me great peace and relief when I am in doubt: "Train up a child in the way he should go: and when he is old, he will not depart from it." Proverbs 22:6.

Calories 221 • Fat 6g • Carbohydrate 29g • Fiber 5g • Sugar 10g • Protein 20g

Spicy Butternut Squash Soup

This is my youngest sister Cara's all-time favorite recipe. I make it especially for her every time she comes to visit. Roasting the squash in the oven first allows the nutty, buttery smell to spread throughout the house, making it feel homey and inviting. It's a great vegetarian supper, too. Since I like a little heat, I'm especially fond of the sweet and spice blend created by the maple syrup and cayenne pepper.

Prep Time: 40 minutes | **Cook Time:** 40 minutes
Serves: 4 | **Serving Size:** 1½ cups

3-pound butternut squash

¼ teaspoon cayenne pepper, plus more for serving

¼ teaspoon ground cumin

⅛ teaspoon paprika

½ teaspoon ground cinnamon

¼ teaspoon salt

¼ teaspoon black pepper

2 tablespoons plus 2 teaspoons extra virgin olive oil

1 cup diced onion

½ cup finely diced carrot

½ cup finely diced celery

2 teaspoons minced garlic

⅛ teaspoon red pepper flakes

4 cups low-sodium vegetable broth (I like Pacific Organic)

½ cup fat-free milk

3 tablespoons sugar-free maple-flavor syrup (I like Maple Grove Farms)

1 teaspoon stevia

Optional Ingredients:

Fat-free milk, to thin the soup

2 tablespoons light sour cream

2 tablespoons coarsely chopped pecans

1. Preheat the oven to 350°F. Line a baking sheet with foil and coat with cooking spray.

2. Quarter the squash lengthwise. Scoop out and discard the seeds.

3. In a small bowl, combine the cayenne, cumin, paprika, cinnamon, salt, and black pepper.

4. Place the cut squash flesh side up on the prepared baking sheet. Drizzle with 2 tablespoons of the olive oil and evenly sprinkle with the spice mixture.

5. Bake until the squash is very soft, 40 to 45 minutes.

6. Meanwhile, in a medium soup pot, heat the remaining 2 teaspoons olive oil over medium heat. Add the onion, carrot, and celery and cook until the onion is translucent, 5 to 8 minutes. Add the garlic and pepper flakes and cook for about 1 minute, or until fragrant.

7. When the squash is cool enough to handle, use a spoon to scrape the flesh off the skin and into the pot. Add the vegetable broth, milk, syrup, and stevia and stir to combine. Cover and simmer for 30 minutes.

skinny sense: I'm a big fan of
cayenne pepper, not just because
I like spice, but because the high
amounts of capsaicin that are
found in the little pepper have been
linked to speeding up metabolism.
That's a great reason to have this
spice as a staple in your pantry.
Sprinkle ground cayenne on almost
any dish from soup to salad and
pasta to poultry.

8. Carefully transfer the soup in batches to a blender (or use an immersion blender) and blend for 1 to 2 minutes, until smooth.

9. If the soup is too thick for your preference after blending, thin out by stirring in additional fat-free milk, a tablespoon at a time, until it reaches the desired consistency.

10. To serve, ladle the soup into bowls and sprinkle with a little cayenne. If desired, garnish each serving with 1/2 tablespoon sour cream and 1/2 tablespoon pecans.

suppertime chat: Name something that you were afraid to try, but after you did you were glad. It could be a food, sport, game, or anything else you've experienced.

Calories 295 • Fat 10g • Carbohydrate 53g • Fiber 10g • Sugar 14g • Protein 6g

Tomato Tortellini Soup

We love tomatoes in my house. My son eats grape tomatoes like they're candy. But usually when eating tomato soup, I find myself preparing something alongside the dish to make it a complete meal. Adding the tortellini to this creamy base brings just enough heartiness to keep it light, yet still satisfying enough for supper.

Prep Time: 10 minutes | **Cook Time:** 20 minutes
Serves: 6 | **Serving Size:** 1⅓ cups, 1 tablespoon Parmesan

½ tablespoon extra virgin olive oil

½ cup diced onion

½ cup chopped carrots

1 tablespoon minced garlic

1 (28-ounce) can crushed tomatoes (I like Hunt's)

1 (14.5-ounce) can no-salt-added diced tomatoes (I like Hunt's)

1 (32-ounce) container low-sodium vegetable broth (I like Pacific Organic)

3 tablespoons tomato paste

2 bay leaves

1 teaspoon dried basil

½ teaspoon dried oregano

1 teaspoon salt

½ teaspoon black pepper

1 tablespoon stevia

½ cup plain 0% Greek yogurt

1 (9-ounce) package refrigerated whole wheat cheese tortellini

¼ cup chopped fresh basil

6 tablespoons shredded Parmesan cheese (I like Sargento Artisan Blends)

1. In a large soup pot or Dutch oven, heat the olive oil over medium-high heat. Add the onion, carrots, and garlic and cook until softened, 2 to 3 minutes.

2. Add the crushed tomatoes, diced tomatoes, vegetable broth, and tomato paste and stir to mix. Season with the bay leaves, dried basil, oregano, salt, pepper, and stevia. Simmer for 12 minutes, stirring occasionally. Discard the bay leaves.

3. Reduce the heat to medium-low. Carefully transfer the soup in batches to a blender (or use an immersion blender) and blend for 1 to 2 minutes, until smooth. Transfer the blended soup back to the pot.

4. Cook the soup mixture over medium-low heat while stirring in the yogurt. Add the refrigerated tortellini to the soup and cook for 6 to 8 minutes, until the tortellini is cooked through.

5. To serve, ladle the soup into bowls and garnish each serving with some fresh basil and 1 tablespoon Parmesan.

Calories 290 • Fat 8g • Carbohydrate 41g • Fiber 9g • Sugar 12g • Protein 15g

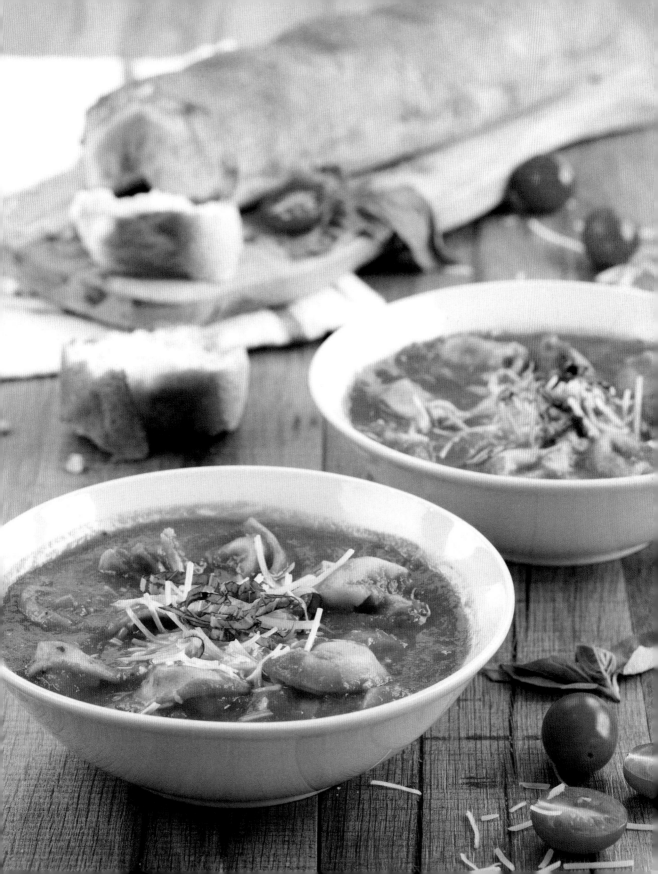

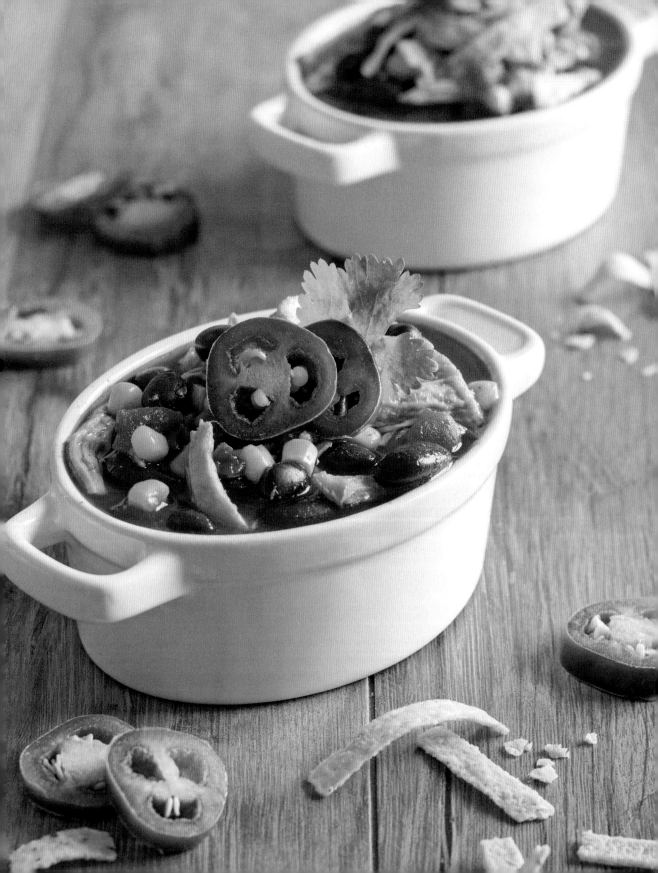

Tortilla Chicken Soup

This is one of my favorite tailgating recipes! It packs the spice, but not the calories. And the longer it simmers, the more flavorful it becomes, so you don't have to worry when your guests want seconds later in the game!

Prep Time: 5 minutes | **Cook Time:** 4 hours on high or 8 hours on low
Serves: 6 | **Serving Size:** 1¾ cups soup, 2 tablespoons tortilla strips

1 pound boneless, skinless chicken breasts

1 small onion, diced

1 (15-ounce) can reduced-sodium black beans, drained and rinsed

1 (12-ounce) bag frozen corn kernels

1 (8-ounce) can tomato sauce

2 (10-ounce) cans Ro*Tel mild diced tomatoes and green chilies

1 (4.5-ounce) can chopped green chilies

1 (1-ounce) packet less-sodium taco seasoning or Make It Homemade (page 299)

1 (32-ounce) container low-sodium chicken broth (I like Pacific Organic)

¾ cup Fresh Gourmet lightly salted tortilla strips

1. Place the chicken in a slow cooker. Add the onion, black beans, corn, tomato sauce, diced tomatoes, green chilies, taco seasoning, and chicken broth and stir to combine. Cover and cook on high heat for 4 hours or on low heat for 8 hours.

2. Remove the chicken and shred. Return the shredded chicken to the slow cooker and mix well.

3. To serve, ladle the soup into bowls. Garnish each serving with 2 tablespoons of tortilla strips.

Suggested Side Dish: Cilantro-Lime Rice (page 271)

no slow cooker, no problem: Combine all of the ingredients in a large soup pot or Dutch oven and cook over low heat, stirring regularly, for 1 hour. Remove the chicken and continue as directed.

quick and easy: Add some low-calorie jalapeño peppers or a squeeze of fresh lime for some added kick and flavor.

Calories 331 • Fat 4g • Carbohydrate 52g • Fiber 7g • Sugar 11g • Protein 25g

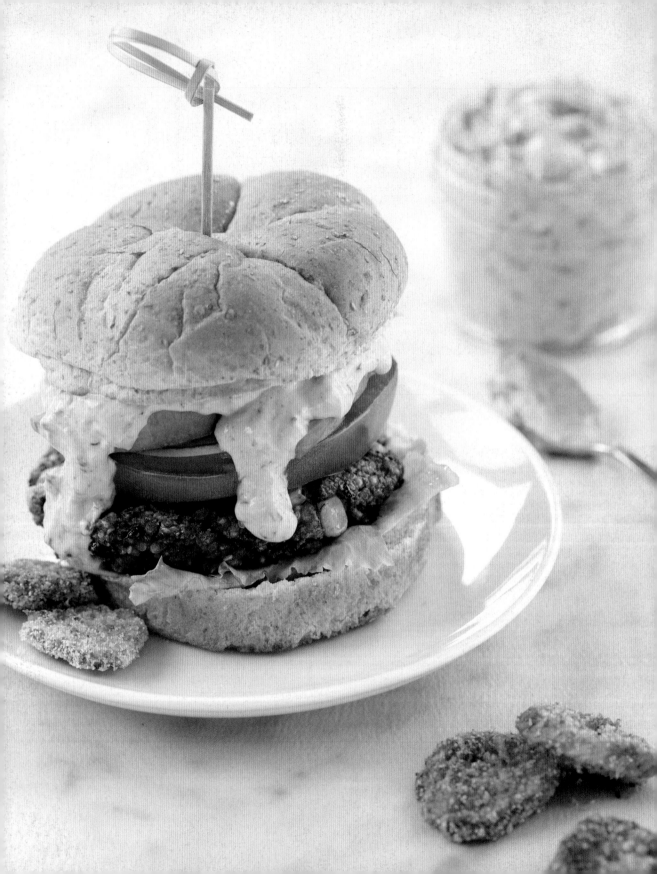

12 SKIP THE MEAT, Y'ALL
VEGETARIAN SUPPERS

Cream Cheese Vegetable Ring

Get ready to wow your guests when you present this beautiful dish. Weaving the crescent rolls together forms an amazing wreath that is festive year-round. This veggie ring is fresh, satisfying, and filling, but oh so light and friendly to the waistline.

Prep Time: 15 minutes │ **Cook Time:** 30 minutes
Serves: 8 │ **Serving Size:** ⅛ of the ring

2 (8-ounce) cans Pillsbury Reduced Fat Crescent Rolls

2 cups small broccoli florets

2 teaspoons extra virgin olive oil

1 small onion, diced

1 cup thinly sliced baby bella (cremini) mushrooms (half of an 8-ounce package)

1 red bell pepper, diced

1 small yellow squash, diced

1 teaspoon garlic powder

¼ teaspoon salt

¼ teaspoon black pepper

4 ounces ⅓-less-fat cream cheese, softened

1 teaspoon chopped fresh basil

1 teaspoon chopped fresh parsley

¼ cup shredded reduced-fat sharp cheddar cheese (I like Sargento)

1 egg

1. Preheat the oven to 350°F. Coat a baking sheet with cooking spray.

2. Unroll both cans of the crescent rolls and separate all of the triangles. On a nonstick baking sheet, assemble the ring by placing the short ends of the triangles together, overlapping each other by about half and leaving about a 5-inch-diameter round opening in the middle. (See photo on page 240 for help.) To guide this shape, turn a bowl that is about 5 inches in diameter upside down in the center of the baking sheet. Place the short ends of the dough triangles along the edge of the bowl to help keep the round shape of the ring. This will create a sun-shaped ring with an open center and with the triangle tips hanging over the edge of the baking sheet.

3. In a microwave-safe bowl, steam the broccoli in the microwave with ¼ cup water for 1 to 2 minutes, until bright green and soft. Drain the excess water.

4. In a large skillet, heat the olive oil over medium heat. Add the onion, mushrooms, bell pepper, and squash and cook until they begin to soften, 5 to 7 minutes. Stir in the garlic powder, salt, and black pepper. Add the cooked broccoli and stir to combine.

(recipe continues)

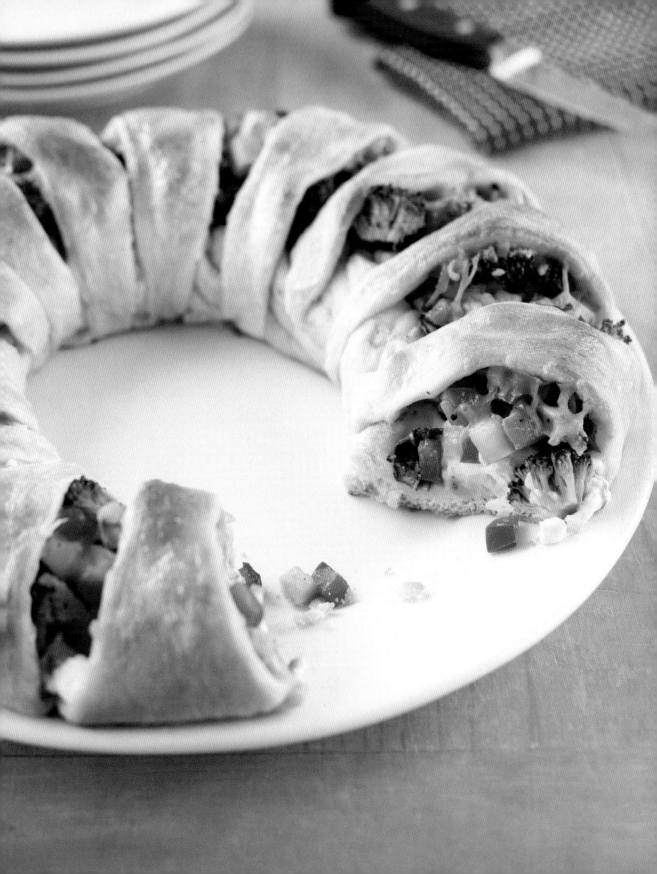

(recipe continued from page 238)

skinny sense: **Adapt for your guests with various fillings for special holidays, especially Christmas using red and green bell peppers, or during Easter using fresh rosemary, to create new, edible holiday traditions.**

5. In a medium bowl, combine the softened cream cheese, basil, and parsley and stir to combine.

6. Spread the cream cheese onto the crescent roll ring, closest to the center edge. Pile the vegetable mixture on top of the cream cheese and then sprinkle with the cheddar cheese. Fold the triangle tips over the filling, and tuck under the bottom of the dough to secure it. Repeat all the way around the ring.

7. In a small bowl, whisk together the egg and ¼ cup of water to make an egg wash. Brush the top of the wreath with the egg wash for browning.

8. Bake until the top is golden brown, 17 to 20 minutes.

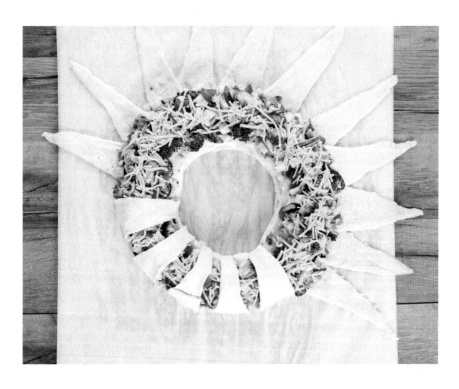

Calories 278 • Fat 12g • Carbohydrate 33g • Fiber 2g • Sugar 9g • Protein 8g

Baked Eggplant Parmesan

As long as I've been cooking, eggplant has just intimidated me. I decided to face my fears, but stay with a traditional recipe. Much to my surprise, I found the eggplant easy to work with, and I'm sure you will, too. Incredibly filling and full of rich flavor, this Italian-inspired supper is bound to become a classic.

Prep Time: 15 minutes | **Cook Time:** 35 minutes
Serves: 6 | **Serving Size:** 1/6 of the casserole

2 medium eggplants

3 egg whites

1½ cups panko bread crumbs

2 teaspoons dried oregano

2 teaspoons dried basil

1 teaspoon salt

¼ teaspoon black pepper

1 (23.25-ounce) jar Prego Light Smart Traditional pasta sauce

6 slices Sargento Ultra Thin sliced provolone cheese, halved

½ cup shredded reduced-fat mozzarella cheese (I like Sargento)

¼ cup shredded Parmesan cheese (I like Sargento Artisan Blends)

suppertime inspiration:
Just like my experience with the eggplant, more often than not our fears regarding many situations in life result from **F**alse **E**vidence **A**ppearing **R**eal. Face your fears in the kitchen and in life with confidence, realizing that it's not as bad as you think!

1. Preheat the oven to 400°F. Line 2 baking sheets with foil and coat with cooking spray. Coat a 13 x 9-inch baking dish with cooking spray.

2. Cut the eggplants crosswise into 1/2-inch-thick slices. Lay the eggplant slices on paper towels to blot out any excess moisture.

3. In a small bowl, whisk the egg whites. In a second small bowl, mix together the panko, oregano, basil, salt, and pepper. Dip the eggplant in the egg whites and allow the excess to drip off. Dredge one side of the eggplant lightly in the panko mixture and arrange crumb side up in a single layer on the prepared baking sheets.

4. Bake until golden brown and fork-tender, 20 to 25 minutes, turning over at halfway mark.

5. Pour a thin layer of the pasta sauce onto the bottom of the prepared baking dish. Layer the eggplant slices to cover the bottom of the dish using about half of the eggplant. Top with all of the provolone, followed by 1/4 cup mozzarella. Repeat the layering using the remaining sauce, the remaining eggplant, and the remaining 1/4 cup mozzarella. Sprinkle the Parmesan evenly on top.

6. Bake until the cheese is bubbling and browned, 15 to 20 minutes. Serve warm.

Calories 237 • Fat 13g • Carbohydrate 34g • Fiber 9g • Sugar 14g • Protein 19g

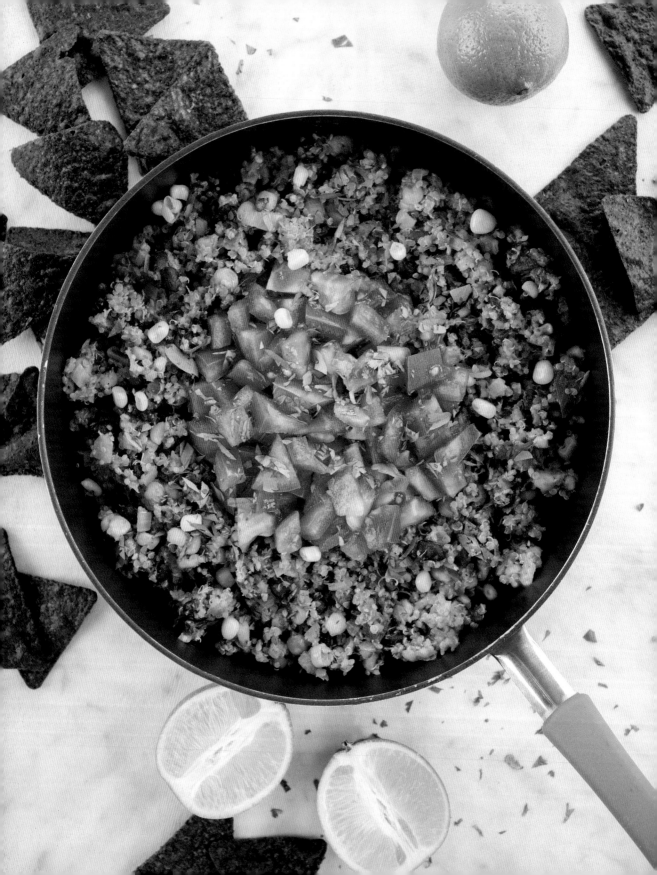

Santa Fe Quinoa Sizzling Skillet

If you are on a mission to minimize cleanup in the kitchen, while providing balanced meals, this skillet could very well become your go-to supper. Truly a one and done! Not only is the whole supper cooked up in one skillet, it also gets served up in one bowl. And by making quinoa the foundation, you ensure a high standard of nutrition.

Prep Time: 5 minutes | **Cook Time:** 25 minutes
Serves: 4 | **Serving Size:** 1⅓ cups

1 teaspoon extra virgin olive oil

1 small onion, diced

2 teaspoons minced garlic

1 (15.25-ounce) can no-salt-added corn kernels (I like Del Monte)

1 (10-ounce) can Ro*Tel Mild Diced Tomatoes and Green Chilies

1 (4.5-ounce) can chopped green chilies

1 tablespoon lime juice

1 cup quinoa, rinsed

1 cup low-sodium vegetable broth (I like Pacific Organic)

3 wedges Laughing Cow Creamy Queso Fresco Chipotle cheese

2 tablespoons chopped fresh cilantro

Optional Toppings:

1 avocado, diced

2 tablespoons light sour cream

2 Roma (plum) tomatoes, diced

1. In a large skillet, heat the olive oil over medium-high heat. Add the onion and garlic and sauté until translucent, 3 to 5 minutes.

2. Add the corn, diced tomatoes, green chilies, lime juice, quinoa, and vegetable broth to the skillet. Stir to evenly combine. Increase the heat to high and bring to a boil. Reduce the heat to medium-low, cover, and simmer until the quinoa is cooked, 20 to 25 minutes.

3. Cut the cheese wedges into small pieces and drop into the skillet, stirring until the cheese is melted.

4. Serve garnished with the cilantro. If desired, add any of the optional toppings.

Suggested Side Dish: Southwest "Fried" Pickles (page 284)

skinny sense: Even if no one in the house is a vegetarian, it's never a bad idea to start a "Meatless Monday" tradition. Not only will you save excess fat and calories, but it's easier on the grocery budget, too!

Calories 306 • Fat 4g • Carbohydrate 51g • Fiber 6g • Sugar 13g • Protein 11g
Nutrition does not include optional toppings.

Butternut Squash Risotto

Until I made this recipe, I thought risotto was a type of rice. Actually, it's a method of preparing rice. Risotto involves cooking rice in broth (I use vegetable broth here) until it develops a creamy consistency. The trick is to ladle the broth in slowly to allow the rice to fully absorb the liquid while stirring the mixture constantly. And the outcome when paired with butternut squash and Parmesan cheese in this supper is creamy, cheesy heaven.

Prep Time: 15 minutes | **Cook Time:** 35 minutes
Serves: 4 | **Serving Size:** 1½ cups

3-pound butternut squash

1 tablespoon extra virgin olive oil

½ teaspoon salt

½ teaspoon ground nutmeg

½ teaspoon black pepper

1 small onion, diced

2 teaspoons minced garlic

1 cup Arborio rice

5 cups low-sodium vegetable broth
(I like Pacific Organic)

⅓ cup shredded Parmesan cheese
(I like Sargento Artisan Blends)

2 tablespoons chopped fresh parsley

quick and easy: Waste not, want not! Roasted butternut squash seeds are a delicious snack or an added garnish for this dish. Preheat the oven to 275°F. Line a baking sheet with parchment paper or foil. Rinse the seeds and remove any strings. Pat dry and spread evenly on the baking sheet. Lightly coat with cooking spray and season with salt and pepper. Bake until the seeds start to pop, about 15 minutes. Remove from the oven and cool before serving.

1. Preheat the oven to 350°F. Coat a baking sheet with cooking spray.

2. Peel the squash, halve, scoop out the seeds (see Quick and Easy), and cut the squash into small chunks.

3. In a large bowl, combine the squash, ½ tablespoon of the olive oil, salt, nutmeg, and pepper. Toss gently to evenly coat the squash.

4. Transfer the squash to the prepared baking sheet. Bake until the squash has softened and is golden brown, 30 to 35 minutes.

5. In a medium saucepan over low heat, add vegetable broth. Keep warm until ready to use.

6. Meanwhile, in a large skillet, heat the remaining ½ tablespoon oil over medium-high heat. Add the onion and garlic and sauté until the onion is translucent, 2 to 3 minutes.

7. Add the rice to the skillet and stir constantly until the rice granules have become clear in color, 3 to 4 minutes.

8. Ladle ½ cup of the vegetable broth into the rice mixture and stir constantly with a wooden spoon until the broth is absorbed. Continue to ladle the vegetable broth in ½-cup increments, stirring

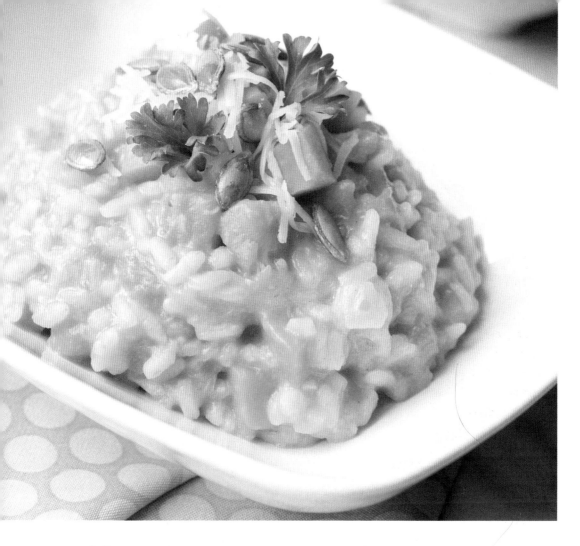

and allowing each ½ cup to absorb into the rice before adding more. The rice should be tender but firm and should start to get creamy. This process should take 20 to 25 minutes and you will add 4 cups of the broth.

9. Add the butternut squash and stir to combine. The consistency should be creamy. If needed, add the remaining 1 cup vegetable broth and stir to combine. Stir in the Parmesan.

10. Serve garnished with the parsley.

skinny sense: When buying squash, make sure the skin is firm and the color is uniform. Can't find butternut squash for your recipe? Acorn squash works just as well.

Calories 413 • Fat 8g • Carbohydrate 81g • Fiber 12g • Sugar 12g • Protein 11g

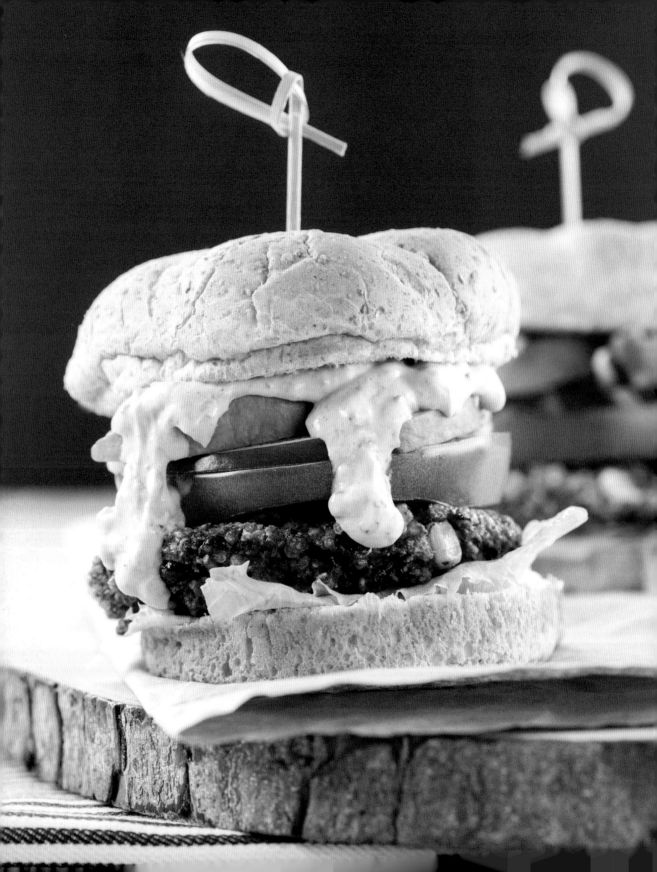

Chipotle Black Bean Burgers

Black bean burgers are jam-packed with vitamins and nutrients, and typically low in fat and calories. Yet, they can be very tricky to prepare. Having a good binding agent is key. Here, the quinoa, bread crumbs, and egg all work together to create a hearty patty with no crumbling. I also like to load mine up with all the fixin's for a super-filling vegetarian supper.

Prep Time: 10 minutes | **Cook Time:** 20 minutes
Serves: 4 | **Serving Size:** 1 burger, ½ tablespoon chipotle mayonnaise

¼ cup quinoa, rinsed

2 cups low-sodium vegetable broth (I like Pacific Organic)

1 (15-ounce) can reduced-sodium black beans, drained

1 teaspoon garlic powder

1 teaspoon onion powder

½ teaspoon ground cumin

½ teaspoon paprika

¼ teaspoon salt

¼ teaspoon black pepper

2 teaspoons lime juice

1 chipotle pepper in adobo sauce, finely chopped

2 teaspoons adobo sauce from the can

1 egg

½ cup plain bread crumbs

½ cup canned low-sodium whole kernel corn, drained

4 whole wheat burger buns, toasted

Chipotle Mayonnaise:

1½ tablespoons light mayonnaise

½ tablespoon light sour cream

½ tablespoon lime juice

½ chipotle pepper in adobo sauce, finely chopped

⅛ teaspoon garlic powder

Optional Ingredients:

4 tomato slices

4 lettuce leaves

4 slices Sargento Ultra Thin Sliced provolone cheese

½ red onion, sliced

½ avocado, sliced

1. Preheat the oven to 375°F. Line a baking sheet with parchment paper.

2. In a medium saucepan, combine the quinoa and vegetable broth. Bring to a boil over medium-high heat, reduce to a simmer, cover, and cook until the seeds are translucent and have "spiraled out," 12 to 15 minutes. Remove from the heat and let stand for 5 minutes to cool.

(recipe continues)

(recipe continued from page 247)

suppertime inspiration:

Being a parent and working full-time is such a balancing act. Sometimes it can feel truly overwhelming. I rely heavily on scripture to carry me through the difficult times. This verse always inspires me to persevere, reminding me that my hard work will soon pay off: "And let us not grow weary of doing good, for in due season we will reap, if we do not give up." Galatians 6:9.

3. In a large bowl, combine the black beans, garlic powder, onion powder, cumin, paprika, salt, pepper, lime juice, chipotle pepper, adobo sauce, egg, and bread crumbs. Mash the mixture together with a fork until incorporated. Fold in the cooked quinoa and corn.

4. Using clean hands, form the mixture into 4 patties. Place the patties on the prepared baking sheet.

5. Bake for 10 minutes, flip over, and bake until the patties are firm, 10 minutes longer. Be careful not to overcook, as the patties will dry out.

6. Meanwhile, to make the chipotle mayonnaise: In a small bowl, whisk together the mayonnaise, sour cream, lime juice, chipotle pepper, and garlic powder. Refrigerate until ready to serve.

7. Serve the burgers on the whole wheat buns with the chipotle mayonnaise. If desired, top the burgers with the optional ingredients.

Suggested Side Dish: Southwest "Fried" Pickles (page 284)

quick and easy: **Remember, veggie burgers are not meat burgers. Since there is so little fat in a veggie burger, they typically cook up quickly and will dry out if overcooked. Pay close attention to cook time.**

Calories 389 • Fat 7g • Carbohydrate 74g • Fiber 11g • Sugar 8g • Protein 16g
Nutrition does not include optional ingredients.

Sweet Potato Frittata

The only difference between omelets and frittatas is that omelets traditionally have the egg mixture cooked and folded around a filling, while a frittata just mixes all the ingredients together. (Personally, I'm more of a frittata girl.) You'll prepare this dish partly on the stovetop first so your potatoes and veggies get a little crispy before blending them together with the eggs and popping it into the oven. Enjoy for brinner or a weekend brunch.

Prep Time: 10 minutes | **Cook Time:** 45 minutes
Serves: 6 | **Serving Size:** ⅙ of the frittata

2 tablespoons walnuts, coarsely chopped

2 teaspoons extra virgin olive oil

1 medium sweet potato, peeled and cut into ½-inch cubes

1 small onion, thinly sliced

1 red bell pepper, thinly sliced

3 cups baby spinach

2 teaspoons apple cider vinegar

5 eggs

4 egg whites

1 teaspoon finely chopped fresh rosemary

1 tablespoon sugar-free maple-flavor syrup (I like Maple Grove Farms)

¼ teaspoon salt

¼ teaspoon black pepper

3 wedges Laughing Cow Creamy Swiss Light cheese, cut into small pieces

1. Preheat the oven to 400°F. Coat a cast iron skillet or other ovenproof skillet generously with cooking spray (see Quick and Easy).

2. In a separate small skillet, toast the chopped walnuts over medium-high heat, stirring occasionally, until the walnuts are fragrant, 4 to 6 minutes. Transfer the walnuts to a plate and set aside.

3. Add 1 teaspoon of the olive oil to the skillet and heat over medium-high heat. Add the sweet potato and stir frequently to brown evenly, 8 to 10 minutes. Remove the sweet potato and set aside.

4. Add the remaining 1 teaspoon oil to the hot skillet. Add the onion and bell pepper and cook for 4 to 6 minutes to soften. Add the spinach and vinegar and cook until the spinach is wilted, about 2 minutes longer.

5. Return the sweet potato to the skillet and stir to evenly combine all of the ingredients. Reduce the heat to low.

6. In a large bowl, whisk together the whole eggs, egg whites, rosemary, syrup, salt, and black

(recipe continues)

(recipe continued from page 249)

quick and easy: If you do not have an ovenproof skillet, transfer the frittata to a standard pie pan before placing it in the oven.

pepper. Whisk thoroughly, making sure to incorporate air into the mixture.

7. Gently pour the egg mixture over the sweet potato mixture in the skillet. Drop the cheese wedge pieces evenly throughout the mixture. Cook the frittata over low heat for 8 to 10 minutes, until the eggs start to set.

8. Transfer the frittata to the oven and bake until the center is completely set, 12 to 15 minutes. Remove from the oven and allow to rest for 3 to 5 minutes.

9. Serve with the toasted walnuts on top.

suppertime chat: If you have kids, you know they're always in the process of learning something: a new sport or a new skill set in school. Often, they (and we) can become overwhelmed, feeling like they'll never get it. Help your child realize their potential by asking, "What is something you couldn't do when you were younger but now you can?" They'll quickly be reminded that there was a time when they couldn't read or ride a bike. But just like learning those skills, they will also learn and conquer new ones now and in the future.

Calories 149 • Fat 8g • Carbohydrate 10g • Fiber 2g • Sugar 4g • Protein 10g

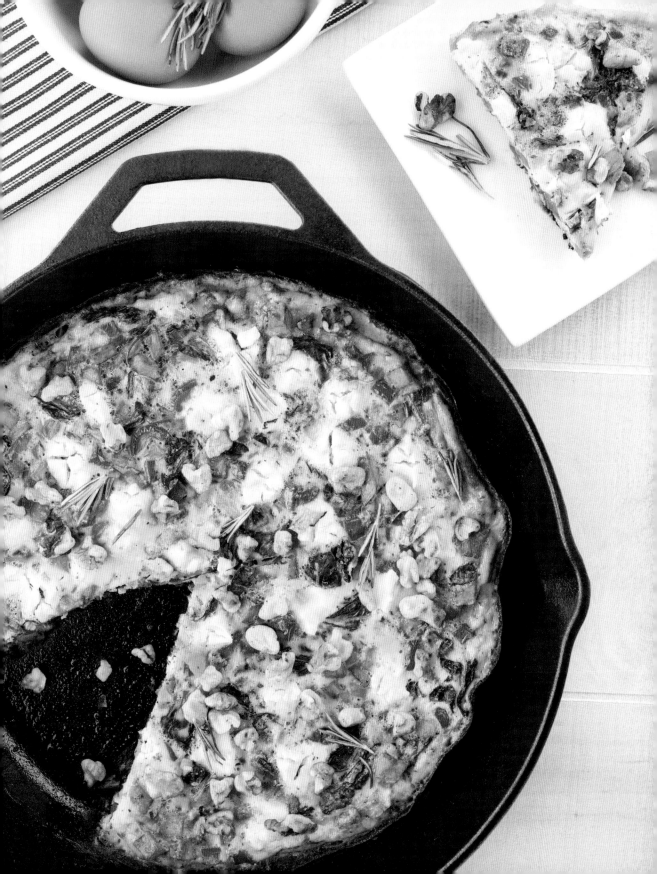

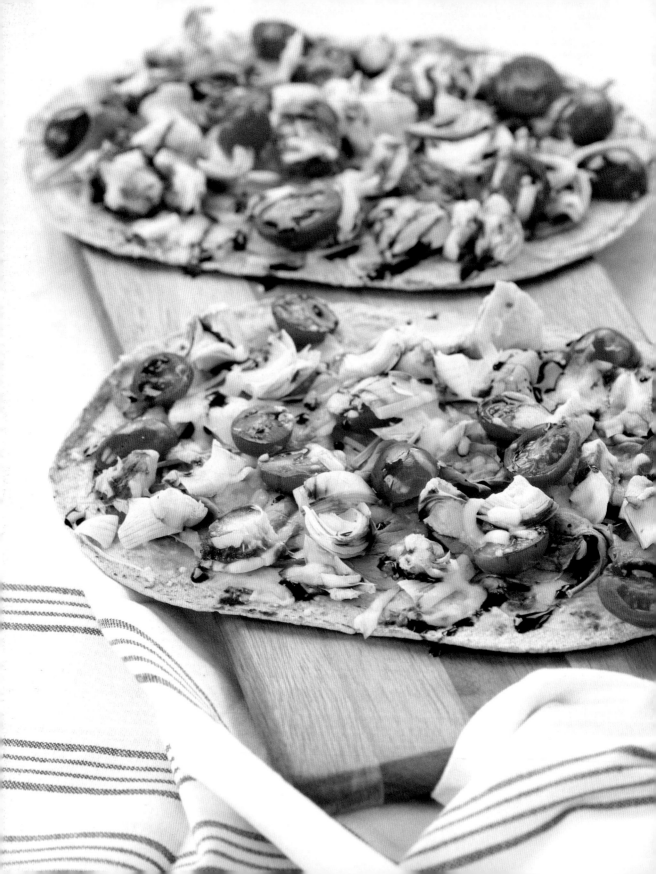

Spinach-Artichoke Flatbread Pizzas

Using flatbread as the foundation for these pizzas ensures a crispy crust that you can feel good about devouring. In this recipe, I finish the pizzas with a balsamic reduction: balsamic vinegar cooked down to a sweet, gooey glaze to drizzle over your flatbread toppings. It's like the "icing on the pizza"!

Prep Time: 5 minutes | **Cook Time:** 25 minutes
Serves: 6 | **Serving Size:** 1 flatbread pizza

1 cup balsamic vinegar

6 Flatout Light Italian Herb flatbreads

¾ cup Prego Light Homestyle Alfredo sauce or Make It Homemade (page 132)

6 cups baby spinach

3 cups grape tomatoes, halved

1 (15-ounce) can quartered artichoke hearts, drained and chopped

¾ cup shredded reduced-fat mozzarella cheese (I like Sargento)

suppertime inspiration:

Dr. Seuss once said, "Sometimes you will never know the value of a moment until it becomes a memory." So, even if sitting down to supper seems insignificant and too difficult, remember, it's the memory you're longing to create.

1. Preheat the oven to 350°F. Line 2 baking sheets with foil.

2. In a small saucepan, bring the balsamic vinegar to a boil over medium heat. Reduce the heat to medium-low and simmer until the balsamic vinegar starts to thicken and has reduced by half, 20 to 25 minutes.

3. Meanwhile, lay out the flatbreads on the prepared baking sheets and coat with cooking spray. Bake for 5 to 6 minutes. Remove from the oven but leave the oven on.

4. Spread 2 tablespoons Alfredo sauce evenly onto each flatbread. Top each with 1 cup spinach, ½ cup grape tomatoes, ¼ cup artichokes, and 2 tablespoons mozzarella.

5. Return to the oven and bake until the cheese is melted, 7 to 9 minutes. Remove from the oven and drizzle the balsamic reduction evenly over each pizza.

Suggested Side Dish: Italian Chickpea Salad (page 278)

Calories 244 • Fat 7g • Carbohydrate 36g • Fiber 11g • Sugar 2g • Protein 14g

Vegetable Ranch Pizza

This is my go-to "girly event" dish. It started several years ago when I made one for a girlfriend for her baby shower. Everyone went wild over the fresh crunchy veggies and the creamy ranch pizza sauce. Not to mention the perfect portion-control slices. This dish is ideal for any other warm-weather get-together. And since it gets served cold, there are no worries about reheating for late arrivals.

Prep Time: 10 minutes, plus 30 minutes chilling time | **Cook Time:** 10 minutes
Serves: 6 | **Serving Size:** ⅙ of the pizza

---

1 (13.8-ounce) can Pillsbury Artisan whole grain pizza dough

1 (.06-ounce) packet ranch dressing mix

¼ cup light sour cream

¼ cup plain 0% Greek yogurt

6 ounces ⅓-less-fat cream cheese, softened

2 teaspoons lemon juice

½ teaspoon garlic powder

2 teaspoons fresh dill

¼ cup diced red onion

1 red bell pepper, diced

½ cup shredded carrots

1 cup coarsely chopped broccoli

1 cup grape tomatoes, halved

1. Preheat the oven to 350°F. Coat a baking sheet with cooking spray.

2. Roll out the pizza dough to fit a 12 x 17-inch baking sheet.

3. Bake the pizza crust for 14 to 16 minutes. Cool and set aside.

4. In a medium bowl, combine the dressing mix, sour cream, yogurt, cream cheese, lemon juice, garlic powder, and dill. Use a handheld mixer to mix the ingredients for 1 to 2 minutes, until smooth.

5. Spread the mixture evenly over the baked pizza crust. Top with the red onion, bell pepper, carrots, broccoli, and tomatoes. Refrigerate for at least 30 minutes before serving.

suppertime inspiration: Although it's natural (and wonderful) to want to improve, don't lose sight of the great qualities God blessed you with. We can spend too much time comparing ourselves with others, frustrated by the skills and qualities they possess that we do not. It's okay if you don't create a new Pinterest board every day and your house isn't a picture out of the Pottery Barn catalog. Maybe you're a whiz with afterschool snacks or make up the best bedtime stories. Spend a little more time this week reminding yourself of the great things about you. The list is longer than you think!

Calories 307 • Fat 14g • Carbohydrate 35g • Fiber 3g • Sugar 6g • Protein 9g

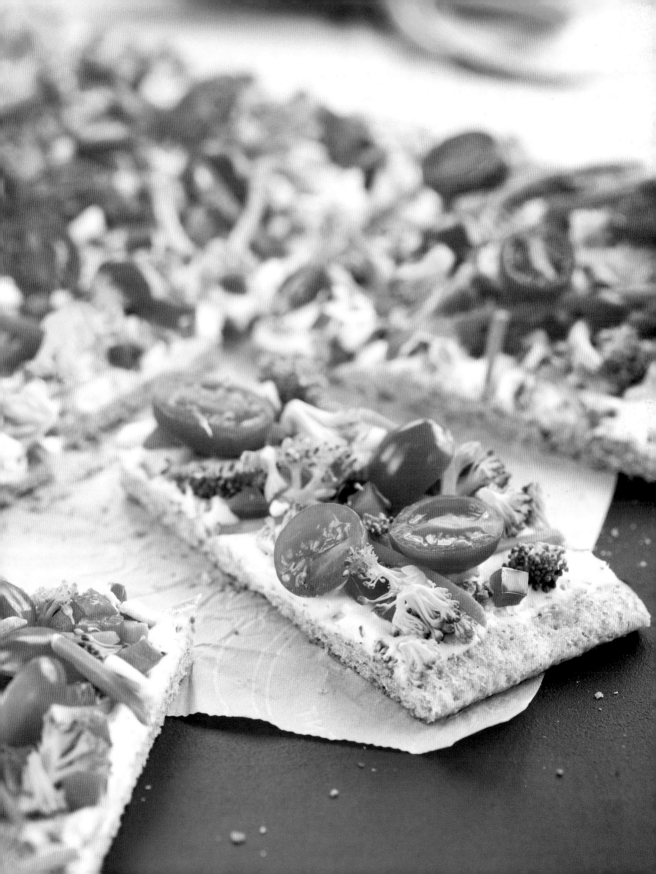

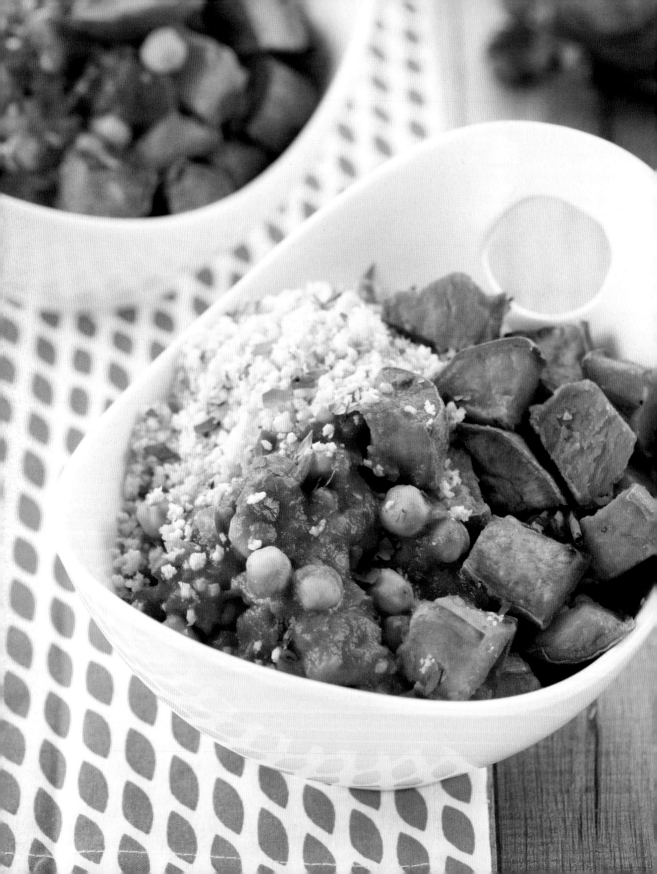

Vegetarian Tikka Masala

While there are many variations, tikka masala is typically a delicious red cream sauce that combines a variety of earthy spices and boasts a unique Indian flavor. Masala spice blend is readily available in most grocery stores alongside other spices like curry and thyme, so the sauce is super easy to make.

Prep Time: 10 minutes | **Cook Time:** 30 minutes
Serves: 4 | **Serving Size:** 1 cup sweet potatoes, 1 heaping cup tikka masala

---

4 medium sweet potatoes, unpeeled and cut into 1½-inch pieces

1 tablespoon coconut oil, melted

1 small onion, diced

1 teaspoon minced garlic

1 serrano chile pepper, minced

1 tablespoon garam masala

¼ teaspoon salt

¼ teaspoon black pepper

1 tablespoon tomato paste

2 (14.5-ounce) cans no-salt-added diced tomatoes (I like Hunt's)

1 (15-ounce) can chickpeas, drained and rinsed

⅔ cup lite coconut milk (I like Thai Kitchen)

2 tablespoons coarsely chopped raw unsalted cashews

¼ cup chopped fresh cilantro

1 lime, cut into 4 wedges (optional)

1. Preheat the oven to 425°F. Coat a baking sheet with cooking spray.

2. In a large bowl, combine the sweet potatoes and ½ tablespoon of the coconut oil and gently toss to evenly coat. Arrange the sweet potatoes on the prepared baking sheet. Roast until tender, about 30 minutes, turning at the halfway mark.

3. Meanwhile, in a large skillet, heat the remaining ½ tablespoon coconut oil over medium-high heat. Add the onion and garlic and cook until the onion is translucent, 3 to 5 minutes. Add the serrano chile, garam masala, salt, and black pepper and stir to evenly coat. Cook for 1 to 2 minutes longer.

4. Add the tomato paste, diced tomatoes, and chickpeas and stir. Bring the mixture to a boil, reduce the heat to medium-low, and simmer, stirring occasionally, for 15 minutes.

5. Pour in the coconut milk and continue to simmer for 6 minutes longer. Taste and adjust the seasonings if needed.

6. To serve, top each portion of sweet potatoes with a heaping cup of tikka masala. Garnish with the cashews and cilantro. If desired, squeeze a lime wedge over each portion.

Suggested Side Dish: Quick Cauliflower Couscous (page 286)

Calories 379 • Fat 9g • Carbohydrate 64g • Fiber 14g • Sugar 17g • Protein 11g

Easy Vegetable Lo Mein

At first, I was unsure about oyster sauce. I gave it a try and now I'm a true fan. It's what gives this lo mein dish its sweet and salty flavor that miraculously mimics my favorite take-out dish while being full of veggies and packed with protein.

Prep Time: 10 minutes | **Cook Time:** 15 minutes
Serves: 4 | **Serving Size:** 2 cups

6 ounces whole wheat spaghetti
　　(I like Barilla)

1 teaspoon extra virgin olive oil

1 small onion, thinly sliced

1 red bell pepper, thinly sliced

1 cup shredded carrots

3 cups broccoli florets

1 (8-ounce) container baby bella
　　(cremini) mushrooms, sliced

1 (7-ounce) jar whole pickled baby
　　corn, drained and sliced in half

¼ teaspoon salt

⅛ teaspoon black pepper

Sauce:

2 teaspoons cornstarch

¾ cup low-sodium vegetable broth
　　(I like Pacific Organic)

2 tablespoons rice vinegar

1 tablespoon sesame oil

1 teaspoon minced garlic

1 tablespoon less-sodium soy sauce

½ tablespoon oyster sauce

2 teaspoons stevia

For Serving:

3 green onions, thinly sliced

1 teaspoon sesame seeds

1. Bring a large pot of salted water to a boil over high heat. Cook the pasta to al dente according to the package directions. Drain and set aside.

2. Heat a wok or large skillet over medium-high heat. Add the olive oil and, when hot, add the onion, bell pepper, carrots, broccoli, mushrooms, and baby corn. Season with the salt and black pepper. Cook, stirring frequently, until the vegetables begin to soften, 8 to 10 minutes.

3. Meanwhile, prepare the sauce: In a small bowl, dissolve the cornstarch in the vegetable broth to make a slurry. Set aside.

4. In a small saucepan, combine the rice vinegar, sesame oil, garlic, soy sauce, oyster sauce, and stevia. Stir to combine and bring the mixture to a boil over medium-high heat. Gradually add in the slurry while stirring the mixture. Reduce the heat to medium-low and simmer, stirring often, until the sauce thickens, 2 to 4 minutes. Remove the sauce from the heat.

5. Transfer the cooked noodles to the wok and mix with the vegetables. Pour the sauce over the noodles and vegetables and toss to coat.

6. To serve, garnish with the green onions and sesame seeds.

Calories 287 • Fat 7g • Carbohydrate 49g • Fiber 9g • Sugar 13g • Protein 13g

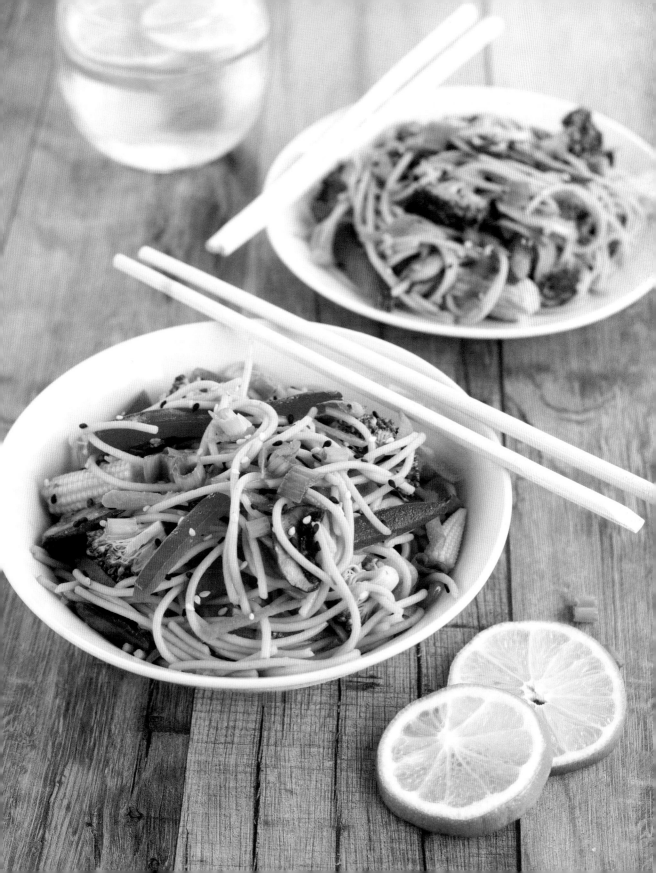

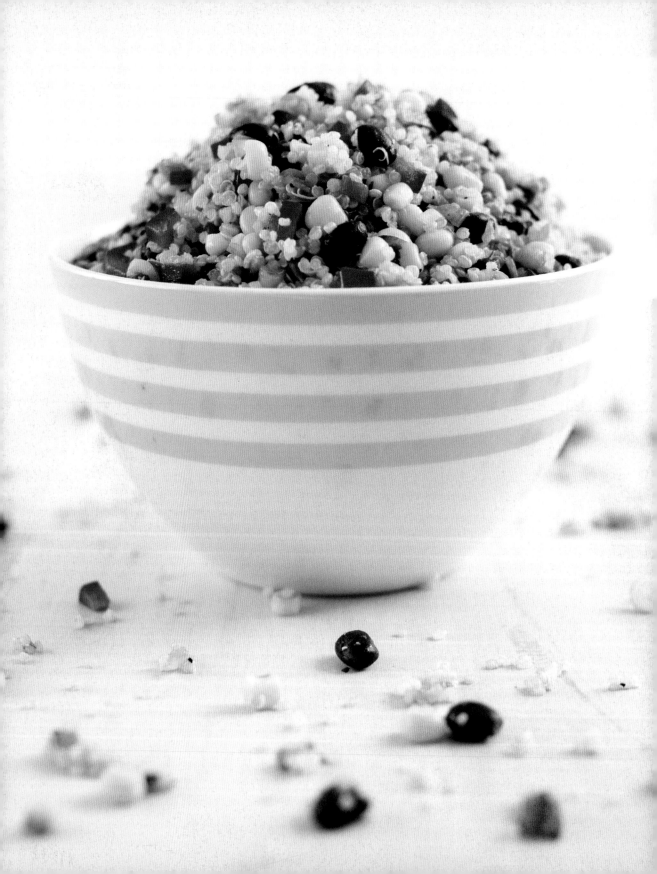

SKINNY SIDE DISHES

Asparagus Fries with Garlic Lemon Aioli

I have found asparagus to be the ideal canvas if you're looking for a new and interesting flavor for french fries. There is very little prep, and the crunchy coating includes flaxseed meal, which adds incredible nutritional value (it's been linked to aiding in weight management, has cancer-fighting properties, and boosts immunity).

Prep Time: 10 minutes | **Cook Time:** 10 minutes
Serves: 4 | **Serving Size:** 7 asparagus spears, 1 tablespoon aioli

---

28 asparagus spears

¼ cup white whole wheat flour

½ teaspoon salt

½ teaspoon black pepper

2 egg whites

¾ cup panko bread crumbs

1 tablespoon flaxseed meal

¼ cup grated Parmesan cheese
(I like Sargento)

Lemon Aioli Dipping Sauce:

3 tablespoons light mayonnaise

½ teaspoon grated lemon zest

1 tablespoon lemon juice

½ teaspoon garlic powder

⅛ teaspoon salt

⅛ teaspoon black pepper

skinny sense: Aioli is a garlicky mayonnaise, superb for dipping foods like fries; but it can also be used as a condiment and is an ideal topping for sandwiches and burgers alike.

1. Preheat the oven to 425°F. Line a baking sheet with foil and coat with cooking spray.

2. Wash the asparagus and trim off the bottoms.

3. In a shallow baking dish, mix together the flour, salt, and pepper. In a separate shallow baking dish, whisk the egg whites. In a third shallow baking dish, or on a plate, mix the panko, flaxseed meal, and Parmesan.

4. To bread the asparagus, roll the spears through the flour mixture and shake off the excess. Next, roll the asparagus through the egg whites and allow the excess to drip off. Third, roll through the panko mixture, and press gently to adhere to the spears.

5. Lay out the asparagus on the prepared baking sheet in a single layer. Bake until golden, 10 to 12 minutes.

6. Meanwhile, prepare the lemon aioli dipping sauce: In a small bowl, whisk together the mayonnaise, lemon zest, lemon juice, garlic powder, salt, and pepper.

7. Serve the asparagus fries with the dipping sauce.

Calories 161 • Fat 6g • Carbohydrate 20g • Fiber 4g • Sugar 3g • Protein 9g

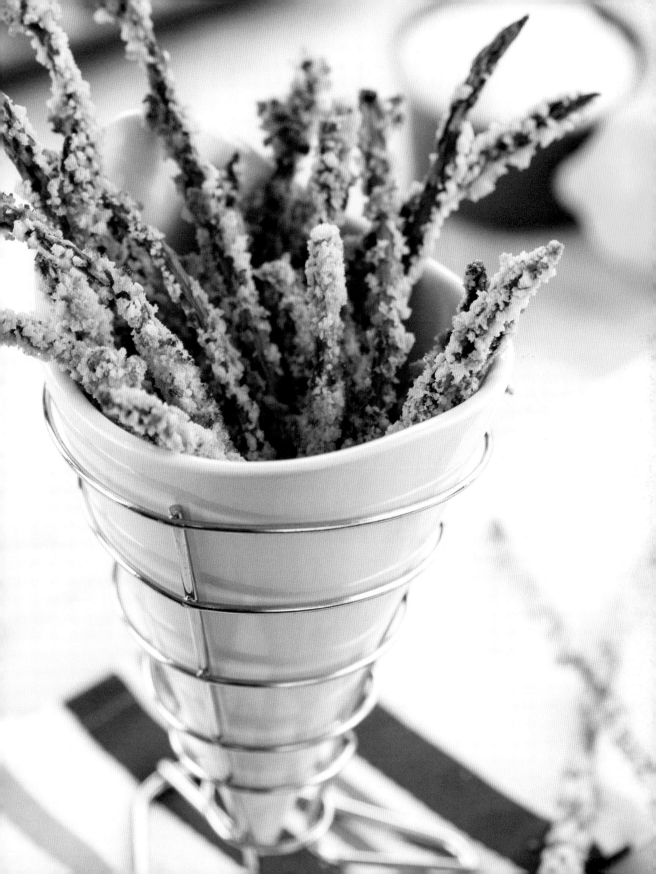

The Creamiest Mac 'n' Cheese Dish You Will Ever Make

I'm beyond proud of this recipe! This mac 'n' cheese will forever be a hit with your kids. So often, in lightened versions of macaroni and cheese, the absence of heavy cream and butter leaves this dish dried out. The combination of Greek yogurt and light sour cream ensures the creamiest mac 'n' cheese around—with far less fat and fewer calories.

Prep Time: 10 minutes | **Cook Time:** 35 minutes
Serves: 12 | **Serving Size:** 2/3 cup

1 (12-ounce) box Barilla Veggie Elbow pasta

1 (10.5-ounce) can Campbell's Healthy Request condensed cheddar cheese soup

½ cup plain 0% Greek yogurt

2 tablespoons light sour cream

¼ teaspoon salt

¼ teaspoon black pepper

½ cup shredded reduced-fat mozzarella cheese (I like Sargento)

½ cup shredded reduced-fat cheddar cheese (I like Sargento)

¼ cup panko bread crumbs

1. Preheat the oven to 350°F. Coat a 13 x 9-inch baking dish with cooking spray.

2. Bring a large pot of salted water to a boil over high heat. Cook the pasta to al dente according to the package directions. Drain.

3. Meanwhile, in a large bowl, combine the cheddar cheese soup, yogurt, sour cream, salt, and pepper and stir to mix well. Fold in the mozzarella and ¼ cup of the cheddar.

4. Add the drained pasta to the cheese mixture and stir until the pasta is evenly coated. Transfer the pasta to the prepared baking dish. Top with the remaining ¼ cup cheddar and the panko.

5. Cover the baking dish with foil and bake for 20 minutes. Remove the foil and bake until the cheese is melted and bubbly, about 5 minutes longer. Serve warm.

Calories 156 • Fat 3g • Carbohydrate 25g • Fiber 1g • Sugar 2g • Protein 7g

Broccoli Mac 'n' Cheese

This is a great way to add veggies to a long-standing kid (and grown-up) favorite. The flavor of the broccoli is enhanced by the rich and creamy combination of Swiss and cheddar cheeses.

Prep Time: 5 minutes | **Cook Time:** 20 minutes
Serves: 12 | **Serving Size:** 2/3 cup

1 (13.25-ounce) box whole wheat elbow pasta (I like Barilla)

4 cups broccoli florets

2 tablespoons unsalted butter

½ cup finely diced onion

2 teaspoons minced garlic

2 tablespoons white whole wheat flour

1½ cups fat-free milk

3 wedges Laughing Cow Creamy Swiss Light cheese

1 cup shredded reduced-fat sharp cheddar cheese (I like Sargento)

1 teaspoon salt

1 teaspoon black pepper

suppertime chat: Spend some time talking about family history. In what country did your family originate? What do you know about your ancestors? Is there anyone famous in your lineage?

1. Bring a large pot of salted water to a boil over high heat. Cook the pasta to al dente according to the package directions. During the last 2 minutes of cook time, add the broccoli. Reserving 1/2 cup of the pasta water, drain the pasta and broccoli and return to the cooking pot. Set aside.

2. Meanwhile, in a large skillet, melt the butter over medium-low heat. Add the onion and garlic and cook, stirring constantly, until the onion has softened, 2 to 3 minutes.

3. Whisk the flour into the butter for about 30 seconds, until the mixture is smooth and smells nutty, making a roux. Increase the heat to medium-high and whisk in the milk. Bring to a boil, making sure to stir constantly. Reduce the heat to low and add the cheese wedges, cheddar, salt, and pepper. Continue to stir the sauce until the cheeses have melted, about 5 minutes. Once the sauce has thickened, remove from the heat.

4. Pour the cheese sauce over the pasta and broccoli and add the reserved pasta water. Stir to evenly combine. Serve warm.

Calories 192 • Fat 5g • Carbohydrate 28g • Fiber 4g • Sugar 3g • Protein 9g

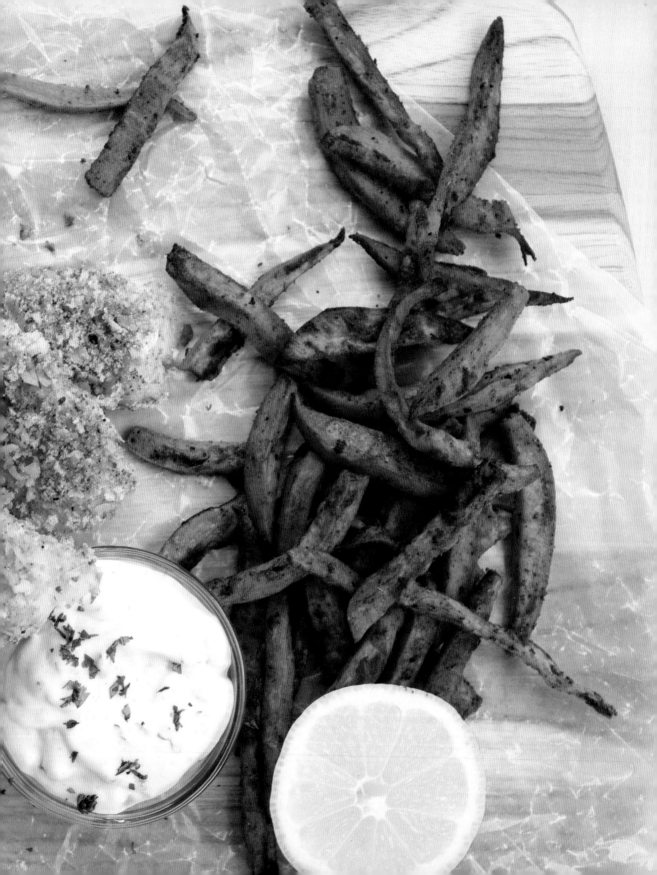

Cajun-Style Sweet Potato Fries

French fries are my all-time favorite side dish. It's a guilty pleasure, I know. But now I've truly found a way to indulge guilt-free with these flavorful sweet potato fries. I make this recipe several times a month, and I love trying out different flavor combinations like sriracha, Parmesan, and fresh rosemary in place of the Cajun seasoning. Get creative and have some fun with this side!

Prep Time: 10 minutes | **Cook Time:** 40 minutes
Serves: 4 | **Serving Size:** 18 to 20 fries

2 large sweet potatoes, peeled and sliced into thin fries

½ tablespoon coconut oil, melted

1 teaspoon cornstarch

1 teaspoon Cajun seasoning or Make It Homemade (page 299)

¼ teaspoon salt

¼ teaspoon black pepper

1 tablespoon chopped fresh parsley

1. Preheat the oven to 400°F. Coat a baking sheet with cooking spray.

2. In a large bowl, combine the sweet potatoes, coconut oil, cornstarch, and Cajun seasoning and toss to evenly coat.

3. Transfer the potatoes in a single layer onto the baking sheet. Bake for 15 to 20 minutes, then turn the fries and bake for 15 to 20 minutes longer, until golden brown and tender.

4. Before serving, season the fries with the salt, pepper, and parsley.

suppertime inspiration: Regularly planning and preparing healthy meals can be quite a stretch with my busy schedule, even though it's just the two of us. A great quote that I discovered a few years ago is "When you feel like quitting, think about why you started." It's a powerful way to get reenergized and refocused.

Calories 74 • Fat 2g • Carbohydrate 14g • Fiber 2g • Sugar 3g • Protein 1g

Carrot and Raisin Salad

This side dish was inspired by one of my son's and my favorite restaurants: Chik-fil-A. They served this amazingly sweet carrot and raisin salad that I ordered until they took it off the menu in 2013. I was so sad. Until now! This is my adaptation and it's tasty, colorful, and easy to pull off. Carrots and raisins balance each other in color, texture, and flavor, and the salad pairs well with any protein. Feel free to swap the raisins for any dried fruit of choice.

Prep Time: 10 minutes
Serves: 4 | **Serving Size:** ¾ cup

1 (10-ounce) bag shredded carrots (see Quick and Easy)

¼ cup raisins

¼ cup walnuts, coarsely chopped

2 tablespoons light mayonnaise

2 tablespoons plain 0% Greek yogurt

2 tablespoons light brown sugar

2 tablespoons fat-free milk

1 teaspoon lemon juice

¼ teaspoon salt

⅛ teaspoon black pepper

1. In a medium bowl, toss the carrots, raisins, and walnuts together.

2. In a small bowl, whisk together the mayonnaise, yogurt, brown sugar, milk, lemon juice, salt, and pepper.

3. Pour the dressing over the carrot mixture and toss to evenly combine. Serve chilled.

quick and easy: Do you have a bag of whole carrots in your crisper drawer that no one is snacking on? Shred them yourself with a grater instead of buying another bag of shredded carrots.

Calories 153 • Fat 7g • Carbohydrate 22g • Fiber 3g • Sugar 16g • Protein 4g

Cauliflower Mashed Potatoes

This is an indulgent side dish without indulging. Homemade mashed potatoes can be high in fat and calories. Using only two potatoes and an entire head of cauliflower gives me the satisfaction of knowing that I'm getting good ingredients but with fewer calories. No one will suspect that you've swapped out the heavy cream for Greek yogurt.

Prep Time: 5 minutes | **Cook Time:** 10 minutes
Serves: 4 | **Serving Size:** 1¼ cups

4 cups low-sodium chicken broth
  (I like Pacific Organic)
2 baking potatoes, peeled and cut
  into 1-inch pieces
1 head cauliflower, cored and
  chopped
¼ cup light sour cream
¼ cup plain 0% Greek yogurt
1 teaspoon salt
Pinch of black pepper

1. In a medium pot, combine the chicken broth, potatoes, and cauliflower. Bring to a boil over medium-high heat and cook until the potatoes are fork-tender, 8 to 10 minutes. Drain and transfer to a large bowl.

2. Use a handheld mixer or potato masher to mash the potatoes and cauliflower. Add the sour cream, yogurt, salt, and pepper and mix or stir for 1 to 2 minutes, until well combined. The potato mixture should be creamy. Serve warm.

suppertime inspiration: Did you know that an "attitude of gratitude" is likely to improve your mental and physical health? Countless studies have proven that those with a grateful heart are happier, are healthier, have more energy, and are less prone to sickness. The next time you feel the urge to complain, take a few seconds to shift your mind-set to an "attitude of gratitude." Your mind and body will thank you!

Calories 109 • Fat 3g • Carbohydrate 16g • Fiber 2g • Sugar 3g • Protein 6g

Cheesy Jalapeño Cornbread

Cornbread as a skinny side? Yes, you read that correctly! I love cornbread and my granny has the most amazing recipe, but there is one problem: It calls for a whole stick of butter! In my quest to make a low-calorie cornbread, I had to make this recipe several times to ensure a moist and crumbly cornbread with just the right amount of sweetness. Enjoy!

Prep Time: 10 minutes | **Cook Time:** 30 minutes
Serves: 12 | **Serving Size:** 1 wedge

1¼ cups yellow cornmeal

½ cup white whole wheat flour

1 tablespoon baking powder

½ teaspoon salt

1½ tablespoons stevia

¼ cup plain 0% Greek yogurt

¼ cup light sour cream

1 cup canned cream-style corn
   (I like Del Monte)

¼ cup unsweetened applesauce

1 egg

1 egg white

¼ cup fat-free milk

¼ cup sugar-free maple-flavor syrup
   (I like Maple Grove Farms)

½ cup shredded reduced-fat sharp
   cheddar cheese (I like Sargento)

1 jalapeño pepper, seeded and
   diced

1. Preheat the oven to 350°F. Coat a cast iron skillet or other ovenproof skillet generously with cooking spray. Place in the oven for 5 minutes to preheat.

2. Meanwhile, in a large bowl, whisk together the cornmeal, flour, baking powder, salt, and stevia.

3. In a medium bowl, mix together the yogurt, sour cream, corn, applesauce, whole egg and egg white, milk, and syrup.

4. Add the wet ingredients to the dry ingredients and stir to combine. Fold in the cheddar and jalapeño.

5. Pour the batter into the preheated skillet. Bake until a toothpick inserted comes out clean, about 30 minutes. Cool for 5 minutes before cutting into 12 equal wedges.

suppertime chat: Share with your children what suppertime was like when you were a kid. Chances are it was much more structured. For me, supper was always at 6 p.m. No one called during suppertime; no one knocked on the door. Suppertime was regarded as "family time." Conveying stories like this will deepen the bond, reminding family members how important time together is.

Calories 115 • Fat 3g • Carbohydrate 19g • Fiber 2g • Sugar 2g • Protein 5g

Cilantro-Lime Rice

This is my go-to side when I'm craving Mexican cuisine. It's the perfect complement to my Carnitas Veggie Bowl (page 158) and the cilantro adds a fresh twist to brown rice.

Prep Time: Less than 5 minutes │ **Cook Time:** 2 minutes
Serves: 4 │ **Serving Size:** 1 cup

2 (8.8-ounce) pouches Uncle Ben's Ready Rice brown rice

2 tablespoons chopped fresh cilantro

½ tablespoon extra virgin olive oil

1 tablespoon lime juice

½ teaspoon salt

1. Microwave the rice according to the package directions.

2. Transfer the cooked rice to a medium bowl. Add the cilantro, olive oil, lime juice, and salt. Stir to combine all the ingredients. Serve warm.

skinny sense: Go brown. Anytime you can trade "brown" for "white," you're packing more vitamins and nutrients into your meals (and typically fewer calories). Try it with sugars, breads, rice, and pasta. For picky eaters, try swapping half white for half brown rice.

Calories 208 • Fat 5g • Carbohydrate 40g • Fiber 3g • Sugar 0g • Protein 6g

Skinny Sweet Potato Biscuits

I had so much fun developing this recipe. Who knew you could make biscuits with sweet potatoes? Just be careful, your hands will get sticky with this one, so be sure to keep them (along with your workspace) well floured.

Prep Time: 15 minutes | **Cook Time:** 25 minutes
Serves: 10 | **Serving Size:** 1 biscuit

1 large sweet potato

2 cups white whole wheat flour

1 tablespoon stevia

2½ tablespoons light brown sugar

1 tablespoon baking powder

½ teaspoon baking soda

½ teaspoon salt

1 teaspoon ground cinnamon

2 tablespoons sugar-free maple-flavor syrup (I like Maple Grove Farms)

3 tablespoons unsweetened applesauce

¾ cup low-fat buttermilk

1. Preheat the oven to 450°F. Line a baking sheet with parchment paper.

2. Wash the sweet potato and then poke the potato several times with a fork. Place it in a microwave-safe bowl and add 2 teaspoons of water to the bowl. Cover with plastic wrap and cut a slit in the top. Microwave for 3 to 5 minutes, until soft and the skin is loose. Let cool.

3. In a large bowl, whisk together the flour, stevia, brown sugar, baking powder, baking soda, salt, and cinnamon.

4. In a separate large bowl, stir together the syrup, applesauce, and buttermilk.

5. Once the sweet potato has cooled, peel and mash well with a fork. Transfer the mashed sweet potato to the wet ingredients and stir to combine.

6. Add the sweet potato mixture to the flour mixture and stir just until the dough comes together, being careful not to overmix.

7. Lightly flour a clean surface and using clean hands, transfer the sweet potato dough to the surface. It is very important to keep the surface covered lightly in flour, as the dough will be sticky. Gently roll the dough out to a 10-inch-

(recipe continues)

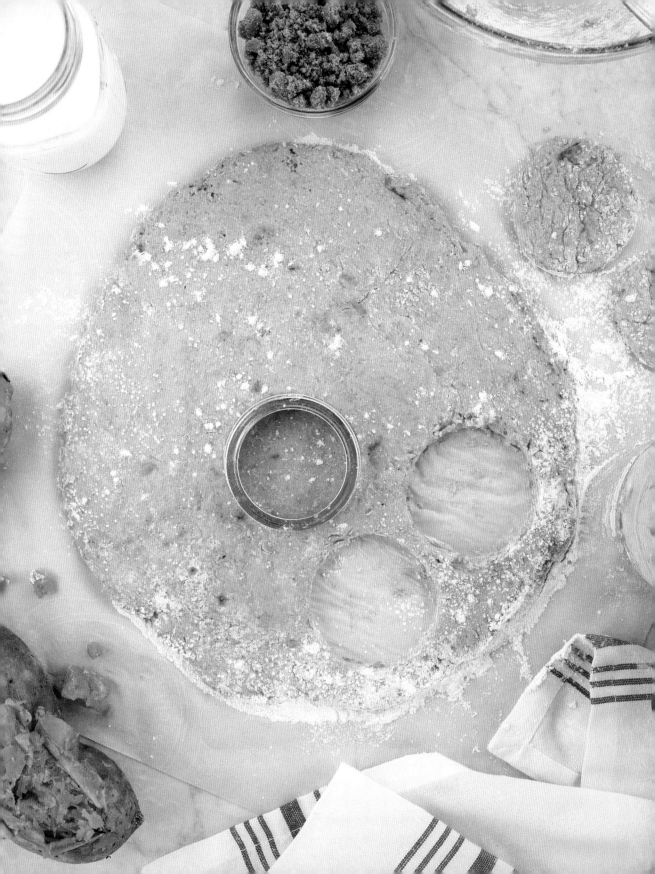

(recipe continued from page 272)

suppertime chat: **Have a family conversation about serving: How can you as individuals, and as a family, serve your extended family, friends, and community? Is there someone you know who needs assistance (or a meal)? This may spark an idea about a service project in the heart of one of your children (or even in your own heart)!**

diameter round about 1/2 inch thick and use a 2½-inch biscuit cutter or the rim of a juice glass to cut out biscuits. Gather the scraps and re-roll to cut out more biscuits. You should get 10 biscuits.

8. Transfer the biscuits to the prepared baking sheet. Bake until slightly browned on the edges, 24 to 28 minutes. Serve warm.

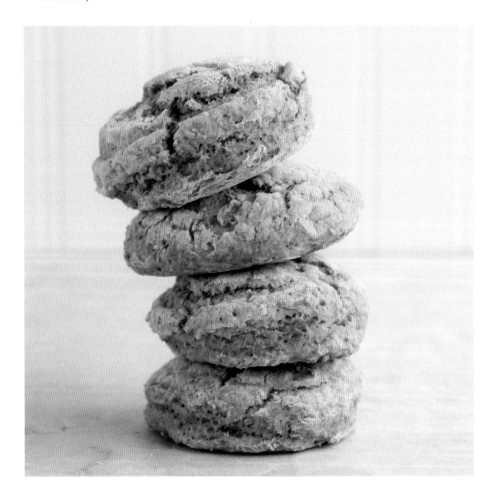

Calories 95 • Fat 1g • Carbohydrate 21g • Fiber 3g • Sugar 4g • Protein 2g

Easy Creamed Spinach

I wanted to make spinach taste a little more flavorful, hoping to convince my five-year-old to eat it. The light cream cheese and Greek yogurt does the trick (without heavy cream), and the total prep and cook time is less than 15 minutes. I like to serve this up alongside my Grilled Red Wine and Balsamic Flank Steak Roll-Ups (page 55).

Prep Time: Less than 5 minutes | **Cook Time:** 8 minutes
Serves: 4 | **Serving Size:** ½ cup

2 (10-ounce) packages frozen chopped spinach, thawed and drained (see Quick and Easy)

1 tablespoon unsalted butter

2 ounces ⅓-less-fat cream cheese, softened

½ teaspoon salt

¼ teaspoon garlic powder

¼ cup grated Parmesan cheese (I like Sargento)

1 tablespoon plain 0% Greek yogurt

1. In a medium saucepan, combine the spinach, butter, cream cheese, salt, garlic powder, and Parmesan and stir to combine.

2. Cook over medium-low heat, stirring occasionally, until heated through, 6 to 8 minutes. Fold in the yogurt and stir to evenly combine. Serve warm.

quick and easy: To thaw spinach quickly (or to prep it ahead of time): Remove the frozen block of spinach from the box and place it in a microwave-safe bowl. Microwave the spinach for 1 to 2 minutes, or until the spinach becomes soft. Place in a fine-mesh strainer and press down with a few paper towels to squeeze out as much water as possible. Set aside.

Calories 145 • Fat 8g • Carbohydrate 5g • Fiber 2g • Sugar 0g • Protein 8g

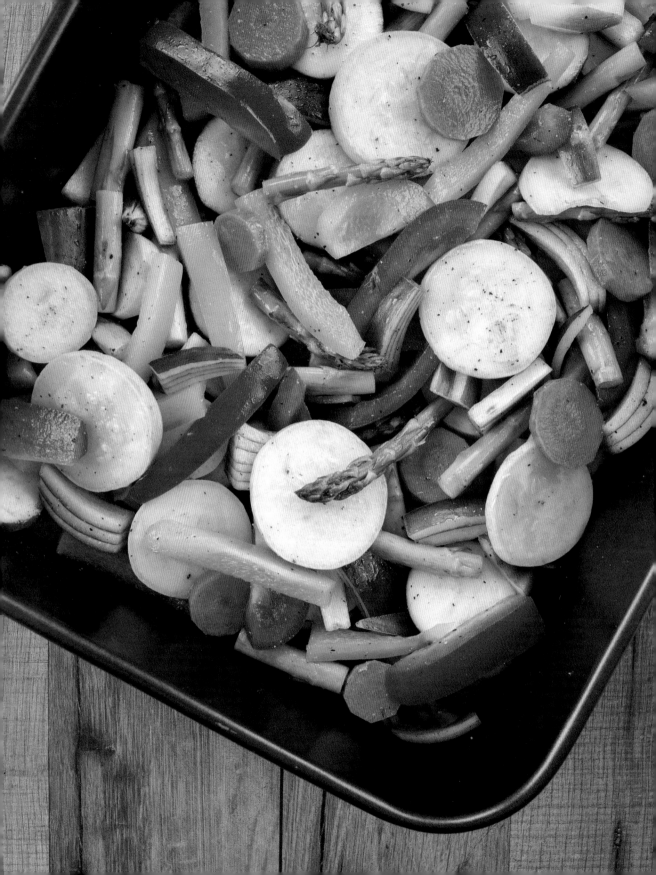

Easy Roasted Vegetables

Sometimes I like to get back to the basics. By simply using a little salt, pepper, and olive oil, you will enhance the color, texture, and flavor of these garden goodies. Enjoy the pure natural goodness of vegetables!

Prep Time: 10 minutes | **Cook Time:** 45 minutes
Serves: 6 | **Serving Size:** Heaping 1½ cups

1 yellow squash, sliced crosswise into ½-inch rounds

1 zucchini, sliced crosswise into ½-inch rounds

1 red onion, sliced

1 pound asparagus, cut into 2-inch lengths

1 red bell pepper, cut into ½-inch chunks

1 yellow bell pepper, sliced

1 carrot, sliced into ¼-inch rounds

½ teaspoon salt

½ teaspoon black pepper

1½ tablespoons extra virgin olive oil

1. Preheat the oven to 350°F. Coat 2 large roasting pans or baking sheets with cooking spray.

2. Place all the vegetables in a single layer in the roasting pans or on the baking sheets.

3. Season the vegetables with the salt and black pepper.

4. Drizzle with the olive oil and lightly toss the vegetables to evenly coat.

5. Bake until the vegetables have started to brown around the edges and are tender, about 45 minutes, turning the vegetables every 15 minutes for even cooking. Serve warm.

make-ahead tip: If you are getting into the habit of having a prep day, this is the perfect recipe. You can even prep these veggies and freeze them. Chopped, frozen veggies will keep several weeks in your freezer in airtight containers or resealable bags.

Calories 90 • Fat 4g • Carbohydrate 13g • Fiber 4g • Sugar 6g • Protein 3g

Italian Chickpea Salad

This salad pairs superbly with virtually any main dish and encompasses the best of the garden. The blend of textures, flavors, and colors bursts on the plate and on your palate. A vegetarian dish boasting protein-dense chickpeas, this stellar side could also be enjoyed as a main dish. It's ideal for any picnic, potluck event, or "what should I bring?" kind of occasion.

Prep Time: 5 minutes | **Cook Time:** 10 minutes
Serves: 8 | **Serving Size:** 1 cup

1 cup orzo pasta

1 (15-ounce) can chickpeas, drained and rinsed

1 (14.5-ounce) can no-salt-added diced tomatoes (I like Hunt's)

2 teaspoons minced garlic

1 small cucumber, diced

½ cup finely diced red onion

½ cup fat-free Italian dressing

1½ tablespoons finely chopped fresh basil

½ teaspoon salt

¼ teaspoon black pepper

1. Bring a large pot of salted water to a boil over high heat. Cook the pasta to al dente according to the package directions. Drain and rinse under cool water to quickly cool down the orzo. Set aside.

2. Meanwhile, in a large bowl, combine the chickpeas, tomatoes, garlic, cucumber, onion, Italian dressing, basil, salt, and pepper. Gently stir until combined.

3. Fold the cooked orzo into the chickpea mixture. Serve chilled.

suppertime chat: Have you ever thought about growing a vegetable or herb garden? Discuss with your family what veggies or herbs they might like to grow. Studies indicate that when kids take part in growing their vegetables, they're much more likely to eat them. Have no fear if you don't own acres of land for your garden. There are many one-pot veggies/herbs that grow just fine on back patios and porches, and there are farming co-ops in cities and suburban areas that you can locate with a quick online search or request at a farmers' market.

Calories 160 • Fat 1g • Carbohydrate 31g • Fiber 5g • Sugar 5g • Protein 3g

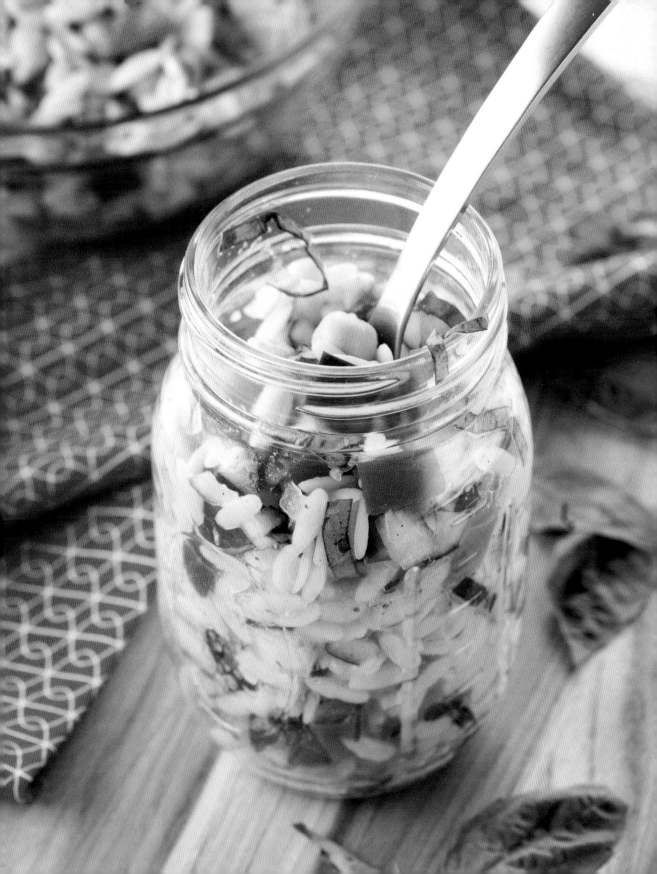

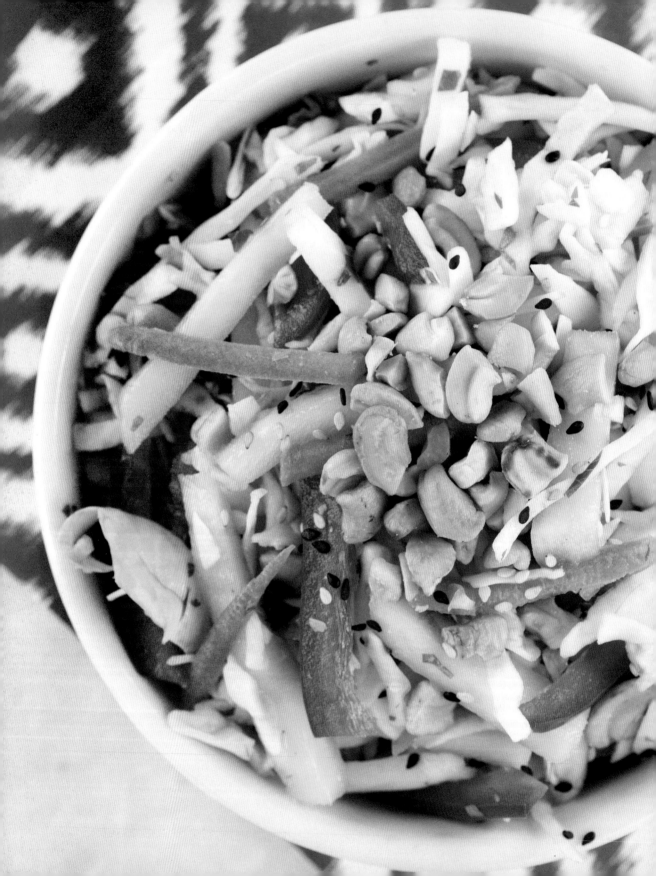

Mango Slaw

I like to mix it up and cook Asian-inspired suppers at least once a month at our house, but I needed a special side dish. Mango is the perfect complement to Asian cuisine, but be careful to buy your mango at the correct ripeness. To tell if a mango is ripe, give it a gentle squeeze on the sides. Ripe mangoes will be slightly soft to the touch, just like avocados and peaches.

Prep Time: 15 minutes, plus 15 minutes chilling time
Serves: 8 | **Serving Size:** ¾ cup

1 mango (see Quick and Easy)

1 (14-ounce) bag coleslaw mix

1 red bell pepper, julienned

3 green onions, thinly sliced

3 tablespoons chopped fresh cilantro

¼ cup lime juice

2 tablespoons rice vinegar

1 tablespoon less-sodium soy sauce

1 tablespoon sesame oil

1 teaspoon stevia

2 tablespoons coarsely chopped raw unsalted cashews

1 teaspoon sesame seeds

1. To cut the mango, slice the fat "cheeks" off the mango on either side of the flat almond-shaped pit. Then slice the 2 thin sides that are left around the pit. Peel the skin off all 4 of these sections and thinly slice the mango.

2. In a large bowl, toss together the mango, coleslaw mix, bell pepper, green onions, and cilantro.

3. In a small bowl, whisk together the lime juice, vinegar, soy sauce, sesame oil, and stevia.

4. Pour the dressing over the coleslaw and toss to mix well.

5. Refrigerate for 15 minutes before serving.

6. Serve garnished with the cashews and sesame seeds.

quick and easy: Feel free to purchase frozen mango for this recipe. To thaw the mango, place 1 cup in a bowl and refrigerate for at least 5 hours before ready to use. Try to stir or turn the fruit a few times while in the refrigerator for an even thaw and drain any juice or water from the mango before using.

Calories 76 • Fat 3g • Carbohydrate 12g • Fiber 2g • Sugar 9g • Protein 2g

Old Bay Deviled Eggs

Deviled eggs are an obvious staple for backyard barbecues. For these eggs, I use lightened versions of most of the ingredients needed in order to substantially cut the fat and calories. But it's the use of Old Bay seasoning that really adds a subtle smoked spice and makes these eggs perfect and not so "devilish."

Prep Time: 15 minutes | **Cook Time:** 25 minutes
Serves: 12 | **Serving Size:** 2 deviled eggs

12 large eggs

3 tablespoons light mayonnaise

3 tablespoons plain 0% Greek yogurt

1 teaspoon yellow mustard

1 tablespoon no-sugar-added pickle relish

1 teaspoon Old Bay seasoning

quick and easy: Make perfect deviled eggs every time using these tips:

- Use eggs that are closer to their expiration date. (Extremely fresh eggs are very difficult to peel.)
- To help center the egg yolks before they are cooked, turn the egg carton on its side at 8 to 12 hours before cooking.

1. In a pot big enough to hold the eggs in a single layer, combine the eggs and enough cold water to cover them completely.

2. Bring the water to a boil over medium-high heat. As soon as it comes to a boil, remove the pot from the heat, cover, and allow to sit for 16 to 18 minutes. Meanwhile, prepare a large bowl of ice and water.

3. Transfer the cooked eggs to the bowl of ice water to cool quickly. Peel the eggs and halve them lengthwise. Remove the yolks from the egg whites. Set aside all of the egg whites and discard 6 of the yolks.

4. In a large bowl, combine the remaining 6 yolks, the mayonnaise, yogurt, mustard, pickle relish, and 1/2 teaspoon of the Old Bay seasoning. Mix until well combined.

5. Spoon the egg yolk mixture into the egg whites evenly. Or to pipe the egg yolk mixture, use a pastry bag fitted with a star tip or a gallon-size resealable bag with one corner cut off.

6. To serve, sprinkle the tops of the eggs with the remaining 1/2 teaspoon Old Bay seasoning. Serve chilled.

Calories 71 • Fat 5g • Carbohydrate 0g • Fiber 0g • Sugar 0g • Protein 6g

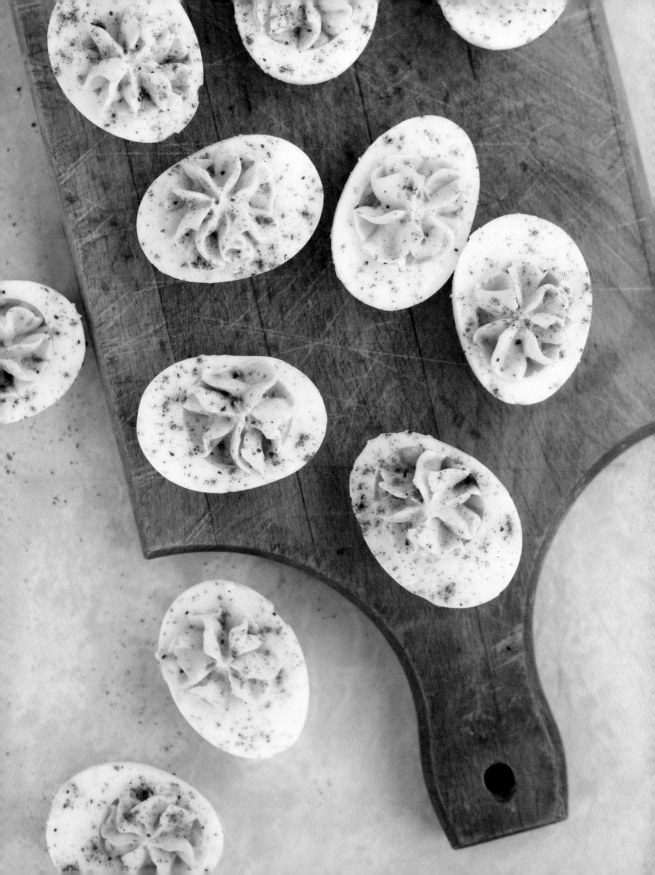

Southwest "Fried" Pickles

I'm obsessed with pickles, and fried pickles have become a huge hit over the last several years. They're as common on restaurant appetizer menus as Buffalo wings and cheese sticks. Knowing the fat and calorie trap they can be, I was determined to find a recipe for oven-fried pickles that could satisfy my craving. What resulted was a Southwestern "fried" pickle with a crispy coating that can be enjoyed as a side or snack anytime.

Prep Time: 10 minutes | **Cook Time:** 10 minutes
Serves: 6 | **Serving Size:** about 10 pickle chips

½ cup yellow cornmeal

½ cup panko bread crumbs

2 tablespoons white whole wheat flour

1 teaspoon chili powder

½ teaspoon ground cumin

¼ teaspoon paprika

¼ teaspoon salt

¼ teaspoon black pepper

2 egg whites

2 tablespoons low-fat buttermilk

2 teaspoons Frank's RedHot Sauce

1 (16-ounce) jar hamburger dill chips

Bolthouse Farms Classic Ranch Yogurt Dressing, for dipping (optional)

1. Preheat the oven to 425°F. Line a baking sheet with foil and coat with cooking spray.

2. In a medium bowl, whisk together the cornmeal, panko, flour, chili powder, cumin, paprika, salt, and pepper. In a separate medium bowl, whisk together the egg whites, buttermilk, and hot sauce.

3. Drain the pickle chips and place in a single layer on paper towels to remove excess moisture.

4. Dip the pickle chips into the egg mixture, then into the panko mixture, pressing the bread crumbs onto the pickle chips. Place on the prepared baking sheet.

5. Coat the pickle chips with cooking spray. Bake for 8 to 10 minutes, turn, and bake for 8 to 10 minutes longer, until golden brown.

6. If desired, serve with ranch dressing for dipping.

Calories 89 • Fat 0g • Carbohydrate 18g • Fiber 1g • Sugar 0g • Protein 3g
Nutrition does not include optional ingredient.

Parmesan-Garlic Quinoa

The more I cook with quinoa, the more I realize how versatile it is. For this particular side dish, feel free to dial the garlic up or down to suit your family's taste buds. This quinoa pairs perfectly with seafood, steak, or chicken.

Prep Time: 5 minutes | **Cook Time:** 15 minutes
Serves: 4 | **Serving Size:** ¾ cup

1 cup quinoa, rinsed

2 cups low-sodium chicken broth
   (I like Pacific Organic)

½ cup grated Parmesan cheese
   (I like Sargento)

3 green onions, thinly sliced

1 teaspoon garlic powder

1 tablespoon extra virgin olive oil

¼ teaspoon salt

¼ teaspoon black pepper

1. In a medium saucepan, combine the quinoa and chicken broth. Bring to a boil over medium-high heat, reduce to a simmer, cover, and cook until the seeds are translucent and have "spiraled out," 12 to 15 minutes.

2. Remove from the heat and fold in the Parmesan, green onions, garlic powder, olive oil, salt, and pepper and mix well until combined. Serve warm.

suppertime chat: Take turns using adjectives to describe everyone at the table. It's a lesson in grammar and compliments—all adjectives must be positive!

Calories 260 • Fat 9g • Carbohydrate 31g • Fiber 3g • Sugar 0g • Protein 13g

Quick Cauliflower Couscous

This simple technique turns a head of cauliflower into a filling bowl of veggie "couscous," or cauliflower rice. The addition of cumin also jazzes up the spice and nutrition level. You'll want to pair this superior side with all of your main dishes.

Prep Time: 10 minutes | **Cook Time:** 7 minutes
Serves: 4 | **Serving Size:** 1¼ cups

1 head cauliflower

1 teaspoon coconut oil

½ teaspoon ground cumin

½ teaspoon paprika

½ teaspoon salt

1. Remove the stem and core of the cauliflower and chop into florets.

2. Add the florets to a food processor and pulse until the cauliflower resembles the consistency of couscous (coarse meal texture).

3. In a large skillet, heat the coconut oil over medium-high heat. Add the cauliflower. Season with the cumin, paprika, and salt and stir to combine. Cook until the cauliflower is heated through, 5 to 7 minutes. Serve warm.

skinny sense: Cumin is a wonderfully warm spice with incredibly earthy undertones. Just be sure to use sparingly, as its sharp flavor can quickly overpower other spices or ingredients in your recipe.

Calories 29 • Fat 1g • Carbohydrate 4g • Fiber 2g • Sugar 1g • Protein 1g

Sweet and Spicy Coleslaw

Coleslaw is definitely a Southern staple. I'm pretty sure it was served with just about every supper growing up. The homemade coleslaw I grew up eating was packed with buttermilk and sugar. Here, I replace those high-fat ingredients with brown sugar and smoky cumin, and just a hint of cayenne pepper. Still a staple, just jazzed up a bit!

Prep Time: 10 minutes │ **Serves:** 6
Serving Size: Heaping 1½ cups

1 red bell pepper, julienned

1 green bell pepper, julienned

1 (16-ounce) bag coleslaw mix

3 tablespoons light mayonnaise

3 tablespoons fat-free milk

2 tablespoons light brown sugar

½ teaspoon ground cumin

⅛ teaspoon cayenne pepper

⅛ teaspoon salt

⅛ teaspoon black pepper

1. In a large bowl, combine the bell peppers and coleslaw mix.

2. In a small bowl, whisk together the mayonnaise, milk, brown sugar, cumin, cayenne, salt, and black pepper.

3. Pour the dressing over the coleslaw mix and toss to evenly cover. Serve chilled.

suppertime chat: Time to gauge the family's knowledge of healthy eating. Name your favorite healthy food and why you like it.

Calories 70 • Fat 2g • Carbohydrate 12g • Fiber 3g • Sugar 8g • Protein 2g

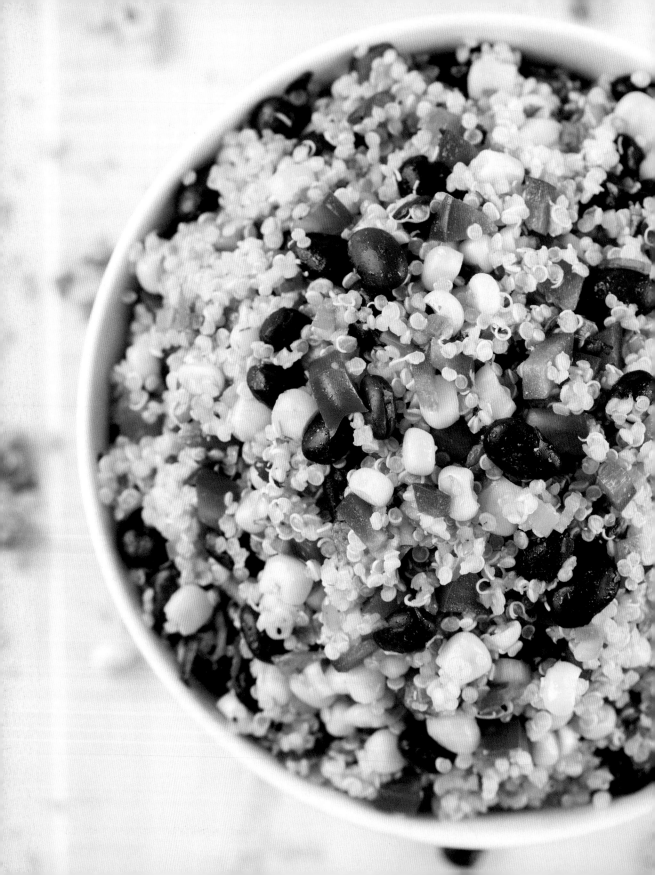

Quinoa Mexi-Lime Salad

This fresh and flavorful dish packs a little heat, yet unlike many salads, the protein-packed quinoa adds satiating power.

Prep Time: 10 minutes | **Cook Time:** 20 minutes
Serves: 8 | **Serving Size:** 1 cup

1¼ cups quinoa, rinsed

2½ cups low-sodium chicken broth (I like Pacific Organic)

1 (15-ounce) can reduced-sodium black beans, drained and rinsed

1 (15.25-ounce) can low-sodium whole kernel corn, drained and rinsed

1 red bell pepper, diced

6 green onions, thinly sliced

¼ cup chopped fresh cilantro

1 jalapeño pepper, seeded and finely diced

⅓ cup lime juice

¼ cup extra virgin olive oil

2 tablespoons red wine vinegar

1 teaspoon ground cumin

½ teaspoon salt

½ teaspoon black pepper

1. In a medium saucepan, combine the quinoa and chicken broth. Bring to a boil over medium-high heat, reduce to a simmer, cover, and cook until the seeds are translucent and have "spiraled out," 12 to 15 minutes. Uncover, fluff with a fork, and set aside to cool for 5 minutes.

2. In a large bowl, combine the black beans, corn, bell pepper, green onions, cilantro, and jalapeño. Add the cooled quinoa and stir to mix all the ingredients well.

3. In a small bowl, whisk together the lime juice, olive oil, vinegar, cumin, salt, and black pepper.

4. Pour the dressing over the quinoa mixture and stir to evenly combine. Refrigerate for at least 1 hour before serving.

suppertime chat: Play the game "two truths and one lie." Each person shares three things about themselves: two of them are true, one is a lie. The other people at the table have to guess which statement is the lie. You're likely to be very surprised at how creative your kids can be.

Calories 248 • Fat 8g • Carbohydrate 38g • Fiber 6g • Sugar 5g • Protein 8g

Rustic Rosemary Root Vegetables

I found a new love in the produce section: parsnips. Similar in shape and texture to carrots, they are just a smidge sweeter. (Bonus: Parsnips are biennials, which means they can actually be found all winter long.) With its creamy color, the parsnip looks gorgeous next to the carrot and red potato in this dish, making it a trio of vitamin and nutrient superstars. Roasting the veggies in the oven with fresh rosemary gives them a rustic and earthy flavor. The key here is to make sure they are cut uniformly to ensure even roasting.

Prep Time: 5 minutes | **Cook Time:** 40 minutes
Serves: 6 | **Serving Size:** 1 cup

1 large parsnip, peeled and cut into
   1-inch pieces

3 large carrots, peeled and cut into
   1-inch pieces

5 medium red potatoes, cut into
   1-inch pieces

1 tablespoon finely chopped fresh
   rosemary

1 tablespoon extra virgin olive oil

1 tablespoon minced garlic

½ teaspoon kosher salt

½ teaspoon black pepper

1. Preheat the oven to 400°F. Line a baking sheet with foil and coat with cooking spray.

2. In a large bowl, toss together the vegetables, rosemary, olive oil, and garlic.

3. Arrange the vegetables in a single layer on the prepared baking sheet. Season with the salt and pepper.

4. Roast until the vegetables are tender and golden brown, about 40 minutes, turning at the halfway mark. Serve warm.

suppertime chat: It's important to make eating healthy fun! My son loves when we play the Rainbow Game (see below). Playing it with him reminds me that eating healthy is an adventure.

the rainbow game: Try eating at least five different colors of produce every day. It can be as simple as a red apple, an orange, purple grapes, green lettuce, and a yellow banana. Or get more creative: green kale, a yellow pepper, a red pomegranate, blueberries, and a purple eggplant. The secret is spending more time in the produce section with a goal of eating the rainbow!

Calories 107 • Fat 3g • Carbohydrate 20g • Fiber 4g • Sugar 4g • Protein 2g

Skillet Corn

I have my aunt Tammy to thank for helping to perfect this family favorite. Longing to re-create my granny's creamed corn, she helped to nail the flavors without piling on the fat and calories. This creamy side is sure to become a long-standing tradition for your family, too!

Prep Time: 5 minutes | **Cook Time:** 15 minutes
Serves: 4 | **Serving Size:** ½ cup

---

5 ears of corn (see Quick and Easy)

½ cup fat-free milk

1 tablespoon stevia

4 ounces ⅓-less-fat cream cheese

1. In a large bowl, use a knife to cut the kernels off the cobs (discard the cobs).

2. In a large skillet, combine the corn and ¾ cup of water. Cook uncovered over medium heat, stirring occasionally, until the water has evaporated and the corn has softened, 8 to 10 minutes.

3. Add the milk, stevia, and cream cheese and mix well to evenly combine. Cook for 5 minutes longer, until heated through and thickened, stirring occasionally. Serve warm.

quick and easy: You can easily swap out fresh corn for frozen corn kernels to save time. You'll need 5 cups frozen corn kernels. Cook as directed.

Calories 190 • Fat 8g • Carbohydrate 25g • Fiber 3g • Sugar 9g • Protein 6g

Sun-Dried Tomato and Pesto Potato Salad

Most summertime picnics have two side dishes that I most always steer clear of: coleslaw and potato salad. The fat and calories (not to mention unknown ingredients) are enough to spoil my appetite. Not anymore! The sun-dried tomatoes and pesto in this recipe make this potato salad the perfect complement to any outdoor barbecue or grill out.

Prep Time: 10 minutes | **Cook Time:** 30 minutes
Serves: 8 | **Serving Size:** ¾ cup

2 pounds red new potatoes, quartered

½ tablespoon extra virgin olive oil

¼ teaspoon salt

¼ teaspoon black pepper

3 tablespoons coarsely chopped walnuts

¼ cup part-skim ricotta cheese

2 tablespoons light mayonnaise

½ cup plain 0% Greek yogurt

½ cup oil-packed sun-dried tomatoes, drained and chopped

2 teaspoons garlic powder

1 teaspoon onion powder

Lightened-Up Pesto:

1 cup fresh basil leaves

1 tablespoon minced garlic

2 tablespoons shredded Parmesan cheese (I like Sargento Artisan Blends)

¼ teaspoon salt

⅛ teaspoon black pepper

2 tablespoons extra virgin olive oil

2 tablespoons walnuts

1. Preheat the oven to 375°F. Line a baking sheet with foil and coat with cooking spray.

2. In a large bowl, combine the potatoes, olive oil, salt, and pepper. Toss gently to evenly coat the potatoes. Transfer the potatoes in a single layer to the prepared baking sheet.

3. Bake until tender, 30 to 35 minutes, turning at the halfway mark. Allow the potatoes to cool to room temperature.

4. Meanwhile, in a dry skillet, toast the walnuts over medium-high heat, stirring frequently, until fragrant and slightly browned, 2 to 4 minutes, watching them carefully so they do not burn. Transfer the walnuts to a plate and set aside.

5. In a medium bowl, combine the ricotta, mayonnaise, and yogurt. Add the sun-dried tomatoes, garlic powder, and onion powder. Stir gently to mix.

6. To make the pesto, combine all the pesto ingredients in a food processor and pulse until well combined. Fold 5 tablespoons of the pesto into the ricotta mixture until well incorporated.

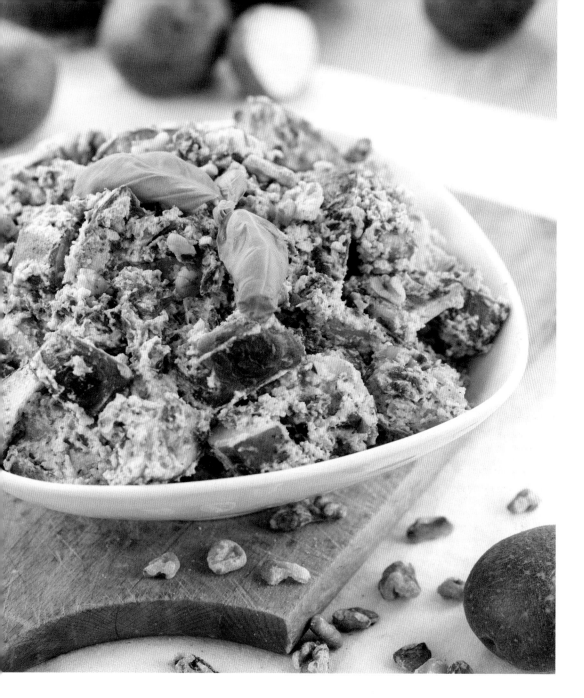

7. Once the potatoes have cooled, add them and the walnuts to the ricotta mixture and toss to evenly coat. Serve at room temperature or chilled.

Calories 223 • **Fat** 12g • **Carbohydrate** 25g • **Fiber** 3g • **Sugar** 4g • **Protein** 6g

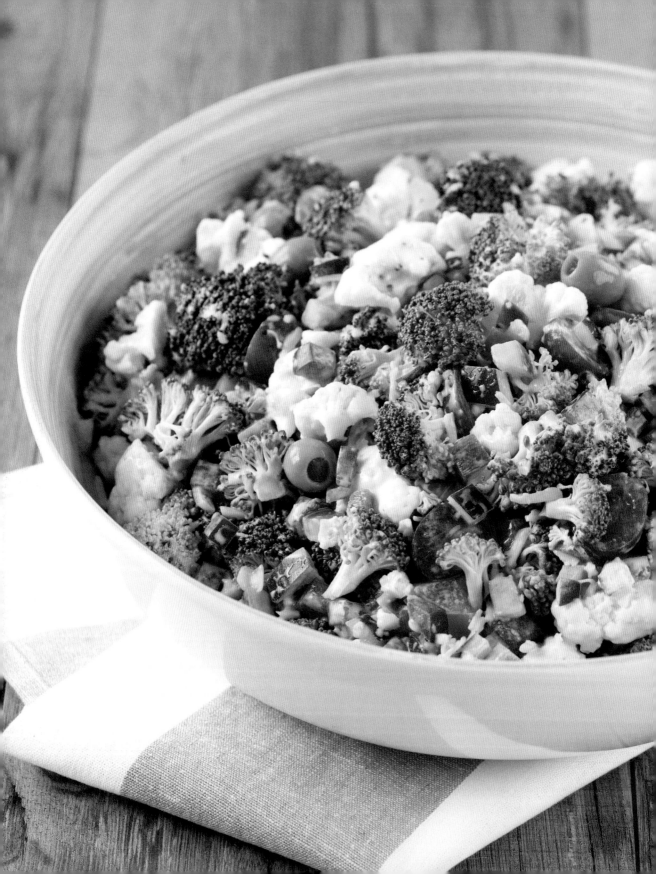

Skinny Broccoli Salad

This light and fresh salad has roots going back more than thirty years in my family! It's an original from my sweet aunt Sherry and a staple on Sunday afternoons after church and all our family get-togethers. I have modified it ever so slightly, just to lighten it up a bit without sacrificing the taste!

Prep Time: 10 minutes
Serves: 12 | **Serving Size:** 1 cup

2 heads broccoli, cut into small florets

1 head cauliflower, cut into small florets

1 red bell pepper, diced

1 green bell pepper, diced

½ small red onion, diced

½ cup reduced-salt green olives

2 cups grape tomatoes, halved

1 cup shredded reduced-fat sharp cheddar cheese (I like Sargento)

1 cup Bolthouse Farms Classic Ranch Yogurt dressing

1. In a large bowl, combine the broccoli, cauliflower, bell peppers, onion, olives, tomatoes, cheddar, and dressing and gently toss.

2. Serve chilled.

quick and easy: Chop the vegetables ahead of time. Make a big batch of this salad at the beginning of the week to serve as a fresh side at suppertime.

suppertime inspiration: Family get-togethers and holiday meals are created with staple recipes that go back for generations. Unfortunately, many of them are loaded with fat and calories! Adopting lighter recipes or modifying current ones are wonderful ways to keep the traditions going while not sacrificing your goals to eat light and balanced! Go ahead, lighten up Aunt Sally's lasagna—your family will thank you!

Calories 106 · Fat 6g · Carbohydrate 9g · Fiber 2g · Sugar 4g · Protein 5g

Southern Sweet Beets

By most people's standards, I'm a little odd when it comes to beets. I can snack on these colorful root veggies and nothing else. Recognizing that not everyone has the same affinity for beets, it was a challenge to reduce their earthy undertones for a wider audience. The use of brown sugar and orange juice tames and sweetens the beets, preserving the foundation of this vitamin- and nutrient-dense taproot.

Prep Time: Less than 5 minutes | **Cook Time:** 10 minutes
Serves: 4 | **Serving Size:** ¾ cup

3 tablespoons Tropicana Trop50 orange juice

2 teaspoons cornstarch

2 tablespoons balsamic vinegar

½ tablespoon unsalted butter

2 tablespoons light brown sugar

1 teaspoon grated orange zest

2 (14.5-ounce) cans no-salt-added sliced beets, drained

⅛ teaspoon salt

1. In a small bowl, stir the orange juice into the cornstarch to make a slurry. Transfer to a medium saucepan and whisk constantly over medium-high heat for 1 minute. Reduce the heat to low and add the vinegar, butter, brown sugar, and orange zest and stir until the sauce starts to thicken, 2 to 3 minutes.

2. Add the beets to the saucepan and stir to evenly coat. Cook over low heat for 4 to 5 minutes to heat through and glaze the beets. Serve warm.

quick and easy: Swap fresh beets for canned beets. Simply peel the fresh beets (to avoid getting beet stains on your hands, wear a cheap pair of latex gloves), place them in a large pot with water to cover, and boil until softened, 35 to 40 minutes. Drain, allow to cool, then slice.

Calories 130 • Fat 1g • Carbohydrate 25g • Fiber 2g • Sugar 18g • Protein 2g

Skinny Fried Apples

The secret in the preparation of this little dish is all in the apple. Be sure to choose good baking apples, like Granny Smith, as choosing the wrong type of apple will leave you with a pan of mush. Also, using a pan that can go from stovetop to oven will save on time and clean up. I love serving these alongside my Country Pork Chops and Gravy (page 170).

Prep Time: 5 minutes | **Cook Time:** 30 minutes
Serves: 6 | **Serving Size:** ¾ cup

1 teaspoon coconut oil

4 Granny Smith apples, peeled and sliced

½ cup reduced-sugar apple juice

2 tablespoons sugar-free maple-flavor syrup (I like Maple Grove Farms)

½ teaspoon vanilla extract

1 teaspoon ground cinnamon

Apple Crisp Topping:

1 tablespoon white whole wheat flour

2 tablespoons brown sugar

2 tablespoons stevia

¼ cup old-fashioned rolled oats

1 tablespoon cold unsalted butter

1. Preheat the oven to 400°F.

2. Heat a skillet over medium-high heat and add the coconut oil. Once heated, add the apple slices, apple juice, syrup, vanilla, and cinnamon and gently stir to mix and evenly coat. Simmer, stirring occasionally, until the apples have started to soften, 12 to 15 minutes. Remove from the heat.

3. Meanwhile, to make the apple crisp topping: In a small bowl, combine the flour, brown sugar, stevia, and oats and stir to combine. Cut in the cold butter with your fingers or a fork until it turns into a coarse crumble.

4. Sprinkle the crumble evenly over the apples. Transfer the skillet to the oven and bake for 10 minutes, until bubbly and golden brown. Serve warm.

skinny sense: I'm a fan of coconut oil for many reasons, but mainly for the medium-chain fatty acids, or MCFAs. These are a great source of energy for the body and they have been known to help boost metabolism, which can help you maintain a healthy weight or even lead to weight loss. This is especially so when combined with exercise and fabulously light side dishes like these skinny fried apples!

Calories 126 · Fat 3g · Carbohydrate 24g · Fiber 4g · Sugar 16g · Protein 1g

Caramelized Brussels Sprouts with Pecans

This is a fantastic way to introduce kids to a vegetable that makes most turn up their noses. I used to stay away from Brussels sprouts because I wasn't a fan of their bitter taste. I now know that it's all in the preparation. These babies are best served right out of the oven: warm, sweet, and crunchy.

Prep Time: 5 minutes | **Cook Time:** 40 minutes
Serves: 6 | **Serving Size:** ¾ cup

2 tablespoons light brown sugar

1 tablespoon extra virgin olive oil

¼ teaspoon salt

⅛ teaspoon black pepper

2 (16-ounce) bags Brussels sprouts

¼ cup pecans, coarsely chopped

1 teaspoon sugar-free maple-flavor syrup (I like Maple Grove Farms)

quick and easy: Uniformity of size is key so that the Brussels sprouts cook up evenly. That's why, if you find especially large sprouts, you should slice them in half during prep.

1. Preheat the oven to 375°F. Line a baking sheet with foil and coat with cooking spray.

2. In a large bowl, mix together the brown sugar, olive oil, salt, and pepper.

3. Trim the Brussels sprouts by cutting off the ends and removing any browned outer leaves. Cut any large sprouts in half (see Quick and Easy).

4. Add the Brussels sprouts to the brown sugar mixture and toss to evenly coat.

5. Transfer the Brussels sprouts to the prepared baking sheet in a single layer. Bake for 35 minutes, making sure to turn at the halfway mark.

6. Meanwhile, in a small bowl, toss the pecans and syrup together to coat evenly.

7. Add the pecans to the Brussels sprouts and bake for 5 minutes longer, until the sprouts have browned and are easily pierced with a fork. Serve warm.

Calories 135 · Fat 6g · Carbohydrate 18g · Fiber 6g · Sugar 7g · Protein 6g

MAKE IT HOMEMADE: SKINNY SEASONINGS

CARIBBEAN JERK SEASONING

Use this homemade seasoning blend as an even replacement for any store-bought blend.

2 tablespoons garlic powder

1 tablespoon onion powder

1 tablespoon dried parsley

½ tablespoon ground allspice

3 teaspoons cayenne pepper

3 teaspoons stevia

1 teaspoon thyme

1 teaspoon black pepper

1 teaspoon salt

½ teaspoon cinnamon

Mix all the ingredients in a small bowl. Store in an airtight container.

CAJUN SEASONING

Use this homemade seasoning blend as an even replacement for any store-bought blend.

3 tablespoons paprika

1½ tablespoons salt

1½ tablespoons black pepper

1 tablespoon garlic powder

1 tablespoon onion powder

1 tablespoon cayenne pepper

½ teaspoon oregano

Mix all the ingredients in a small bowl. Store in an airtight container.

ITALIAN SALAD DRESSING MIX

Use 2 tablespoons of this mix in place of any store-bought packet.

1½ tablespoons garlic powder

1½ tablespoons onion powder

1 tablespoon stevia

2 tablespoons dried parsley

1 tablespoon dried oregano

½ teaspoon dried thyme

2 teaspoons dried basil

1 tablespoon salt

2 teaspoons black pepper

Mix all the ingredients in a small bowl. Store in an airtight container.

TACO SEASONING

Use 2 tablespoons of this seasoning in place of any store-bought packet.

3 tablespoons chili powder

3 teaspoons cumin

1 teaspoon garlic powder

1½ teaspoons paprika

½ teaspoon red pepper flakes

½ teaspoon cayenne pepper

2½ teaspoons salt

2 teaspoons black pepper

Mix all the ingredients in a small bowl. Store in an airtight container.

ACKNOWLEDGMENTS

To my mom, there are no words to express my gratitude. Thank you for the countless hours of playing with Easton when I needed to run to the grocery store, plan and cook recipes, or work on my forever long to-do list. Thank you for your prayers and for always believing in me.

Dad, Amanda, and Cara, thank you for your support, your love, and your willingness to be taste testers for the many recipes in this book. Your constructive criticism and feedback gave me the confidence to share my recipes with families everywhere.

Liz, Sarah, and Jen . . . may you never forget the days that we all spent together at my house and the fun times that we shared while working on this project. Thank you for being honest with me and for pushing me to be the best that I can be throughout this entire process. I am so proud of the recipes and the photography that came out of my little kitchen.

To my literary agent, Kari, thank you for your willingness to take a chance on me and for believing in me from the beginning, long before this project ever began.

To my editor, Cara, thank you for sending the email that would change my life and open the door for one of my dreams to come true.

To my wonderful team at William Morrow and A. Larry Ross, thank you for your support and fantastic ideas.

Julie House, thank you for stepping out in faith on this journey with me. God connected us and I will be forever grateful for our friendship. Through our many conversations and your inspired words, my story would come to life and be shared beautifully throughout the pages of this book.

To my dear Easton, you bring so much joy to my life and I am blessed by your love. I smile knowing that I get to share these recipes and create suppertime memories with you every day.

To Audrey and the entire Skinny Mom team, thank you for your dedication and hard work in making sure that all of the day-to-day tasks of the company, the social media sites, and everything with the website were taken care of while I was working on this project. To Tori, thank you for never giving up on me and for caring about every single detail of this book.

To Jessica Penner, RD, thank you for the hard work and diligence you spent on making sure that all of the recipes in this book have accurate and trustworthy nutritional values.

To Granny, Aunt Tammy, Aunt Von, and Aunt Sherry, thank you for teaching me how to cook and for sharing family recipes that would serve as inspiration for many of the recipes in this book.

Finally, to my Lord and Savior, thank you for never giving up on me. I live my life for you and may everything I do be to glorify your name and show love to others.

UNIVERSAL CONVERSION CHART

Oven temperature equivalents

250°F = 120°C   350°F = 180°C   450°F = 230°C

275°F = 135°C   375°F = 190°C   475°F = 240°C

300°F = 150°C   400°F = 200°C   500°F = 260°C

325°F = 160°C   425°F = 220°C

Measurement equivalents

Measurements should always be level unless directed otherwise.

$\frac{1}{8}$ teaspoon = 0.5 mL

$\frac{1}{4}$ teaspoon = 1 mL

$\frac{1}{2}$ teaspoon = 2 mL

1 teaspoon = 5 mL

1 tablespoon = 3 teaspoons = $\frac{1}{2}$ fluid ounce = 15 mL

2 tablespoons = $\frac{1}{8}$ cup = 1 fluid ounce = 30 mL

4 tablespoons = $\frac{1}{4}$ cup = 2 fluid ounces = 60 mL

$5\frac{1}{3}$ tablespoons = $\frac{1}{3}$ cup = 3 fluid ounces = 80 mL

8 tablespoons = $\frac{1}{2}$ cup = 4 fluid ounces = 120 mL

$10\frac{2}{3}$ tablespoons = $\frac{2}{3}$ cup = 5 fluid ounces = 160 mL

12 tablespoons = $\frac{3}{4}$ cup = 6 fluid ounces = 180 mL

16 tablespoons = 1 cup = 8 fluid ounces = 240 mL

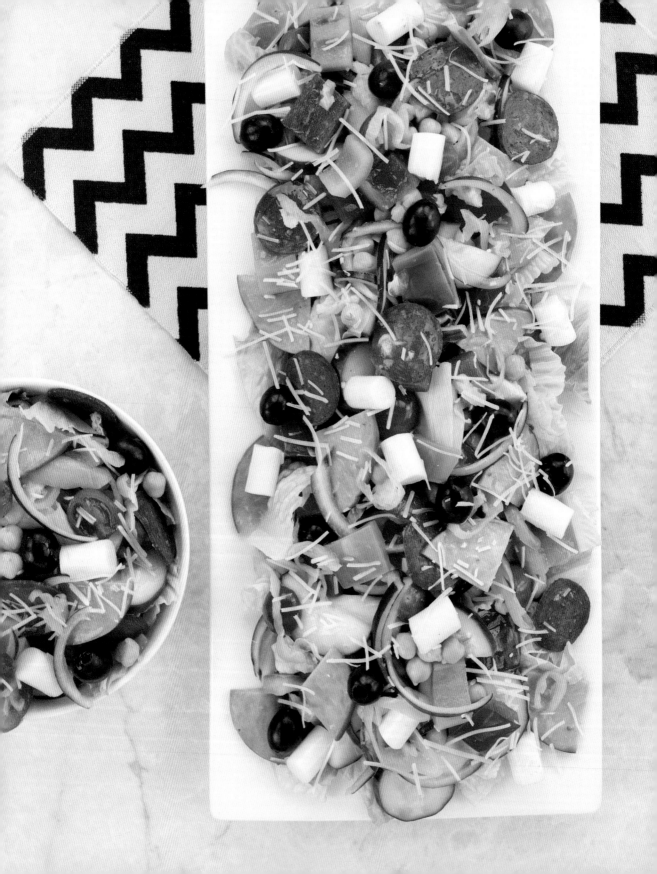

INDEX

ABOUT THE AUTHOR

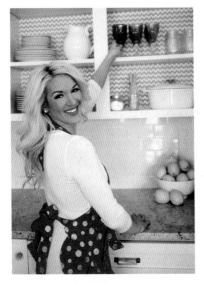

BROOKE GRIFFIN grew up in Corbin, Kentucky, a small town in one of the poorest counties in the state, and is the oldest of three girls. Sunday suppers were a staple of her childhood, and she fondly remembers squeezing into her granny's tiny country house after church along with her large extended family to eat home-cooked meals and pray.

After being the first person in her family to graduate from college, Brooke went on to realize her childhood dream of cheerleading in the NFL. Shortly after winning the title of Fitness Universe Champion in 2009, Brooke gave birth to her son, Easton Jack. After rediscovering her faith amid a time of personal struggle, Brooke founded SkinnyMom.com, which now reaches more than 6 million women each month, giving moms the "skinny" on healthy eating and living.

Brooke has appeared in national magazines, including *Oxygen, Women's Fitness, Maxim, Redbook, GQ, Natural Muscle, American Cheerleader,* and *American Baby,* and on national television, including on ESPN, ABC, NBC, Fox, Fox Sports, and *20/20.*